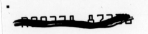

D0812551

Conformationally Directed
Drug Design

ACS SYMPOSIUM SERIES 251

Conformationally Directed Drug Design

Peptides and Nucleic Acids as Templates or Targets

Julius A. Vida, EDITOR
Bristol-Myers Company

Maxwell Gordon, EDITOR
Bristol-Myers Company

Based on a symposium sponsored by
the Division of Medicinal Chemistry
at the 186th Meeting
of the American Chemical Society,
Washington, D.C.,
August 28–September 2, 1983

American Chemical Society, Washington, D.C. 1984

Library of Congress Cataloging in Publication Data

Conformationally directed drug design.
  (ACS symposium series, ISSN 0097–6156; 251)

  Includes bibliographies and indexes.

  1. Chemistry, Pharmaceutical—Congresses.
2. Peptides—Congresses. 3. Nucleic acids—Congresses.
4. Structure–activity relationship (Pharmacology)—
Congresses. 5. Stereochemistry—Congresses.

  I. Vida, Julius A., 1928–   . II. Gordon, Maxwell,
1921–   . III. American Chemical Society. Division of
Medicinal Chemistry. IV. American Chemical Society.
Meeting (186th: 1983: Washington, D.C.) V. Series.
[DNLM: 1. Nucleic acid conformation—Congresses.
2. Protein conformation—Congresses. 3. Chemistry,
Pharmaceutical—Congresses. QU 58 C7487 1983]

RS401.C66   1984   615′.31   84–2921
ISBN 0–8412–0836–0

FOREWORD

The ACS Symposium Series was founded in 1974 to provide
a medium for publishing symposia quickly in book form. The
format of the Series parallels that of the continuing Advances
in Chemistry Series except that in order to save time the
papers are not typeset but are reproduced as they are submitted by the authors in camera-ready form. Papers are reviewed under the supervision of the Editors with the assistance
of the Series Advisory Board and are selected to maintain the
integrity of the symposia; however, verbatim reproductions of
previously published papers are not accepted. Both reviews
and reports of research are acceptable since symposia may
embrace both types of presentation.

CONTENTS

PREFACE

TRADITIONAL MEDICINAL CHEMICAL RESEARCH has involved the testing of drugs on whole animals or isolated organ systems for a desired end result. The drugs themselves were usually arrived at empirically through screening, or they represented analogs of compounds previously found to show the desired activity.

In the new era of medicinal chemistry, drug design is based on the structure of effector molecules or receptor sites. Thus, cimetidine was designed to be a specific histamine antagonist, captopril was designed to inhibit the angiotensin-converting enzyme, and so forth. Using powerful new developments in immunology, molecular biology, computer modeling, and recombinant techniques, scientists can study receptor sites from the point of view of three-dimensional structure and can design antagonists specific to the action of drugs or transmitter substances at those sites. In particular, the conformation of biopolymers and their tertiary structures is amenable to X-ray analysis or other powerful techniques for determining structure.

Many studies report the use of peptide and nucleic acid conformation as a tool for drug design. Analogs of somatostatin having greater potency and stability than the prototype have been designed from a model of the prototype. In one study the design of an affinity label for creatine kinase demonstrated how such information could be used in the search for agents directed at an enzyme's active site.

One series of investigations has shown that a rational, conformationally based approach to analog design requires supplementary information, over and above simple sequence data. One tool was the introduction of highly constrained transannual bridges to construct specific antagonists of active peptides. In other studies free synthetic peptides have proven to be powerful reagents for inducing specific tolerance to preselected regions of a protein and for preparing antibodies having specificities for preselected protein regions.

In this volume many investigators report on their own studies in conformationally directed drug design. The common theme of all the chapters is the importance of the conformational structure of peptide and nucleic acid in the design of drugs that are either peptide- or nucleic-acid-based or that interact with peptides or nucleic acids. We anticipate that at the present rate of progress significant therapeutic advances will result from these investigators' efforts. We are grateful to the authors for their contributions and for the privilege of collaborating with them on the publication of this volume.

JULIUS A. VIDA
MAXWELL GORDON
Bristol–Myers Company
New York, New York

January 1984

Virus–Receptor Interactions

BERNARD N. FIELDS

Department of Microbiology and Molecular Genetics, Harvard Medical School, and Department of Medicine (Infectious Disease), Brigham and Women's Hospital, Boston, MA 02115

MARK I. GREENE

Department of Pathology, Harvard Medical School, Boston, MA 02115

In this discussion we have considered certain protein-protein interactions determined by the binding of reovirus hemagglutinin with cell receptors. A specific epitope on the reovirus hemagglutinin identified by the G5 monoclonal antibody is critical for binding reovirus type 3 to cell surface receptors. Monoclonal anti-idiotypic reagents have been generated which resemble the virus in terms of its ability to interact with cell receptors. The monoclonal anti-idiotype interacts with the monoclonal antibodies of the G5 neutralization epitope specificity. This idiotype-anti-idiotype system mimics the protein-protein interaction observed with binding of the virus hemagglutinin to cell surface receptor. Hence anti-idiotypes are anti-receptor. Such anti-receptor antibodies might also be used in the development of vaccines for certain pathogenic organisms since the anti-idiotypic antibodies resemble the ligand.

The mammalian reoviruses are segmented double-stranded RNA viruses (1). Of the various proteins of reovirus, the hemagglutinin appears to play a predominant role in determining tropism of the virus for different cell tissues. This has been appreciated as a consequence for the genetic analysis of the reovirus serotypes (2). For example, reovirus type 3 has a tropism for neuronal cells but spares ependymal cells. Reovirus type 1, on the other hand, has a tropism for ependymal cells and spares neuronal cells damage (3). Recombinant viruses have been developed which have all the genes of type 3 except for the gene encoding the hemagglutinin of type 1, (this recombinant is termed 3.HA1). Similarly, viruses have been developed which have all the

0097–6156/84/0251–0001$06.00/0
© 1984 American Chemical Society

genes for type 1 except the gene encoding the hemagglutinin
of type 3 (this recombinant is termed 1. HA3). Use of these
viral recombinants has shown that the viral hemagglutinin
specifies tropism for the neuronal and ependymal cells
discussed above.

The hemagglutinin is also a major immunogen in terms of
the immune response (4). The greater portion of the
cytolytic T cell response is directed at the reovirus
hemagglutinin in association with histocompatibility proteins
(5). Thus animals immunized with reovirus type 3 generate
cytolytic T cells which have the capacity to lyse and infect
histocompatibility matched reovirus type 3 infected targets
but not a reovirus type 1 infected target. Similarly, 1.HA3
infected targets are lysed whereas 3.HA1 infected targets are
not lysed appreciably. The targets can be protected from
lysis with antibodies directed to the hemagglutinin or by
anti-H-2 antibodies (6).

Antibody response; structural characteristics

At the level of the B cell the antibody response to the
hemagglutinin has been studied in great detail. The response
is markedly oligoclonal with a cluster of HA specific
immunoglobulins with a PI of between 6.9 and 7.1 (7). The
antibody response to the hemagglutinin of type 3 is also
typified by the presence of a structural determinant known as
a shared or cross-reactive idiotypic determinant (Figure 1)
expressed in many of the antibodies with specificity for the
type 3 hemagglutinin. The idiotype has been identified by
rabbit antibodies direct at anti-hemagglutinin
immunoglobulins. The anti-idiotype-idiotype interaction is
inhibitable by free hemagglutinin. Hence the idiotype (see
below) is associated with the antigen conbining site of the
immunoglobulin protein. Hence in the response to
hemagglutinin a homogeneous structurally similar antibody
response is induced (8).

Hemagglutinin topography

A panel of monoclonal antibodies has been developed and used
to analyze various regions of the hemagglutinin (9,10).
Three distinct epitopes have been defined for the reovirus
type 3 hemagglutinin. (Figure 2) One region is important for
neutralization. Similarly, distinct monoclonal antibodies
determine the spatially separate hemagglutinin inhibition
epitope, and other antibodies distinguish a third region
which has not yet been functionally defined. Of interest in
the screening of these monoclonal antibodies was the fact
that one of them, termed G5, expresses similar cross-reactive
idiotypic determinants as antibodies with hemagglutinin

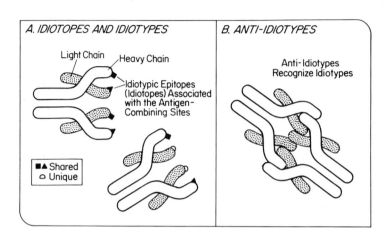

Figure 1.   A general scheme of idiotypes and anti-idiotypes. Depicted here are immunoglobulin proteins whose antigen-combining site expresses unique conformations or epitopes, that are termed idiotopes.   A collection of idiotopes constitute what is termed idiotype.   Some idiotypes are shared by many immunoglobulins with the same antigenic specificity.

Anti-idiotypes are antibodies with specificity for idiotypes.   The antibodies can be made in the same species or in other species.   Often the interaction of anti-idiotypes to idiotypes is inhibited by free antigen.

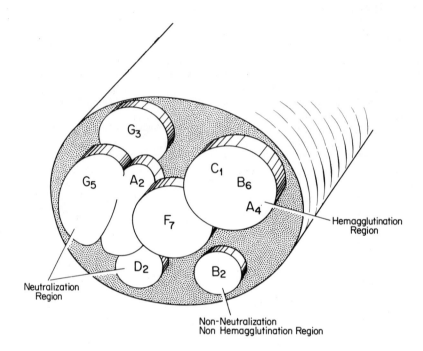

Figure 2.   Topography of the reovirus hemagglutinin.
Depicted here in this cartoon is a representation of various
domains of the reovirus hemagglutinin.   Some domains are
overlapping whereas others are separate and unique from all
the rest.   The G5 domain appears to be the most relevant to
the immune response and also for tropism.

specificity (9). Studies focusing on the G5 region of the
hemagglutinin protein have indicated that this epitope is
important in the tropism of the virus. Immunoselection of
variant reoviruses by using G5 antibody has shown that
viruses that resist neutralization by G5 are attenuated and
show altered tropism (11).

Monoclonal anti-idiotypes resemble ligand

The network theory of N. Jerne (12) proposes that antibodies
themselves can act as antigens and provoke the synthesis of
anti-antibodies in the host animal. The immunogenic portions
of the antibody molecule as suggested above results from the
structure in and around the antigen combining site and are
referred to as idiotypes. As discussed, immunoglobulins that
recognize these sites are referred to as anti-idiotypes. We
reasoned that if the binding site of the reovirus type 3
hemagglutinin on cell receptors and on antibodies to the
hemagglutinin were similar, antibodies made against the
binding site of one protein (such as the G5 monoclonal) might
recognize the binding site of other proteins (such as somatic
cell receptors). To test this idea, by repeatedly priming
BALB/c mice with G5 monoclonal cells, we were able to
generate syngeneic monoclonal anti-idiotype reagents. The
analysis of the interaction of the monoclonal anti-idiotype
binding with the monoclonal G5 antibody revealed that this
interaction was determined through the antigen-combining
site. When monoclonal anti-hemagglutinin antibodies were
assessed for their ability to bind radiolabeled purified
hemagglutinin protein in the presence of monoclonal-anti-
idiotype, there was marked inhibition (8). Thus, the
monoclonal anti-idiotype and hemagglutinin bind to the same
region of the antigen-combining site of G5 antibodies. This
indicates that the monoclonal anti-idiotype functionally
resembles the hemagglutinin neutralization domain epitope.
We have analyzed further the protein-protein interactions
which are important in viral receptor binding by a variety of
approaches. Many of these approaches have in common the use
of monoclonal anti-idiotype. For example, it has been
possible to show that reovirus type 3 binds to a subset of
murine cells or to a panel of lymphoid lines that have been
maintained in vitro. Exposure of monoclonal anti-idiotype to
the cell lines at the time of exposure to mammalian reovirus
blocks the binding of reovirus type 3 (13). Monoclonal anti-
idiotype is thus capable of interfering with viral
interaction with the mammalian reovirus receptor on these
cell lines. These observations suggest that monoclonal anti-
receptor antibodies might represent a new approach for
preventing virus binding, an event necessary for infection.

Monoclonal anti-idiotypic reagents were also assessed
for their ability to prime for cellular immunity to mammalian
reoviruses. We reasoned that if the anti-idiotype resembled
the viral hemagglutinin enough to recognize the surface
receptors, it might stimulate antibodies that in turn
recognize the viral hemagglutinin. Such a result would
indicate that anti-idiotype could serve as a potential
vaccine (4). In order to evaluate whether the monoclonal
anti-idiotypic reagent could be used as a vaccine in a
syngeneic system, BALB/c mice were immunized with 200
microliters of clarified ascites fluid derived from animals
bearing the anti-idiotypic hybridoma. Animals were
challenged in the footpad 5 days later with virus. Animals
primed with anti-idiotype developed a T cell-dependent
inflammatory response in vivo to mammalian reovirus type 3,
type 1.HA3, and not to type 1 or type 3 HA1. Thus these
results suggest that monoclonal anti-idiotypes resemble the
viral hemagglutinin biologically and might be of use in the
immunization against certain pathogenic agents. (Figure 3)

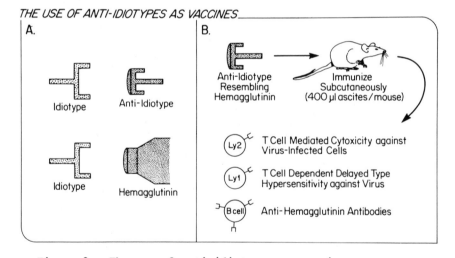

Figure 3. The use of anti-idiotypes as vaccines.

The anti-idiotypes in the reovirus system resemble

hemagglutinin neutralization domains. Functionally shown

here is the consequence of administering monoclonal anti-

idiotypic proteins to mice. A variety of reovirus specific

immune reactivities are induced.

Literature Cited

1. Joklik W.K. Reproduction of reoviridal. In "Comprehensive Virology" (H. Fraenkel-Conrat and R. Wagner, eds.) 1974, New York: Plenum Press, Vol. 2, pp 231-334.
2. Fields B.N. 1982. Arch. Virol. 71:95-107
3. Weiner H.L., Drayna D., Averill D.R. Jr. and Fields B.N. 1977. Proc. Natl. Acad. Sci. U.S.A. 74:5744.
4. Fields B.N. and Greene M.I. Nature 1982 300:19.
5. Finberg R., Weiner H.L., Fields B.N., Benacerraf B. and Burakoff S.J. 1979 Proc. Natl. Acad. Sci. U.S.A. 76:442.
6. Finberg R, Spriggs D.R. and Fields B.N. 1982. J. Immunol. 129:2235.
7. Nepom J.T., Weiner H.L., Dichter M.A., Spriggs D., Gramm C.F., Powers M.L., Fields B.N. and Greene M.I. 1982 .J. Exp. Med 155:155.
8. Noseworthy J.H., Fields B.N., Dichter M.A., Sobotka, C., Pizer E., Perry L.L., Nepom, J.T. and Greene M.I.J. Immunol. 1983, in press.
9. Burstin S.J., Spriggs D.R. and Fields B.N. 1982 Virology 117:146.
10. Spriggs D.R., Kaye K. and Fields B.N. 1983 Virology 12:71.
11. Spriggs D.R. and Fields B.N. 1982 Nature 297:68.
12. Jerne N.K. 1974 Ann. Immunol. (Inst. Pasteur) 125c:373.
13. Unpublished data.

RECEIVED November 15, 1983

Design of Peptide Superagonists and Antagonists
Conformational and Dynamic Considerations

VICTOR J. HRUBY

Department of Chemistry, University of Arizona, Tucson, AZ 85721

The design of conformationally restricted peptide
analogs can provide a rational approach to peptide
hormone and neurotransmitter analogs as potential
drugs and pharmaceuticals. This requires the development of a conformational model with limited conformational alternatives and testing this model
with conformationally restricted analogs. We have
applied this approach to the design of a number of
peptide hormone and neurotransmitter analogs with a
number of useful properties for potential drugs.
1) Conformationally restricted oxytocin analogs
with prolonged in vivo antagonist activities which
can also block prostaglandin release; 2) Highly
conformationally restricted cyclic analogs of
enkephalin which are highly potent and have exception δ receptor selectivity; 3) α-Melanotropin analogs, both cyclic and linear, some with superagonist potency, others with superprolonged in vitro
(days) and in vivo (weeks) activities, and others
which are completely stable to serum enzymes.

Peptide hormones and neurotransmitters are primary agents of communication between different cell types in the body of complex
living systems including man. Thus, analogs of natural peptide
hormones and neurotransmitters with appropriate properties have
exceptional potential as drugs. Despite this potential and the
need for peptide drugs, development has been slow. Why?
     In general, a suitable peptide drug should have one or more
of the following properties: 1) it should have high specificity
for a single receptor type; 2) it should be stable in the biological milieu; 3) it should have long lasting activity; 4) it
should be highly potent; 5) if possible, it should be orally
active.
     Though peptide hormones and neurotransmitters tend to

0097–6156/84/0251–0009$06.00/0

possess very high potency, they generally possess chemical and physical properties which make rational design of drugs difficult.

1. Many peptide hormones and neurotransmitters are small, conformationally flexible molecules. Thus, their conformational properties are difficult to determine, and the statistical distribution of their conformations are highly dependent on the environment. Furthermore, it is difficult to determine which, if any, of the conformations in solution are related to their biological activity at a receptor.

2. Since peptide hormones and neurotransmitters act as biological switches, evolutionary development has tended to lead to peptides which have a short duration of biological activity at target tissue and which are rapidly degraded in the biological milieu.

3. Closely related to 1. and 2. are problems related to events occurring at the receptor. Biological information transfer for peptide hormones and neurotransmitters appears to involve two separate but closely related events: a) receptor recognition or binding; followed by b) biological transduction leading to activation of the biological response (1-5). In view of the general properties of the peptides outlined in 1. and 2., it is difficult to define which of the multitude of conformational properties of the peptide are important to these two events and other aspects of the biological response. In addition, biological activities of peptide hormones generally are mediated by a variety of other allosteric factors (6). Thus, one must choose well defined assay conditions so that potency values, efficacy, and other parameters of biological activity can be meaningfully compared and then utilized for rational structure-function analysis.

4. Finally, many peptide hormones and neurotransmitters have a number of physiologically and/or pharmacologically relevant receptors. In general, development of a suitable peptide drug would require that the analog have high specificity for the tissue in question so that undesirable side reactions would be minimized. Furthermore, the conformational and stereostructural properties of the peptide receptors are generally very poorly understood and thus, at least for the time being, it will be necessary to develop design strategies that do not require extensive knowledge of the three dimensional structure of the receptor.

In an effort to overcome some of these difficulties and to provide the beginnings of a rational approach to the design of hormone analogs, we have utilized conformational and topographical restriction of peptide hormone and neurotransmitter structures. In this approach, we have attempted to make use where possible of classical structure-function studies, to interpret the results from these studies in terms of specific conformational parameters which may be involved in the observed rela-

tions of structure to biological activity, and from this to develop a conformational model which can be examined and tested. We
have previously discussed the biological considerations and
bioassay studies which are critical to such an approach (4, 5,
7). In particular, we would emphasize the need to obtain full
dose-response curves and a careful assessment of potency differences and efficacy differences based on these full dose-
response relationships. This is critical if one is to develop
insight into those features of structure and conformation which
are critical to receptor recognition and those which are critical
to transduction (2, 8). Such insight is essential in the development of antagonists, superagonists, etc.

In addition, any rational approach to peptide hormone and
neurotransmitter design must ultimately depend on the application
of physical-chemical principles of conformation and structure,
the use of various spectroscopic methods (especially nuclear magnetic resonance, circular dichroism, and Raman spectroscopies,
X-ray analysis where possible, etc.), and an understanding of the
nature of a hormone-receptor interaction in physical-chemical
terms. Here again the use of conformationally restricted peptide
structures is critical (4, 5, 7, 9-13). Recently we have
discussed some of the potential advantages of such an approach
(13, 14). Of particular importance for peptide drug design are
the following: 1) receptor specificity can be increased for peptides having several sites of action; 2) increased potency will
result if the conformation relevant to receptor binding is
stabilized; 3) peptides generally will be more stable to enzymatic degradation; 4) conformational and structural features important to binding and transduction can be more precisely
determined; 5) appropriate conformational strictions can lead to
inhibitors; and 6) conformational properties determined in solution are more likely to have relevance to the receptor-bound conformation.

In this paper, we will discuss how we have utilized this
approach for a) the development of linear and cyclic melanotropin
analogs which superagonist potency; b) the development of cyclic
enkephalin analogs with high receptor specificity; c) the development of oxytocin antagonists with prolonged *in vivo*
activities; and d) the development of α-melanotropin analogs with
prolonged *in vitro* and *in vivo* biological activities and complete
enzymatic stability.

Development of Conformationally Constrained α-Melanotropin Superagonists

As discussed above, the development of peptide analogs with high
potency requires an understanding of those features of structure
and conformation which are critical for receptor binding and compatible with receptor transduction. Superpotency can result by
maximizing the conformational and stereoelectronic structural

features which are complimentary to biological recognition and
transduction. We believe that some of the α-melanotropin analogs
we have developed are approaching maximum complimentarity.

α-Melanotropin (α-MSH) is a linear tridecapeptide, Ac-Ser-
Tyr-Ser-Met-Glu-His-Phe-Arg-Trp-Gly-Lys-Pro-Val-NH_2 found in the
pars intermedia of the vertebrate pituitary and in various parts
of the brain. It is the hormone responsible for melanosone
dispersion (skin darkening) and for integumental melanogenesis
(melanin production) (15, 16). In addition, considerable evidence has accumulated that α-MSH is implicated in fetal development, in CNS functioning related to attention, facilitated
memory, and other behaviors, in thermoregulation, in sebum production and in other activities (16,17). In view of these
interesting activities at diverse receptor sites, its linear conformationally flexible nature, and extensive structure function
studies (18,19), we felt that it presented an excellent peptide
to examine by the above approach.

Our starting point was an interesting, earlier biological
observation that when α-MSH was heat-alkali treated, it led to a
complex diastereoisomeric mixture which was highly active and
displayed prolonged activity (20,21). We hypothesized that race-
mization had resulted in specific conformational effects which
were critical to the biological activity of the hormone.
Quantitative characterization of the chemical effects of heat-
alkali treatment (22), conformational considerations (23), and
other considerations led us to suggest that [Nle^4,-D-Phe^7]-α-MSH
might possess the increased biological potency and prolonged
biological activities associated with the heat-alkali treated
hormone. Indeed, (Table I) [Nle^4, D-Phe^7]-α-MSH was found to be
about 60 times more potent than the native hormone in the frog
skin system, five times more potent than α-MSH in the lizard skin
system, and 25 times more potent than α-MSH in the mouse melanoma
adenylate cyclase assay system (23). These results led us to
investigate whether fragment analogs might retain exceptional
biological potency. We first prepared the analog in which the D-
Phe-7 residue is replaced by the L-amino acid residue, i.e.,
[Nle^4]-α-MSH (3, Table I). In the lizard skin assay system, this
analog retains nearly the same high potency of the 1-13 D-Phe-7
analog, but in the frog skin system the compound is only 1/26th
the potency of the D-Phe-7 1-13 analog 2. Interestingly, the
Nle^4, 4-13 fragment analog 4 (Table I) is nearly as active as the
Nle-4 1-13 analog 3 in the frog skin system and in the lizard
skin system (24). These results demonstrate that the N-terminal
tripeptide is important to the potency of α-MSH in the frog skin
system but is of little importance in the lizard skin system
(24). We then prepared the "active site" analogs 5 and 6 (Table
I) (25). Indeed, Ac-[Nle^4,D-Phe^7]-α-MSH_{4-10}-NH_2 is the most
potent linear analog thus far known in the lizard skin system.
Further studies with the 4-11 analogs 7 and 8 (Table I) and the
5-11 analogs 9 and 10 (Table I) (26) illustrate the critical

Table I.   Relative in Vitro Potencies of α-MSH Analogs on Frog
(Rana pipiens) Skin and Lizard (Anolis carolinensis)
Skin Assays[a]

Compound	Frog Skin Assay	Lizard Skin Assay
1. α-MSH	1.0	1.0
2. [Nle^4,D-Phe^7]-α-MSH	60.0	5.0
3. [Nle^4]-α-MSH	2.3	1.5
4. Ac-[Nle^4]-α-MSH$_{4-13}$-NH$_2$	1.0	1.0
5. Ac-[Nle^4,D-Phe^7]-α-MSH$_{4-10}$-NH$_2$	0.02	10.0
6. Ac-[Nle^4]-α-MSH$_{4-10}$-NH$_2$	0.002	0.06
7. Ac-[Nle^4]-α-MSH$_{4-11}$-NH$_2$	0.002	1.0
8. Ac-[Nle^4,D-Phe^7]-α-MSH$_{4-11}$-NH$_2$	0.20	8.0
9. Ac-[D-Phe^7]-α-MSH$_{5-11}$-NH$_2$	0.01	1.0
10. Ac-α-MSH$_{5-11}$-NH$_2$	0.0002	0.004
11. [Cys^4, Cys^{10}]-α-MSH	10-100[a]	~4.0
12. Ac-[Cys^4, Cys^{10}]-α-MSH$_{4-13}$-NH$_2$	10-100[a]	0.6
13. Ac-[Cys^4, Cys^{10}]-α-MSH$_{4-11}$-NH$_2$	0.12	0.12
14. Ac-[Cys^4, Cys^{10}]-α-MSH$_{4-10}$-NH$_2$	0.07	0.003
15. Ac-α-MSH$_{4-10}$-NH$_2$	0.0003	0.004

[a]All potencies are relative to α-MSH in dose-response assays.
Relative potency = conc. of α-MSH at 50% response/conc. of peptide at 50% response. The cyclic peptides 11 and 12 have much
higher minimal effective dose potencies (~10,000) in the frog
skin system.

importance of the 5 and 11 positions to α-MSH potency in the frog
system and the relative unimportance of the 11 position to the
lizard system in some cases but not others.
    As discussed previously, the biological results with the
D-Phe-7 analogs in frog skin system suggested to us that the very
high potency of these analogs had their basis in specific conformation features. Since our goal has been to develop a conformational model consistent with the biological activity data and
then to test this model by appropriate conformational restric-
tions, we decided to examine this approach in the frog skin
system. Important considerations were the following: 1) as previously mentioned, we considered it likely that residue 7 directs
the correct biologically active conformation at the frog skin
receptor system; 2) since D-amino acid residues in peptides can
stabilize reverse turn conformations (27), we hypothesized that a
reverse turn in the vicinity of the Phe-7 position might stabi-

lize the biologically active conformation; 3) application of conformational calculations and Chou and Fasman analysis (28) of
conformational tendencies suggested that the tetrapeptide
fragment His-Phe-Arg-Trp in α-MSH had a reasonable tendency to
exist in a reverse turn conformation (23); 4) structure-function
studies suggested a conformational proximity between the Lys-11
residue and some structural moiety in the central region of α-MSH
(perhaps Glu-5 or His-6); 5) model building indicated that conformations of α-MSH could be built which incorporated the Phe-7
residue as part of a β-turn, a C_7 turn, or a γ-turn. A schematic
representation of the proposed reverse-turn bioactive conformation of α-MSH at the frog skin receptor is shown in Figure 1.
    From the above considerations and model building, we
observed that Met-4 and Gly-10 were in reasonable proximity of
one another in several conformations. Furthermore, we wished to
prepare a cyclic analog to test our model, and noted that replacement of the Met-4 (side chain = $-CH_2-CH_2-S-CH_3$) and Gly-10
(side chain = H) residues by a Cys^4, Cys^{10} bridged cyclic
disulfide residue (side chains = $-CH_2-S-S-CH_2-$) would correspond
to a "pseudo-isosteric" replacement. Thus we prepared [$\overline{Cys}^4$,
$\overline{Cys}^{10}$]-α-MSH (11, Table I) and found that it was a superagonist
in both the frog skin and lizard systems. For example, we have
obtained biological activity at concentrations as low as 10^{-15}
molar (about 10,000 more potent than α-MSH) (28). However, the
responses are variable and true dose-response curves are only
seen in the 10^{-13}M to 10^{-10}M range. The reasons for this potency
variability relative to α-MSH are unclear, but may reflect
variations in compartmentalization and/or receptor sensitivity
which may be variable with season and from animal to animal.
Interestingly, the cyclic 4-13 analog 12 (Table I) retains its
superpotency in the frog skin but not the lizard skin systems.
The 4-10 cyclic analog 14 (Table I) is quite inactive in both
systems, but relative to the linear pseudo-isosteric analog 15
much more so in the lizard skin system (29). Addition of Lys-11
to the cyclic 4-10 analog to give analog 13 leads to a large
increase in potency in the lizard but not the frog skin system
(30).

Development of Cyclic Enkephalin Analogs with High Receptor Specificity

Examination of the data in Table I and other data not reported
here provides evidence that conformation restriction (in this
case cyclization) favors specificity at one physiological receptor type over another. For example, in the cyclic 4-13 analog
(12, Table I) about a 60-fold relative specificity preference for
the frog skin system is seen, but it is actually more than that
due to the 5- to 10-fold greater absolute potency of α-MSH in the
frog skin system.
    In our investigations, we were anxious to examine the possi-

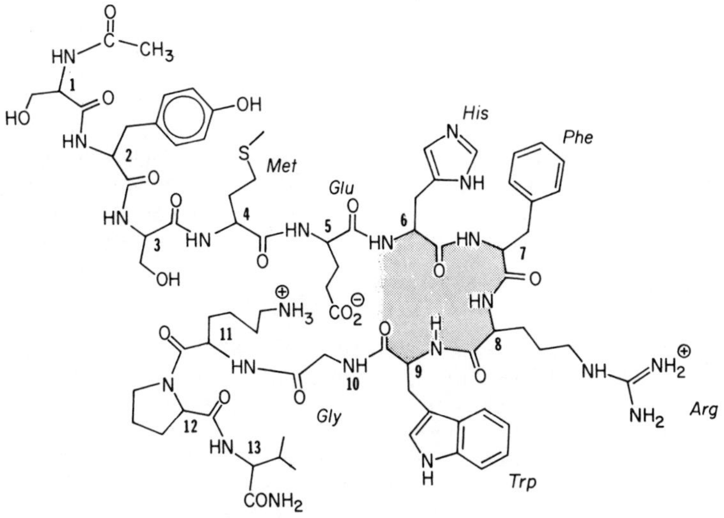

Figure 1. Schematic representation of a proposed reverse turn conformation of α-MSH at the frog skin receptor. Reproduced with permission from Ref. 50. Copyright 1982, Zoological Society.

bility that conformational restriction could lead to high receptor selectivity in other systems. The enkephalin molecules,
[Met[5]]-enkephalin (H-Tyr-Gly-Gly-Phe-Met-OH) and [Leu[5]]-
enkephalin (H-Tyr-Gly-Gly-Phe-Leu-OH) seemed particularly
intriguing from several viewpoints. First, since their discovery
and structure determination (31), they have been studied extensively for their structure-activity relationships and virtually
all analogs have been linear peptide. Conformational properties
have been examined using almost exclusively the native hormones
and linear analogs. Not surprisingly, there are many con-
flicting models of solution and receptor-bound geometries (for
recent reviews see 32,33). Second, these peptides appear to
interact with several subclasses of opoid receptors, the most
commonly accepted being the mu (μ), delta (δ), and kappa (κ)
receptors (34-36). The physiological roles for these receptors
are not well understood. Third, structure-function studies had
not led to many reported analogs with high receptor selectivity.
Therefore, we decided to investigate the possibility of developing cyclic, conformationally-restricted enkephalin analogs
which would possess high receptor selectivity.

On examination of the structures of the enkephalin and the
structure-activity relationships published by late 1980, we were
struck by two observations. First, highly potent enkephalin analogs could be prepared by substituting Gly-2 by a large variety
of D-amino acids, and Met-5 (or Leu-5) could be replaced by a
large variety of L- or D-amino acid and lead to a potent enkephalin analog. Second, the Gly-2, Met-5 combination is highly remi-
niscent of the Met-4, Gly-10 situation in α-MSH.

Examination of the literature revealed that Sarantakis had
prepared and patented [D-Cys2,L-Cys5]-enkephalins (37), and
shortly thereafter Schiller and co-workers also prepared these
compounds and examined extensively their biological activities
(38). In previous studies with oxytocin antagonist analogs (see
below), we had demonstrated (3,4,7,10,39) that increased rigidity
can be conferred on medium-sized disulfide-containing peptide
rings if half-cystine is replaced by half-penicillamine. These
considerations led us to prepare a number of D-Pen-2, D(L)-Cys-5
cyclic enkephalinamide (40) and enkephalin (41) analogs
(compounds 18-21, Table II). These compounds turned out to have
considerable δ receptor selectivity as measured by comparison of
inhibitory potencies in the guinea pig ileum (μ receptor) vs.
mouse vas deferens (δ receptor), and receptor binding affinities
in the rat brain (Table II). Examination of the D-Cys-2,
D(L)-Pen-5 cyclic enkephalins 23 and 22 (Table II) showed they
retained high δ selectivity in the former assay, but less so in
the latter assay (42).

These results led us to prepare the bis-penicillamine cyclic
analogs 24 and 25 (Table II). These highly conformationally
restricted cyclic analogs are extraordinarily δ receptor specific
(43), being more selective than any previously reported δ selec-

Table II.   Receptor Binding Affinities of Enkephalin Analogs for [^{3}H]-Labelled Naloxone ([^{3}H]NAL) and [^{3}H]-Labelled [D-Ala^2,D-Leu^5]Enkephalin ([^{3}H]DADLE) in Rat Brain Homogenates[a]

Analog	IC$_{50}$(nm) [^{3}H]NAL	IC$_{50}$(nm) [^{3}H]DADLE	μIC$_{50}$ / δIC$_{50}$	IC$_{50}$(GPI) / IC$_{50}$(MVD)
16. [D-Cys^2,L-Cys^5]EA	9.4	30.2	0.31	—
17. [D-Cys^2,D-Cys^5]EA	5.2	15.4	0.34	—
18. [D-Pen^2,L-Cys^5]EA	73.4±15	3.35±0.15	21.9	32.4
19. [D-Pen^2,D-Cys^5]EA	162 ±35	7.20±1.8	22.6	6.9
20. [D-Pen^2,L-Cys^5]E	178 ±16	11.7 ±1.2	15.2	666.0
21. [D-Pen^2,D-Cys^5]E	157 ±74	26.0 ±0.5	6.0	215.0
22. [D-Cys^2,L-Pen^5]E	52.7±2.3	5.4 ±0.1	9.8	53.2
23. [D-Cys^2,D-Pen^5]E	22.2±2.8	3.5 ±0.8	6.3	513.0
24. [D-Pen^2,L-Pen^5]E	3710 ±740	10.0 ±0.2	371.0	1088.0
25. [D-Pen^2,D-Pen^5]E	2840 ±670	16.2 ±0.9	175.0	3164.0
26. [D-Ala^2,D-Leu^5]E	16 ±5.0	3.9 ±0.7	4.1	—
27. [D-Ser^2,Leu^5,Thr^6]E	88 ±6.0	5.73±0.42	15.4	333.0
28. [D-Thr^2,Leu^5,Thr^6]E	36.3±3.8	6.40±0.60	5.7	173.0

[a]Also shown are δ receptor selectivities as measured by comparison of inhibitory potencies (IC$_{50}$) of enkephalin analogs in the guinea pig ileum (GPI) and mouse vas deferens (MVP) assays. E = enkephalin; EA = enkephalinamide.

tive analogs. Conformational analysis of these analogs should
provide critical insight into the biologically active conformation of enkephalins at δ receptors, and aid in the further
development of δ selective enkephalin agonists and antagonists.
In addition, we are beginning to unravel the physiological significance of δ receptors. For example, we have recently
demonstrated, using the δ selective analog 20 (Table II), that δ
receptors in the brain can mediate analgesia but do not affect
gut transit, while in the spinal cord δ receptors appear to
affect both functions (44).

Development of Conformationally Constrained Oxytocin Antagonists with Prolonged in Vivo Activities

We have extensively investigated the conformation-activity relationships of oxytocin (H-Cys-Tyr-Ile-Gln-Asn-Cys-Pro-Leu-Gly-NH$_2$)
antagonists based on the antagonist [Pen^1]-oxytocin (4,5,7). On
the basis of these studies, we have proposed a conformational
model for antagonist activity (4,5,7), and suggested the conformational and dynamic features of these analogs critical for
binding and for preventing transduction (5,7). A key result was
our finding from NMR, CD, and Raman studies that the geminal
dimethyl groups of the Pen-1 residue greatly stabilized the conformation of the 20-membered ring and the disulfide dihedral
angle at about 115° with a right-handed chirality. Furthermore,
it was found that the side chain moieties at positions 2 and 5
are restricted such that one or both side chains cannot orient
over the 20-membered disulfide-containing ring. Recently, we
have concentrated our efforts in two directions. The first is
directed toward testing and refining our conformational model for
Pen-1 analogs and to improve their antagonist potency. This
aspect of our work will not be discussed. The second is directed
toward developing antagonist analogs with prolonged in vitro and
in vivo biological activity. Most previous approaches to prolong
the bioactivity of peptide hormones or neurotransmitters have
involved the use of D-amino acids, N-methylamino acids, or N or C
terminal blocking groups. We have suggested (44) that prolongation of biological activity might also be a receptor-related
event, and therefore may be a function of structural and conformational features of the peptide important to the receptor-
hormone complex in the transduced (biologically active) state, or
to a bound complex in a non-biologically active (inhibitory)
state. If this hypothesis has merit, it should be possible to
design conformational and dynamic features into a molecule which
are primarily important to the transduced state for an agonist or
the non-biologically active but bound state for an inhibitor.

Our approach to testing this hypothesis and developing oxytocin antagonists with prolonged in vivo activity has been to
further restrict the conformations of side chain groups at positions believed to be important for binding in the antagonist

bound state. Earlier observations led us to investigate modifications of side chain groups at positions 4, 7, and 8 in conjunction with lipophilic residues in position 2. The results of some of these studies are summarized in Table III. As previously reported (45), the use of a β-branched amino acid Thr at position 4 of Pen-1 oxytocin analogs increases their potency (31, Table III) as does the Phe-2 substitution (33, Table III). The dehydroproline analog 32 (Table III) is considerably more potent an antagonist than [Pen^1]-oxytocin but when used in conjunction with the Phe-2 and Thr-4 substitutions produces a slightly less potent antagonist analog 34 than the analog with a Pro in position 7 (33, Table III). However, when the ornithine-8 substitution first introduced by Manning and co-workers (46) was used in conjunction with the Thr-4 substitution, a series of analogs were obtained with exceptionally prolonged in vitro and in vivo activities. As we previously suggested (7), these results also sup-

Table III.   Antagonist Potencies of Oxytocin Analogs in the Rat Uterus Assay

Compound	pA$_2$[a]
29. [Pen^1]Oxytocin	6.86
30. [Pen^1,Leu^2]Oxytocin	7.14
31. [Pen^1,Thr^4]Oxytocin	7.55
32. [Pen^1,Δ^{3,4}Pro^7]Oxytocin	7.11
33. [Pen^1,Phe^2,Thr^4]Oxytocin	7.68
34. [Pen^1,Phe^2,Thr^4,Δ^{3,4}Pro^7]Oxytocin	7.5[b]
35. [Pen^1,Phe^2,Thr^4,Δ^{3,4}Pro^7,Orn^8]Oxytocin	∼7.5[b,c] prolonged
36. [Pen^1,Tyr(OMe)^2,Thr^4,Orn^8]Oxytocin	prolonged[b,c]
37. [Pen^1,Phe(Me)^2,Thr^4,Orn^8]Oxytocin	prolonged[b,c]

[a]pA$_2$ values represent the negative log to the base 10 of the average concentration (M) of an antagonist which will reduce the response of the uterine horn 2X units of pharmacologically active compound (agonist) to X units of the agonist.
[b]Rockway, T.W.; Ormberg, J.; Chan, W.Y.; Hruby, V.J., unpublished results.
[c]These compounds have very prolonged (minutes to hours) in vitro and in vivo antagonist activities. In some cases (compounds 36 and 37) it was not possible to obtain even an estimate of the in vitro antagonist potencies (pA$_2$). In other cases (compounds 34,35) the estimates are lower limits and represent only estimates since due to the prolonged activity, true equilibrium measurement cannot be made.

port the idea that the binding mode of antagonist analogs to oxytocin receptors is different than oxytocin agonists. This is particularly relevant in this case since in the agonist series, substitution of Leu-8 by Orn-8 leads to a large decrease in agonist potency. Moreover, we believe these results provide support for our hypothesis that structural and conformational features can be designed into an antagonist molecule that are unrelated to receptor recognition (binding potency), but rather are related to specific features related to the peptide-receptor complex in its inhibitory state. We currently are examining the conformational features which may be important for prolonged activity. Further impetus for these studies have been provided by our findings that compounds 31 and 33 (Table III) have antiprostaglandin-releasing effects in pregnant rats and pregnant human myometrial tissue (47,48). Clearly, long-acting analogs have great potential as tocolytic agents for the treatment of preterm labor. Furthermore, we believe that our hypothesis regarding design of antagonist analogs with prolonged activity offers a potentially useful approach to peptide drug design.

Development of α-Melanotropin Analogs with Prolonged In Vitro and In Vivo Biological Activities

As discussed earlier, heat-alkali treatment of α-MSH results in a complex diastereoisomeric mixture which displays prolonged activity. One might anticipate that this prolonged activity would simply be the result of the presence of peptides with D-amino acids. However, our hypothesis that prolongation may also result from structural and conformational properties of the peptide when it is part of the peptide-receptor complex, prompted us to investigate the conformational and structural requirements for prolongation of α-MSH activity. We reasoned that if our hypothesis were correct, prolongation should be manifested in two differential effects: 1) there should be no necessary relationship between potency and prolongation of activity; and 2) prolongation for a particular analog need not be manifested at all physiological receptors for the hormone. Our recent results fully support these ideas.

For reasons discussed earlier, we predicted that [Nle^4,D-Phe^7]-α-MSH, 2 (Table I), would have prolonged activity in addition to its superpotency. Indeed, this was the case in the in vitro frog and lizard skin bioassays systems. Thus, when the skins exposed to the analog were thoroughly washed with melanotropin-free Ringer solution and then incubated in peptide-free assay medium, the skins remained dark for several hours (23). Similar treatment of the skins which had been darkened with the native hormone led to rapid return to the light unstimulated color. We next examined whether prolonged effects could be observed in vivo. A single injection of 2 into frogs (Rana pipiens) led to skin darkening for several weeks (49) (Figure 2).

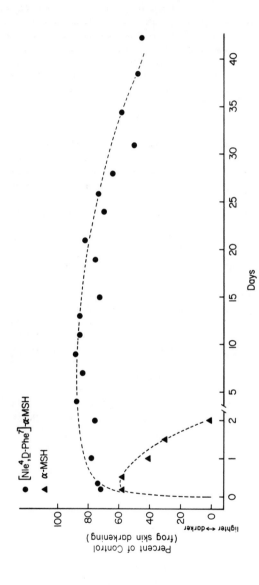

Figure 2. Long-term effect of single injection of [Nle^4,D-Phe^7]-α-MSH (●) on darkening of the frog R. pipiens showing the transient darkening effects of α-MSH (▲). Modified figure 1 from Ref. 49 by permission of the AAAS. Copyright 1981.

A remarkable aspect of this skin darkening was that over this long time there was only a small amount of skin lightening, suggesting that there was little loss (down regulation) of receptor-hormone complex during this time period. Morphological examination revealed that the vast majority of skin darkening was due to melanocyte dispersion, a direct receptor-related event. These findings suggest that [Nle^4,D-Phe^7]-α-MSH binds to its receptors in a non-reversible manner in the transduced state, or that it produces a receptor system which is "frozen" in the transduced state. This peptide should provide a powerful tool for studying the transduced state of the melanotropin receptor system. In fact, we have already used this analog to demonstrate the absolute requirement for Ca^{+2} for transduction in the lizard skin system (49).

These results led us to investigate the relationships between biological potency and prolonged activity, the structural and conformational requirements of prolonged activity, and the differential requirements for prolongation in the frog and lizard systems. Some results are summarized in Table IV, and demonstrate a number of points. First, there is no obvious relationship between biological potency and prolongation of biological activity. This is particularly clear in the frog skin system where highly potent analogs (2, Table IV) show prolonged activity, but so do very weak analogs such as Ac-[Tyr^4]-α-MSH$_{4-10}$-NH$_2$ (38, Table IV) (26). On the other hand, the relatively potent 4-10 α-MSH analog, Ac-[Nle^4,D-Phe^7]-α-MSH$_{4-10}$-NH$_2$ (5, Table IV), produces only minor prolongation of activity in the frog skin system (25). However, the 4-11 analog 8 (Table IV) has the same extraordinary prolonged activity of the full 1-13 Nle-4,D-Phe-7 analog 2.

As for the importance of conformational restriction to prolongation, thus far we have examined only the 1-13 and 4-13 cyclic analogs 11 and 12 in the frog system (Table IV). These highly potent analogs have minimal prolonged in vitro activity (28). From this study it appears quite certain that the structural and perhaps conformational requirements for potency (receptor recognition) are different than the requirements for prolongation. We believe these results support our hypothesis that prolongation of biological activity is amenable to design based on structural and conformation consideration. Two other pertinent observations support this conclusion. First, prolongation activity for a particular hormone at a particular receptor type does not necessarily lead to prolongation at another receptor. This is most clearly illustrated by two examples in Table IV. Ac-[Nle^4,D-Phe^7]-α-MSH$_{4-10}$-NH$_2$ has extended prolonged activity in the lizard system but is barely prolonged in the frog system. On the other hand, Ac-α-MSH$_{5-11}$-NH$_2$ has prolonged activity in the frog system but has no prolonged activity whatsoever in the lizard receptor system. Clearly, these two physiologically similar receptor systems have quite different structural

Table IV. Relative Potency and Prolongation of Selected α-Melanotropin Analogs in the In Vitro Frog and Lizard Systems[a]

Compound	Potency in Frog	Prolongation in Frog	Potency in Lizard	Prolongation in Lizard
1. α-MSH	1.0	No	1.0	No
2. [Nle^4,D-Phe^7]-α-MSH	60.0	Yes	5.0	Yes
5. Ac-[Nle^4,D-Phe^7]-α-MSH$_{4-10}$-NH$_2$	0.02	Weak	10.0	Yes
6. Ac-[Nle^4]-α-MSH$_{4-10}$-NH$_2$	0.002	Medium	0.06	N.D.[b]
7. Ac-[Nle^4]-α-MSH$_{4-11}$-NH$_2$	0.002	No	1.0	No
8. Ac-[Nle^4,D-Phe^7]-α-MSH$_{4-11}$-NH$_2$	0.16	Yes	8.0	Yes
9. Ac-[D-Phe^7]-α-MSH$_{5-11}$-NH$_2$	0.01	No	1.0	No
10. Ac-α-MSH$_{5-11}$-NH$_2$	0.0002	Yes	0.004	No
38. Ac-[Tyr^4]-α-MSH$_{4-10}$-NH$_2$	0.0002	Yes	0.0006	N.D.
11. [Cys^4, Cys^{10}]-α-MSH	10-100[c]	Yes	~4.0	N.D.
12. Ac-[Cys^4, Cys^{10}]-α-MSH$_{4-13}$-NH$_2$	10-100[c]	Yes	0.6	N.D.

[a] All potencies are relative to α-MSH which is defined as equal to 1.
[b] N.D. = Not determined.
[c] Minimal effective dose potency ~10,000. See Table I.

and probably conformational requirements for prolonged biological
activity. Secondly, one might suggest that prolongation of
biological activity is primarily a function of enzymatic stability of these analogs. We have examined the stability of these
compounds to serum enzymes and to trypsin and chymotrypsin as
measured by their biological activities. We have found, for
example, that all D-Phe-7 α-melanotropin analogs are stable to
these enzyme systems. Yet the D-Phe-7 analog Ac-[D-Phe^7]-α-MSH$_{5-}$
$_{11}$-NH$_2$ does not have prolonged activity at either the frog or the
lizard receptor system.

Conclusions

In our research over the past several years we have attempted to
utilize chemical and physical principles related to conformation
and structure to develop a rational approach to the design of
biologically active peptide hormones and neurotransmitters. It
is critical in this approach that intensive biological data over
the full dose-response range be available so that critical evalu-
ations can be made of those conformational and stereostructural
features related to recognition (binding), transduction
(biological activity) and prolongation (long term biological
response). Conformational restriction via covalent cyclization,
transannular steric effects, side chain rigidization, backbone
conformational stabilization, etc. are applicable for such studies. The success of any such endeavor will depend ultimately on
the careful and synergistic utilization of the biological assay
data and physical-chemical studies of the conformational and
dynamic properties of the native hormone and well chosen analogs.
The development of this approach is clearly in its infancy, but
it appears to have considerable potential for future development.

Acknowledgments

The author is deeply grateful to his colleagues and co-workers
without whose diligent work and creative ideas this report could
not be written. In particular, he thanks Professors Mac Hadley,
H. Yamamura, T. Burks and W. Chan, whose astute biological studies and observations and strong collaborative interactions have
been so critical to the development of these ideas, and his stu-
dents and postdoctoral associates Wayne Cody, Paul Darman, Robin
Hurst, James Knittel, Jean-Paul Meraldi, Henry Mosberg, Todd
Rockway, Tomi Sawyer, Brian Wilkes, and Young Yang and others who
contributed so much of their ideas and experimental ability to
this research. The support of the U.S. Public Health Service
and the National Science Foundation is particularly acknowledged.

Literature Cited

1.   Van Rossum, J.M.; Ariens, E.J.   Arch. Int. Pharmacodyn.
     1962, 136, 385-413.

2. Rudinger, J. in "Drug Design"; Ariens, J., Ed.; Academic: New York, 1971; Vol. 2, pp. 319-419.
3. Schwyzer, R. Ann. N.Y. Acad. Sci. 1977, 297, 3-25.
4. Hruby, V.J. in "Perspectives in Peptide Chemistry"; Eberle, A.; Geiger, R.; Wieland, T., Eds.; S. Karger: Basel, 1981, pp. 207-220.
5. Hruby, V.J. in "Topics in Molecular Pharmacology"; Burgen, A.S.V.; Roberts, G.C.K., Eds.; Elsevier/North Holland: Amsterdam, 1981, pp. 99-126.
6. Rodbell, M. Nature 1980, 284, 17-22.
7. Hruby, V.J.; Mosberg, H.I. in "Hormone Antagonists"; Agarwal, M.K., Ed.; Walter de Gruyter: Berlin, 1982, pp. 433-474.
8. Hruby, V.J. Molecul. Cellul. Biochem. 1982, 44, 49-64.
9. Marshall, G.R.; Bosshard, H.E.; Vine, W.H.; Glickson, J.D.; Needleman, P. in "Recent Advances in Renal Physiology and Pharmacology"; Wessen, L.G.; Fanelli, G.M., Eds.; University Park Press: Baltimore, 1974, pp. 215-256.
10. Meraldi, J.-P.; Yamamoto, D.; Hruby, V.J.; Brewster, A.I.R. in "Peptides: Chemistry, Structure, and Biology"; Walter, R.; Meienhofer, J., Eds.; Ann Arbor Sci. Publ.: Ann Arbor, 1975, pp. 803-814.
11. Veber, D.F.; Holly, F.W.; Paleveda, W.J.; Nutt, R.F.; Bergstrand, S.J.; Torchiana, M.; Glitzer, M.S.; Saperstein, R.; Hirschmann, R. Proc. Natl. Acad. Sci. USA 1978, 75, 2636-2640.
12. Marshall, G.R.; Gorin, F.A.; Moore, M.L. Annu. Rep. Med. Chem. 1978, 13, 227-238.
13. Hruby, V.J. Life Sciences 1982, 31, 189-199.
14. Hruby, V.J., Knittel, J.J.; Mosberg, H.I.; Rockway, T.W.; Wilkes, B.C.; and Hadley, M.E. in "Peptides 1982"; Blaha, K.; Malon, P., Eds.; Walter de Gruyter: Berlin, 1983, pp. 19-30.
15. Hadley, M.E.; Bagnara, J.T. Amer. Zool., Suppl. 1 1975, 15, 81-96.
16. "Peptides of the Pars Intermedia"; Evered, D.; Lawrenson, G., Eds.; CIBA FOUNDATION SYMPOSIUM 81, Pitman Medical: London, 1981.
17. O'Donohue, T.L.; Dorsa, D.M. Peptides 1982, 3, 353-395.
18. Medzihradszky, K. in "Recent Developments in the Chemistry of Natural Carbon Compounds"; Bognar, R.; Bruckner, R.; Szantay, C.S., Eds.; Publ. House Hung. Acad. Sci.: Budapest, 1976, pp. 119-250.
19. Hruby, V.J.; Wilkes, B.C.; Cody, W.L.; Sawyer, T.K.; Hadley, M.E. Peptide Protein Rev. 1983, in press.
20. Smith, P.E.; Graeser, J.B. Anat. Rec. 1924, 27, 187.
21. Bool, A.M.; Gray, G.H., II; Hadley, M.E.; Heward, C.B.; Hruby, V.J.; Sawyer, T.K.; Yang, Y.C.S. J. Endocrinol. 1981, 88, 57-65.

22. Engel, M.H.; Sawyer, T.K.; Hadley, M.E.; Hruby, V.J. Anal.
     Biochem. 1981, 116, 303-311.
23. Sawyer, T.,.; Sanfilippo, P.J.; Hruby, V.J.; Engel, M.H.;
     Heward, C.B.; Burnett, J.B.; Hadley, M.E. Proc. Natl.
     Acad. Sci. USA 1980, 77, 5754-5758.
24. Hadley, M.E.; Wilkes, B.C.; Sawyer, T.K.; Hruby, V.J.,
     unpublished results.
25. Sawyer, T.K.; Hruby, V.J.; Wilkes, B.C.; Draelos, M.T.;
     Hadley, M.E.; Bergsneider, M. J. Med. Chem. 1982, 25,
     1022-1027.
26. Wilkes, B.C.; Sawyer, T.K.; Hruby, V.J.; Hadley, M.E. Int.
     J. Peptide Protein Res. 1983, in press.
27. Chandrasekaran, R.; Lakshminarayanan, A.V.; Pandya, U.V.;
     Ramachandran, G.N. Biochim. Biophys. Acta 1978, 303, 14-27.
28. Sawyer, T.K.; Hruby, V.J.; Darman, P.S.; Hadley, M.E.
     Proc. Natl. Acad. Sci. USA 1982, 79, 1751-1755.
29. Knittel, J.J.; Sawyer, T.K.; Hruby, V.J.; Hadley, M.E. J.
     Med. Chem. 1983, 28, 125-129.
30. Cody, W.L.; Knittel, J.J.; Hruby, V.J.; Hadley, M.E.,
     unpublished results.
31. Hughes, J.; Smith, T.W.; Kosterlitz, H.W.; Fothergill, L.A.;
     Morgan, B.A.; Morris, H.R. Nature 1975, 258, 577-579.
32. Miller, R.J.; Cuatrecasas, P. Vitamins and Hormones 1978,
     36, 297-382.
33. Olson, G.A.; Olson, R.D.; Kastin, A.J.; Coy, D.H. Peptides,
     1982, 3, 1039-1072.
34. Lord, J.A.H.; Waterfield, A.A.; Hughes, J.; Kosterlitz, H.W.
     Nature 1977, 267, 495-499.
35. Wolozin, B.L.; Pasternak, G.W. Proc. Natl. Acad. Sci. USA
     1981, 78, 6181-6185.
36. Chang, K.-J.; Cuatrecasas, P. J. Biol. Chem. 1979, 254,
     2610-2618.
37. Sarantakis, D. U.S. Patent 4 148 789, 1979.
38. Schiller, P.W.; Eggimann, B.; DiMaio, J.; Lemieux, C.;
     Nguyen, T.M-D. Biochem. Biophys. Res. Commun. 1981, 101,
     337-343.
39. Meraldi, J.-P.; Hruby, V.J.; Brewster, A.I.R. Proc. Natl.
     Acad. Sci. USA 1977, 74, 1373-1377.
40. Mosberg, H.I.; Hurst, R.; Hruby, V.J.; Galligan, J.J.;
     Burks, T.F.; Gee, K.; Yamamura, H.I. Biochem. Biophys. Res.
     Commun. 1982, 106, 506-512.
41. Mosberg, H.I.; Hurst, R.; Hruby, V.J.; Galligan, J.J.;
     Burks, T.F.; Gee, K.; Yamamura, H.I. Life Sciences, 1983,
     32, 2565-2569.
42. Mosberg, H.I.; Hurst, R.; Hruby, V.J.; Gee, K.; Akiyama, K.;
     Yamamura, H.I.; Galligan, J.J.; Burks, T.F. Life Sciences,
     in press, 1983.
43. Mosberg, H.I.; Hurst, R.; Hruby, V.J.; Gee, K.; Yamamura,
     H.I.; Galligan, J.J.; Burks; T.F. Proc. Natl. Acad. Sci.
     USA, in press, 1983.

44. Porecca, F.; Mosberg, H.I.; Hurst, R.; Hruby, V.J.; Burks, T.F. Life Sciences, in press, 1983.

45. Hruby, V.J.; Mosberg, H.I.; Hadley, M.E.; Chan, W.Y.; Powell, A.M. Int. J. Peptide Protein Res. 1980, 16, 372-381.

46. Bankowski, K.; Manning, M.; Seto, J.; Haldar, J.; Sawyer, W.H. Int. J. Peptide Protein Res. 1980, 16, 382-391.

47. Chan, W. Y.; Powell, A.M.; Hruby, V.J. Endocrinology 1982, 111, 48-54.

48. Chan, W.Y.; Hruby, V.J. in "Peptides: Structure and Function"; Hruby, V.J.; Rich, D.H., Eds.; Pierce Chem. Co.: Rockford, 1983, in press.

49. Hadley, M.E.; Anderson, B.; Heward, C.B.; Sawyer, T.K.; Hruby, V.J. Science 1981, 213, 1025-1027.

50. Sawyer, T. K.; Hruby, V. J.; Hadley, M. E.; Engel, M. H. Amer. Zool. 1983, 23, 529-40.

RECEIVED November 15, 1983

Localization and Synthesis of Protein Antigenic Sites

Use of Free Synthetic Peptides for the Preparation of Antibodies and T-Cells of Preselected Specificities

M. ZOUHAIR ATASSI

Department of Biochemistry, Baylor College of Medicine, Houston, TX 77030

Intensive research in the author's laboratory had culminated in the determination and synthesis of all the antigenic sites of myoglobin in 1975 and of lysozyme in 1978 and more recently those of serum albumin and of human hemoglobin. These investigations provided the first unique insight into the molecular features responsible for the immune recognition of protein antigens and the factors which determine and regulate the antigenicity of the sites. But moreover, these studies have charted chemical strategies for investigation and synthetic duplication of protein binding sites. Furthermore, the concept of 'surface-simulation' synthesis, introduced and developed during determination of the antigenic structure of lysozyme, has provided a dimension of unlimited versatility for the synthetic mimicking of any type of protein binding sites. Binding sites representing other protein activities (including antibody combining sites) have been mimicked synthetically in our laboratory by this concept.

Recently we have shown that synthetic peptides can be successfully employed in their free form for the preparation of antibodies (both polyclonal and monoclonal) with specificities to preselected protein regions. Antibodies can even be prepared against regions that are not antigenic, when the native protein is used as immunogen, by immunization with the appropriate free synthetic peptide. Free synthetic peptides have also proved to be powerful reagents for preparation of T-cells of preselected specificity and for inducing specific tolerance to preselected regions of a protein. These immunogenic properties should afford important and simple tools for basic immunological investigations and, in

0097–6156/84/0251–0029$11.75/0
© 1984 American Chemical Society

disease related antigens and invasive agents (e.g.,
viruses, bacteria, toxins, allergens, etc.), for
therapeutic and diagnostic purposes.

Localization and Synthesis of Protein Antigenic Sites

Introduction

The first step in the biological activity of a protein involves
binding with a target molecule to form a complex. This complex
could be transient (e.g. enzyme-substrate complexes) or extremely
stable (e.g. haptoglobin-hemoglobin complex) or anywhere between
these two extremes. Most of the approaches for studying protein
binding sites have been limited to observing the site (e.g.
affinity labels, nuclear magnetic resonance, x-ray crystallography). Our efforts have been focused not only on observing
protein binding sites but on devising strategies for synthetic
mimicking of the sites. The ability to synthetically mimic
protein activities affords the potential for manipulation of
these activities.

The first protein binding sites to be precisely delineated
chemically and then synthesized were the antigenic sites of
sperm-whale myoglobin (Mb) (1). The great majority of antigens
associated with immune disorders and invasive agents (viruses,
bacteria, allergens, toxins, etc.) are attributed to protein
molecules. Thus knowledge of the molecular features responsible
for the antigenicity of proteins lies at the basis of understanding in molecular terms the cellular events of the immune response. Furthermore, charting a strategy for such undertakings
will be critical for the ultimate manipulation of these functions. Localization and synthesis of antigenic sites on invasive
agents should afford valuable synthetic vaccines (2) which will,
in principle, be expected to have little or no side effects.

The elucidation of the entire antigenic structure of a
protein had frustrated many attempts because of considerable
chemical and technical problems and these have already been discussed by this author in detail (1,3). It was not until 1975
that the first complete protein antigenic structure was precisely
determined (1). In fact, studies in this laboratory have given
the first protein antigenic structures to be determined in their
entirety. These were the antigenic structures of Mb in 1975 (1)
and of hen egg lysozyme in 1978 (4). Also, we have recently
localized and synthesized all the antigenic sites of the α- and
β-chain of human adult Hb (5-7) and the major antigenic sites of
serum albumin (8-11). Our determination of the antigenic
structure of Mb answered many questions relating to the molecular
immune recognition of native proteins with surprising accuracy
(1). These conclusions were soon confirmed with lysozyme (4) and

have since become established concepts that have been confirmed with a variety of other proteins.

This article focuses mainly on the immunology of proteins whose complete antigenic structures have been chemically localized and synthetically confirmed. These are Mb, lysozyme, Hb and serum albumin. The antigenic sites of many other proteins are now being investigated.

Chemical Strategy for the Determination and Synthesis of Antigenic Sites

a. General Chemical Strategy

The antigenic structure of a protein cannot be determined by the exclusive application of a single approach. A strategy was, therefore, developed (12) which relied on five approaches. This strategy enabled the precise determination of the entire antigenic structure of Mb (1) and was subsequently equally as effective in scoring a similar achievement with lysozyme (4). These approaches were: (1) to study the effect of conformational changes on the immunochemistry of the protein; (2) to study the immunochemistry and conformation of chemical derivatives of the protein, specifically modified at appropriate amino acid locations; (3) to isolate and characterize immunochemically-reactive fragments that can quantitatively account for the total reaction of the native protein; (4) to study the effect of chemical modification at selected amino acid locations on the immunochemistry and conformation of immunochemically reactive peptides; (5) after narrowing down each of the antigenic sites by approaches (1-4) to a region of conveniently small size, the final delineation would rely on studying the immunochemistry of synthetic peptides corresponding to many overlaps around this region. It is critical to note that each of these chemical approaches has advantages as well as shortcomings (1,3,13). It is also necessary to stress here that none of these approaches by itself is capable of yielding the full antigenic structure. We invariably used the results from one approach to confirm and/or correct those from the others. The complete structure is a composite, logical coordination of all the information.

It should be noted that the above strategy, although first employed in the delineation of protein antigenic sites, is applicable, with appropriate adaptations, to the precise delineation and chemical synthesis of other types of protein binding sites. The introduction of the concept of surface-simulation synthesis (14,15) has provided a methodology by which in principle any type of protein binding site can be mimicked synthetically after careful chemical characterization.

b. Comprehensive Synthetic Approach for Continuous Antigenic Sites

The study of overlapping peptide fragments is a key approach in the delineation of protein antigenic structures (12,1). This approach, when systematically employed, can yield valuable information on the number and locations of antigenic sites and their relative contributions to the total protein activity. In practice, however, this approach has severe shortcomings (13). These include the relatively limited number of reproducible cleavage procedures for proteins, the inadvertent scission within an antigenic site usually affording inactive or only slightly active peptides, the chemical modification frequently occurring at internal locations within a chemical-cleavage fragment and any traces of contamination of an isolated peptide. Furthermore, the distribution of residues whose peptide bonds are potentially susceptible to cleavage in the protein does not permit the desired overlapping peptides to be obtained. These were indeed the reasons why the strategy developed for the determination of protein antigenic structures employed five distinct chemical approaches (12,1).

In spite of the complexity of each chemical approach, however, the molecular details of the antigenic sites of Mb and lysozyme were derived (1) by such a strategy and have been immensely valuable in furthering our comprehension of immune recognition processes. As will be seen in the following sections, the antigenic sites of Mb and lysozyme consist of discrete surface portions of their respective native molecules. Each site comprises five to seven amino acid residues that come into close proximity either through direct peptide linkage, such as the 'continuous' antigenic sites of Mb (1), or in a more complex manner, through polypeptide-chain folding, such as the 'discontinuous' sites of lysozyme (4). In view of the structural alternatives in their architecture (continuous or discontinuous sites; ref. 16), the determination ab initio of the antigenic structures of other proteins should anticipate both alternatives. The logical progression, therefore, is first to localize and characterize the more readily identifiable continuous antigenic sites, with attention later paid to discontinuous sites.

Any approach that could facilitate the localization of continuous antigenic sites would certainly diminish the overall effort required for complete immunochemical characterization. Thus, with this goal in mind, and in order to circumvent the aforementioned problems and render the determination of protein antigenic structures more feasible within a reasonable time, we have devised (5) a novel comprehensive synthetic approach designed to yield the full antigenic profile of the protein under study. This approach consists of the direct synthesis and examination of the immunochemical activities of a series of overlapping peptides having uniform size and overlaps and that encompass the entire primary structure of the protein, from the beginning to the end. We have employed this approach to determine the antigenic sties on the α- and β-chains of human adult Hb (5-7).

Comparative Analysis of Protein Antigenic Structures

Derivation of the antigenic structures of Mb and lysozyme in each case spanned numerous publications. A concise review of our determination of the antigenic structure of Mb has appeared (1) and a very comprehensive account of the derivation has also been published (3). The climax of our studies on the antigenic structure of lysozyme can be found in the papers dealing with the synthesis of the three antigenic site of lysozyme (14,15,17-19) which quantitatively accounted for its entire antigenic reactivity and the work has already been reviewed (4). The main features of the antigenic structures of Mb (Figures 1 and 2) and of lysozyme (Figures 3-5) will be outlined very briefly below. Also, the antigenic sites of the α-chain of Hb (6), and the six major antigenic sites of serum albumin (8-11) (Fig. 7) will be given.

Myoglobin has five antigenic sites, each comprising a conformationally distinct continuous surface region of the polypeptide chain, and are situated on: (Site 1) residues 16-21 + 1 or 0 residue on one side only of this segment depending on the antiserum. This antigenic site exhibits a certain degree of "shift" or "displacement" and minor variability in size (limited to ± 1 residue only) from one antiserum to the next. Its location in the three-dimensional structure is on the bend between helices A and B: (Site 2) residues 56-62, on the bend between helices D and E. This antigenic site has exhibited no variablity in size with the antisera so far studied; (Site 3) residues 94-99 on the bend between helices F and G; (Site 4) residues 113-119, on the end of helix G and only part of the bend GH; (Site 5) residues 146-151 (+ lysine 145 with some antisera). This antigenic site is situated on the end of helix H and part of the randomly-coiled C-terminal pentapeptide. The covalent structures of the five antigenic sites are shown in Figure 2.

The findings that purely conformational changes in Mb will influence its reaction with antisera to the native protein (20,21) and the immunochemical results on numerous peptide fragments have enabled us to conclude (20) that the antibody response is directed against the native three-dimensional structures of proteins. These conclusions, initially derived with early course antisera were shown, in more recent studies from this laboratory (22) to apply to antisera obtained up to a year after the initial immunization.

Through the application or appropriate adaptations of the general chemical strategy outlined above, we found that lysozyme has three antigenic sites, each constituting spatially adjacent residues (which are otherwise distant in sequence) that occupy a

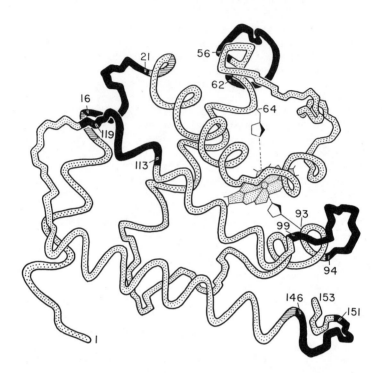

Figure 1. A schematic diagram showing the mode of
folding of Mb and its antigenic structure. The solid
black portions represent segments which have been
shown to comprise accurately the antigenic sites of
the protein. The striped parts, each corresponding to
one amino acid residue only, can be part of the
antigenic sites with some antisera. The dotted portions represent parts of the molecule which have been
shown exhaustively to reside outside antigenic sites
(1).

```
            15   16                        21    22
Site 1:  (Ala)-Lys-Val-Glu-Ala-Asp-Val-(Ala)

            56                    62
Site 2:  Lys-Ala-Ser-Glu-Asp-Leu-Lys

            94                    99   100
Site 3:  Ala-Thr-Lys-His-Lys-Ile-[Pro]

            113                   119   120
Site 4:  His-Val-Leu-His-Ser-Arg-His-[Pro]

            145                   151
Site 5:  (Lys)-Tyr-Lys-Glu-Leu-Gly-Tyr
```

Figure 2. Structure of the synthetic Mb peptides representing the five antigenic sites of Mb (1). The residues in brackets are not actual parts of the antigenic sites (in the case of sites 3 and 4, a C-terminal proline residue was added for ease of synthesis). Residues in parentheses are not required as part of the antigenic sites in all antisera.

discrete area on the surface topography of the protein (for
review, see ref. 4). Although we had proposed the existence of
this type of protein antigenic site quite early (23), we subsequently found that they did not exist in Mb (1) and it was in
lysozyme that the first such sites were identified (14). The
need for the chemical verification of such sites led us to introduce (14,15) the concept of surface-simulation synthesis. By
this concept, the spatially adjacent surface residues constituting a protein binding site are linked directly via peptide bonds
with appropriate spacing and directionality. Our introduction
of the concept of surface-simulation synthesis enabled us to
precisely delineate, and chemically synthesize, the three antigenic sites of lysozyme (for review, see ref. 4). Furthermore,
surface-simulation synthesis afforded a powerful new concept in
protein molecular recognition that provided for the first time a
novel and versatile chemical strategy for the synthesis of any
type of protein binding sites (14,4,24,25).
     The highlights of the antigenic structure of lysozyme are
outlined here. Native lysozyme has three antigenic sites (4).
The identities of the sites are shown in Figure 3 and their locations in the three-dimensional structure of lysozyme can be seen
in Figures 4 and 5.
     Determination of the antigenic structures of Mb and lysozyme
has permitted the definition in precise molecular terms of the
antibody recognition of protein antigens. Many of the general
conclusions relating to antigenic structures of proteins which
we had derived from the precise definition of the antigenic
structure of Mb (12,1) are applicable to lysozyme equally as well
(4). These include: The small size and sharp boundaries of the
antigenic sites, their presence only in a limited number, their
surface locations, their sensitivity to changes in the conformation and to changes in the environment of the site (e.g. amino
acid substitutions in nearby residues), their independence of the
immunized species and the variation of their immunodominancy with
the antiserum and many other features. For a detailed discussion
of these general conclusions, see refs. 1 and 3).
     The sizes of the lysozyme antigenic sites in their extended
forms (Figure 3) are 30, 27, and 21 Å, respectively (4). These
resemble the dimensions of the extended antigenic sites of Mb
(Figure 2) which range between 19 and 23 Å (1). Since the antigenic sites of a protein are not in the extended form, the actual
dimensions of the sites in their folded shapes will be smaller
than the values given. Nevertheless, the sizes of the antibody
combining sites needed for binding with antigenic sites on either
of the two proteins will have to be somewhat larger than the combining sites found for haptens by X-ray crystallography (26,27).
     Examination of the antigenic sites of lysozyme reveals that
they are very rich in basic amino acids. This was also seen in
Mb, but we caution against premature generalizations. Obviously,
interactions with antibody are predominantly polar in nature (as

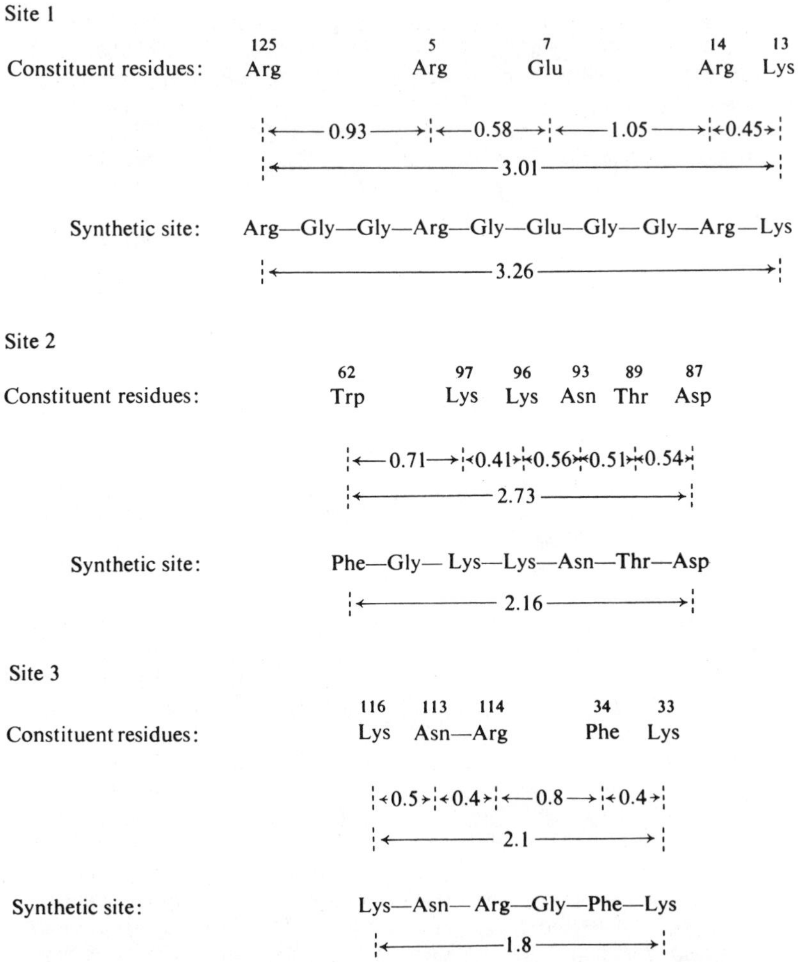

Site 1

	125		5	7		14	13
Constituent residues:	Arg		Arg	Glu		Arg	Lys

$|{\longleftarrow} 0.93 {\longrightarrow}|{\longleftarrow} 0.58 {\longrightarrow}|{\longleftarrow} 1.05 {\longrightarrow}|{\leftarrow}0.45{\rightarrow}|$

$|{\longleftarrow}\hspace{3cm} 3.01 \hspace{3cm}{\longrightarrow}|$

Synthetic site: Arg—Gly—Gly—Arg—Gly—Glu—Gly—Gly—Arg—Lys

$|{\longleftarrow}\hspace{3cm} 3.26 \hspace{3cm}{\longrightarrow}|$

Site 2

	62	97	96	93	89	87
Constituent residues:	Trp	Lys	Lys	Asn	Thr	Asp

$|{\longleftarrow} 0.71 {\longrightarrow}|{\leftarrow}0.41{\rightarrow}|{\leftarrow}0.56{\rightarrow}|{\leftarrow}0.51{\rightarrow}|{\leftarrow}0.54{\rightarrow}|$

$|{\longleftarrow}\hspace{2cm} 2.73 \hspace{2cm}{\longrightarrow}|$

Synthetic site: Phe—Gly— Lys—Lys—Asn—Thr—Asp

$|{\longleftarrow}\hspace{2cm} 2.16 \hspace{2cm}{\longrightarrow}|$

Site 3

	116	113	114	34	33
Constituent residues:	Lys	Asn—Arg		Phe	Lys

$|{\leftarrow}0.5{\rightarrow}|{\leftarrow}0.4{\rightarrow}|{\longleftarrow} 0.8 {\longrightarrow}|{\leftarrow}0.4{\rightarrow}|$

$|{\longleftarrow}\hspace{2cm} 2.1 \hspace{2cm}{\longrightarrow}|$

Synthetic site: Lys—Asn— Arg—Gly—Phe—Lys

$|{\longleftarrow}\hspace{2cm}1.8 \hspace{2cm}{\longrightarrow}|$

Figure 3. The three antigenic sites representing the entire antigenic structure of lysozyme. The diagram shows the spatially adjacent residues constituting each antigenic site and their numerical positions in the primary structure. The distances (in nm) separating the consecutive residues and the overall dimension of each site (in its extended form) are given, together with the dimension of each surface-simulation synthetic site. The latter assumes an ideal C -to-C distance of 0.362 nm. The precise boundary, conformational, and directional definitions of the sites are described in the text. The three sites account quantitatively for the entire (96 to 100%) antigenic reactivity of lysozyme.
Reproduced with permission from Ref. 75.

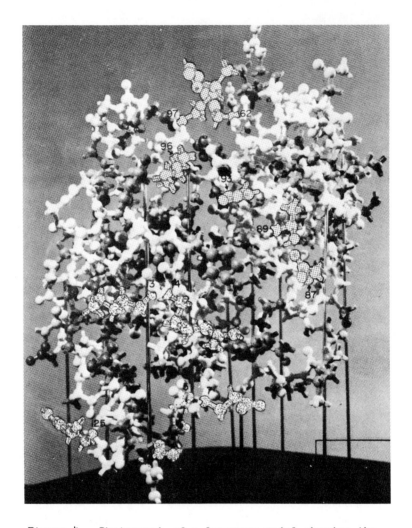

Figure 4. Photograph of a lysozyme model showing the
relative positions of the residues constituting
antigenic sites 1 and 2. The side chains of the
residues in the sites are outlined, those making up
site 1 are speckled areas, while those constituting
site 2 are shown as dotted areas to avoid confusion.
The preferred direction of site 1 (at least by
surface-simulation synthesis) is Arg-125 to Lys-13.
Site 2 also had a preferred direction (Trp-62 to
Asp-87).
Reproduced with permission from Ref. 75, as modified
from color in Adv. Biol. Med., 1978, 98, 41.

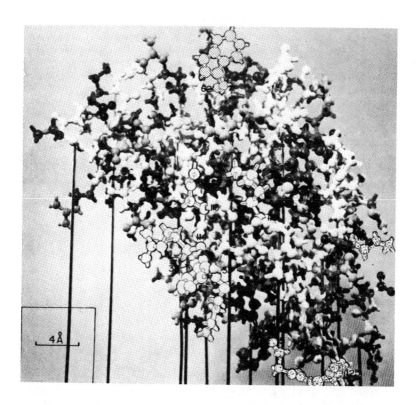

Figure 5. Photograph of a lysozyme model showing the
position of antigenic site 3 on the molecule relative
to sites 1 and 2. The side chains of the residues
comprising the sites are outlined. The residues
constituting site 3 are shown as striped areas. This
view is taken by rotating the model 125° anticlockwise
on the vertical axis relative to the view shown in
Figure 5. From this perspective only parts of site 1
can be seen, which are the residues Lys-13, Arg-5, and
Arg-125 (speckled areas). Of site 2, only Trp-62 can
be seen (dotted areas). Site 3 showed the same directional preference (Lys-116 to Lys-33) toward rabbit
and goat antisera.
Reproduced with permission from Ref. 75, as modified
from color in Adv. Biol. Med., 1978, 98, 41.

to be expected from the surface location of protein antigenic
sites) with considerable stabilizing effects being contributed
by hydrophobic interactions and some hydrogen bonding (1,4).
However, it should be emphasized that the hydrophilicity and
exposure of the lysozyme and myoglobin antigenic sites cannot be
the only underlying factor for their antigenic expression (4).
    In spite of the aforementioned points of resemblance between
the antigenic structures of Mb and lysozyme, the antigenic sites
of these two proteins are radically different in structural terms
(4). The five antigenic sites of Mb are each made up of residues
that are directly linked to one another by peptide bonds (1).
In contrast, in lysozyme each of the three antigenic sites constitutes spatially adjacent surface residues that are mostly
distant in sequence reacting with antibody as if they are in
direct peptide linkage (4). An important question here is what
are the factors which determine the type of the site? An un-
equivocal answer to this question cannot be formulated at this
stage. Perhaps it can be tentatively concluded that an important
factor in determining the type of the antigenic site may be
dependent to a great extent on the stabilization or otherwise of
the structure by internal disulfide cross-links (14,15). A more
definitive understanding of this subject must await knowledge of
the antigenic structures of several proteins.
    Even though we had suggested quite early in our work (23) the
existence of protein antigenic sites which are made up of spatially adjacent surface residues that are distant in sequence,
their identification in lysozyme and precise definition chemically and synthetically (14,15,17,18) is the first such example
in protein immunochemistry. A common feature of these two types
of antigenic sites is that they occupy exposed regions on the
surface topography of the respective protein, and this has
invariably been the situation with other protein sites such as
Hb (6,7), cytochrome c (28) and influenza virus Hemagglutinin
(29,30). It should be stressed that the antigenic sites of these
proteins are sensitive to conformational changes in the respective protein, with those of lysozyme showing, as expected, a much
higher sensitivity. Accordingly, it is totally inadequate to
identify the antigenic sites of Mb and Hb by the terms "linear",
"sequential" or "primary" or some such terms, while identifying
the antigenic sites of lysozyme by the terms "spatial", "conformational;, etc. We have proposed (4,16), that antigenic sites
of the type seen in Mb and Hb be named "continuous" antigenic
sites which implies that they consist of conformationally distinct continuous surface portions of the polypeptide chain. For
antigenic sites of the type seen in lysozyme, the term "discontinuous" antigenic sites will be most appropriate (16). A "discontinuous site" is made up of conformationally (or spatially)
contiguous surface residues that are totally or partially not in
direct peptide bond linkage.

In Hb, the antigenic sites of the α-chain (Figure 6) and the β-chain, which have been localized by synthesis, all reside in exposed parts of the individual subunit (31, 5-7). This, as already mentioned, led to the conclusion that Hb is recognized predominantly at the level of its individual subunits (5,6), and that its antigenic sites occur mostly (but not exclusively) at molecular locations that coincide with the regions obtained from a structural extrapolation of the Mb antigenic sites to Hb (6). These findings afforded further confirmation of our concept of structurally inherent antigenic sites (31,32).

The antigenic sites of serum albumin have not yet been narrowed down to their precise boundaries (8-11). The peptide regions shown in Figure 7 are not intended to imply that the entire region constitutes an antigenic site, but rather that the site falls within that region. Nevertheless, it can be readily seen, even at this level of delineation, that the antigenic sites of serum albumin exhibit the expected characteristics of having discrete boundaries and being limited in number, sensitive to conformational and environmental changes independent of the immunized species, and variable in immunodominancy with the antiserum (8-11).

In albumin, the status of exposure of its antigenic sites is not known. Unfortunately, the three-dimensional structure of a serum albumin has not yet been determined. Therefore, it is not possible to correlate the locations of the antigenic sites with the shape of the protein molecule. Three of the antigenic sites (sites 1 to 3 in Figure 7) occupy continuous portions of the polypeptide chain of albumin and are, therefore, "continuous" antigenic sites. The other three antigenic sites (sites 4 to 6) are each localized around a disulfide bond and belong to the type termed "discontinuous" antigenic sites. However, by analogy with Mb, lysozyme and Hb, it would be expected that the antigenic sites of serum albumin also occupy exposed structural locations. The predominance of polar and hydrophilic amino acids in the albumin antigenic sites (Figure 7) tends to support this expectation.

Significantly, the location of the antigenic sites on a given protein is independent of the immunized species. Thus, rabbits, cats, goats, and mice antibodies to native lysozyme recognize the same three antigenic sites (33). Antibodies produced in rabbit, goat, pig, cat, mouse (outbred) and chicken against sperm-whale Mb recognize the same five antigenic sites on Mb (34). The same antigenic sites on serum albumin are recognized by rabbit and mouse antisera against this protein (8,9). The antigenic sites localized on the α- and β-chains of Hb are similarly recognized by rabbit, goat, and mouse antibodies against Hb (5,6,7). The antigenic sites thus far localized and confirmed by synthesis on influenza hemagglutinin are similarly recognized by human, rabbit, goat and mouse anti-influenza antibodies (29,30).

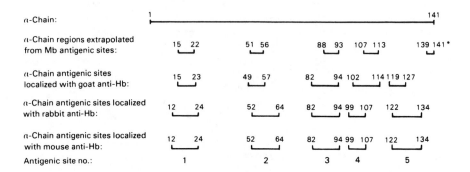

Figure 6. Schematic diagram of the α chain of Hb, chain regions that have been extrapolated from the five antigenic sites of sperm whale Mb, and the antigenic sites of the α chain that were localized to Hb with goat, rabbit, and mouse antisera. The numbers refer to the locations of the residues in the α chain. The asterisk indicates that, owing to differences in the sizes of the polypeptide chains of Mb and the subunit, the antigenic site 5 of Mb (residues 145-151) does not really have a full structural counterpart in the α chain. Reproduced with permission from Ref. 6.

Site 1:

```
      137                                    146
BSA:  Tyr-Leu-Tyr-Glu-Ile-Ala-Arg-Arg-His-Pro
      138                                    147
HSA:  Tyr-Leu-Tyr-Glu-Ile-Ala-Arg-Arg-His-Pro
```

Site 2:

```
      328                                    337
BSA:  Phe-Leu-Tyr-Glu-Tyr-Ser-Arg-Arg-His-Pro
      329                                    338
HSA:  Phe-Leu-Tyr-Glu-Tyr-Ala-Arg-Arg-His-Pro
```

Site 3:

```
      526                                    535
BSA:  Ala-Leu-Val-Glu-Leu-Leu-Lys-His-Lys-Pro
      527                                    536
HSA:  Ala-Leu-Val-Glu-Leu-Val-Lys-His-Lys-Pro
```

Site 4:

```
      168                                              179
BSA:  Gln-Ala-Glu-Asp-Lys-Gly-Ala-Cys-Leu-Leu-Pro-Lys
      170                                              181
HSA:  Gln-Ala-Ala-Asp-Lys-Ala-Ala-Cys-Leu-Leu-Pro-Lys
```

Site 5:

```
      308                        314 359         362
BSA:  Ala-Glu-Asp-Lys-Asp-Val-Cys Cys-Ala-Lys-Asp
                                 S—S
      309                        315 360         363
HSA:  Val-Glu-Ser-Lys-Asp-Val-Cys Cys-Ala-Ala-Asp
                                 S—S
```

Site 6:

```
      559                        565 556         553
BSA:  Ala-Asp-Asp-Lys-Glu-Ala-Cys Cys-Lys-Asp-Val
                                 S—S
      560                        566 557         554
HSA:  Ala-Asp-Asp-Lys-Glu-Thr-Cys Cys-Lys-Glu-Val
                                 S—S
```

Figure 7. Structure and location of the six regions of bovine serum albumin (BSA) and of human serum albumin (HSA) that we have shown to carry antigenic sites. It is not implied that the antigenic sites comprise the entire size of the regions shown, but rather that they fall within these regions. Reproduced with permission from Refs. 9, 10, and 11.

Comments on attempts to predict location of protein antigenic sites.

Recenty, based on the foregoing qualitative observations (1,4,35), an empirical approach was suggested (36) which, by linear analysis of the protein sequence in relation to a hydrophilicity index using the Chou and Fasman (37) method, attempted to correlate antigenic sites with hydrophilicity maxima. However, such a relationship is not supported by what we know about protein antigenic structures. For example, in the classical case of Mb analysis has revealed that only two (out of five) antigenic sites coincide with hydrophilicity maxima and, furthermore, other hydrophilicity maxima are not antigenic. The antigenic structure of Mb was first to show that all antigenic sites are exposed, but not every exposed region constitutes an antigenic site. Thus exposure is not a sufficient criterion for antigenicity. Furthermore, antigenic sites are not necessarily in highly hydrophilic locations. Hydrophobic interactions frequently provide major contributions to the binding energy (1). For example, in the case of the α-chain of Hb, the two most immunodominant locations (6) are not hydrophilic maxima. A strongly immunogenic location on influenza virus hemagglutinin has recently been reported (29) which is entirely hydrophobic and in fact the synthetic peptide comprising this region (HA2 1-11, Figure 8) is so hydrophobic that it is insoluble in aqueous solvents. Two regions that may be 'expected' to be antigenic on cytochrome c on basis of hydrophilicity (regions 60-65 and 89-94) have been found not to be antigenic sites by synthetic peptides around these regions (28). Recent determination of the antigenic structure of ragweed allergen Ra3 has localized by synthesis four antigenic sites with IgG and IgE antibodies (38), none of which coincided with that predicted (36) on the basis of hydrophilicity. Clearly, application of hydrophilicity analysis of the linear sequence for prediction of protein antigenic sites is not supported by the findings because it does not take into account the influences of the three-dimensional structure. It is very common, for example, for hydrophobic regions to become exposed by virture of the three-dimensional folding of the protein. It is well to caution here that the sequence and three-dimensional features that confer immunogenicity on given parts or surface areas of a protein molecule are still not too clear. Undue speculation is inadvisable at this stage.

In the recent literature, there appears to have occurred a confusion as to what is a protein antigenic site. This term has always been used to describe a region of a protein antigen that is recognized (by antibodies and/or T-cells) in the immune response to the whole protein. However, it has long been known that any peptide from a given protein, if immunized as a conjugate on an appropriate large carrier, will stimulate the formation of anti-peptide antibodies. This even applies to peptides

```
                                  1                                          11
HA2 (1-11)   Type A:   Gly-Leu-Phe-Gly-Ala-Ile-Ala-Gly-Phe-Ile-Glu

             Type B:   Gly-Phe-Phe-Gly-Ala-Ile-Ala-Gly-Phe-Ile-Glu
```

Figure 8. Antigenic sites in the fusion region of
influenza virus hemagglutinin of strains A and B. The
sites have been localized and their antigenic activity
confirmed by synthesis and reactivity with rabbit,
goat, and mouse antivirus and antihemagglutinin
antibodies. Also, each of the peptides bound considerable amounts of anti-influenza antibodies from
sera of human individuals after influenza attack.
Reproduced with permission from Ref. 29.

representing regions that are not antigenic when the whole
protein is used as immunogen. As previously pointed out (39),
"antibodies obtained by immunization with a peptide (coupled or
free) corresponding to a surface region of a protein can recognize that region in the protein, even though that region itself
is not part of an antigenic site when the intact protein is used
as an immunogen". Thus, it is necessary not to confuse this fact
with protein antigenic sites which define the regions that are
immunogenic when the whole protein is the antigen.

Regions outside the Antigenic Sites

The exhaustive strategies on which the immunochemical analyses
were based, probed in detail every part of a given protein molecule for its immunochemical reactivity and permitted the determination of the contribution of each part of the protein molecule
to the overall immune response against that protein. As already
mentioned, the amounts of antibodies that can be bound by the
synthetic antigenic stes of Mb (Tables I, II, and III) and the
synthetic antigenic sites of lysozyme (Table IV and Figure 3)
account for the bulk (usually over 98%) of the total antibodies
against the respective protein in a given antiserum. But, how
much antibody is directed against regions outside these antigenic
sites.

In studies on Mb (1) and lysozyme (4) a 'general background
response' to regions between their respective antigenic sites was
found to account for 0.2-1.4% of the total antibodies to these
proteins. Also, Takagaki et al. (40) have reported the detection
of antibodies to a continuous region of hen egg-white lysozyme
(residues 28-54) that account for about 0.1-1% of the total anti-
lysozyme antibodies. In very recent studies (6,7) employing the
overlapping synthetic peptide approach, peptides that were seem-
ingly inactive in binding of ^{125}I-labelled anti-Hb antibodies
in a titration assay were further studied by attempting to
isolate, from adsorbents of these peptides, antibodies specific
for Hb. By using large excesses of unlabelled immune IgG, traces
of Hb-specific antibodies could be isolated (6) from that of peptide 1-15. Although the amount of these antibodies were not
quantified, they accounted for less than 1-2% of the specific
antibodies, since no binding could be detected in the titration
assay with the immunoadsorbent of this peptide. This indicates
the presence of a trace antibody response directed to this region
of the α-chain, and suggests that other apparently inactive regions of the α-chain may also be recognized by amounts of antibodies below the detection level of these methods. Similarly, a
subpopulation of anti-Hb antibodies directed against the region
α129-141 have been isolated (41), but which represented less than
1% of the total anti-Hb antibodies. Also, recent studies with
synthetic reference non-antigenic regions of serum albumin revealed the presence of trace antibody binding accounting for

Table I. Specificity of serum antibodies obtained by immunization with free synthetic antigenic sites of Mb

Serum Antibody[b]	Antibodies bound (cpm) to Mb and to peptides[a]					
	Site 1	Site 2	Site 3	Site 4	Site 5	Mb
Anti-site 1	16,737 ± 711	0	0	0	0	17,398 ± 1586
Anti-site 2	0	16,859 ± 1457	0	0	0	20,784 ± 2214
Anti-site 3	0	0	17,881 ± 1163	0	0	20,117 ± 1973
Anti-site 4	0	0	0	16,437 ± 695	0	21,455 ± 1305
Anti-site 5	0	0	0	0	19,246 ± 611	20,632 ± 2358
Prebleed[c]	0	0	0	0	0	0

[a] Values represent means (± S.E.M.) of 3-4 replicate analyses (by direct solid phase RIA) and have been corrected for binding to baseline control antigens. Peptide-BSA conjugates were employed in the binding assay. Baseline control antigen for peptide-BSA conjugates was peptide 121-127-BSA conjugate. Baseline control antigen for Mb was BSA. No binding was detected against a control protein hen egg white lysozyme. Values not significantly >0 by Student's T-test (P<0.05) reported as 0.

[b] Serum antibodies were obtained by immunization with free peptide in complete Freund's adjuvant.

[c] Prebleed sera was a pooled sera obtained from the mice before they were injected with any synthetic peptides.

Table is from Schmitz et al. (ref. 54), by permission.

Table II.   Serum antibodies obtained by immunization with free synthetic peptides representing surface regions that are non-immunogenic in whole Mb

Peptide/Protein[b]	Antibodies Bound (CPM)[a]	
	Anti-Peptide 1-6 Antisera[c]	Anti-Peptide 121-127 Antisera[c]
Site 1	0	0
Site 2	0	0
Site 3	0	0
Site 4	0	0
Site 5	0	0
Peptide 1-6	26,050 ± 2,281	0
Peptide 121-127	0	17,082 ± 3,282
Mb	33,058 ± 2,983	29,608 ± 1,542

a Values represent Mean (± S.E.M.) of 3-4 replicate (by direct solid phase RIA) and have been corrected for binding to baseline control antigen BSA. Values not significantly >0 by Student's T-test (P<0.05) reported as 0. No significant binding was detected using prebleed sera preparations obtained from the mice prior to immunization. Representative data shown.

b Peptides were conjugated to BSA before use in RIA.

c Serum antibodies were obtained by immunizations with free peptide emulsified in complete Freunds' adjuvant.

Table is from Schmitz et al. (43), by permission.

Table III. Example of antibodies against influenza virus elicited by immunization with <u>free</u> synthetic antigenic sites

Antigen	Harvest Day	Antibody bound (Δ cpm $\times$ 10^{-3})	
		Virus (A/port Chalmer's)	Virus (X-31)
Peptide 1-11 of HA2 strain A	51	9.72	9.60
	80	40.64	39.71
	108	43.29	46.59
	125	64.68	61.32
		HA (B/Hong Kong)	Virus B/Hong Kong
Peptide 1-11 of HA2 strain B	66	11.99	11.19
	108	16.32	17.30
	125	24.41	25.86

Antibody binding to HA or to virus was determined by direct solid phase RIA. Lysozyme and bovine serum albumin were used to correct for non-specific binding (3% or less). Values are means of triplicate with varied ± 1.4% or less.

Binding studies were carried out with antiserum dilution of 1/1000.

Table is from Atassi and Webster (29), by permission.

TABLE IV. Comparison of the response profiles in selected mouse strains following immunization with free peptides or with intact Mb

	Response and its level following:				
	Immunization with Mb[a]		Immunization with free synthetic peptides[b]		
Mouse Strain	High	Low	High	Intermediate	Low
B10.R11(72NS)	No response to Mb or peptide	No response to Mb or peptide	--	Sites 1,2,4,5	Site 3 peptides 1-6, 121-127
C57B1/10.J	Site 4	Sites 1,2,3,5 Mb	--	Site 1 peptide 121-127	Sites 2,3,4,5 peptide 1-6 121-127
B10.A(2R)	Mb, Sites 1,2,4	Sites 3,5	--	--	Sites 1,2,3,4,5 peptides 1-6, 121-127
B10.A(5R)	Mb, Sites 1,2	Site 5	--	Sites 2,3,5	Site 1,4 peptides 1-6 121-127
B10.D2/n	Mb, Sites 1,2 3,5	Site 4	Sites 1,2,3,4 Peptide 121-127	Peptide 1-6	Site 5

a This is a summary of the findings when the mouse strains shown are each immunized with Mb and the responses subsequently tested with the synthetic peptides. Upon immunization with Mb, no response is detectable to peptides 1-6 and 121-127 in any of these strains.

b The column represents a summary of the findings when a given mouse stain is immunized with each of the synthetic peptides (shown in Figures 2 and 10) in their free form.

Table is from Young et al. (55), by permission.

0.5-1.1% of the anti-protein antibodies in the antisera (9,11).
Thus the presence of trace antibody responses to regions inter-
spersed among immunodominant sites would appear to be a general
phenomenon for protein antigens.

Although the regulation of the relative immunodominance of
antigenic sites in proteins is poorly understood, it was suggested (35) that the methodology for producing monoclonal antibodies
introduced by Kohler and Milstein (42) should permit amplifica-
tion in vitro of what would ordinarily constitute trace antibody
responses in vivo. The specificities and regulation of such
responses could then be more readily studied. This prediction
(35,6) has recently been confirmed by the description of two
monoclonal anti-Mb antibodies whose specificities were directed
to regions that are either outside the five antigenic sites of
Mb or that are displaced from a site (43,44). One of these monoclonal exhibited specificity to the synthetic peptide 121-127 and
the other, although essentially reacting with site 2, exhibited
a specificity displacement to the left by two residues so that
it required residues 54 and 55 as part of the site. Interestingly, such antibodies were below the detection level in the antisera of the parent mice (whose spleens were used for fusion) by
immunoadsorbent titrations of ^{125}I-labelled antibodies with
peptide adsorbents.

Free Synthetic Peptides as Immunogens

It has long been thought in Immunology that small peptides, of
only a few amino acids, are not antigenic in the free form. Consequently, in order to elicit antibodies against a small peptide
from a given protein, it is standard practice to couple the peptide to a large carrier, (e.g. bovine serum albumin, poly-L-
lysine, keylimpet hemocyanin) prior to immunization (see 45, for
review).

Having determined the antigenic structure of Mb (1), we have
carried out detailed studies designed to investigate the antigenicity of the synthetic antigenic sites and selected putative
non-antigenic surface regions of Mb in their free form (i.e.
without coupling to a carrier), and the effect of peptide size
on antigenicity.

Antibodies were preselected submolecular specificities evoked by immunization with FREE peptides

Initially we investigated whether immunization of H-2^d and H-2^s
mice (two high responder strains to Mb; refs. 46,47) with free
synthetic peptides of increasing length and carrying site 5
(Figure 9) could evoke antibodies that will react with native Mb
(48). Thus immunization with peptides of 22 amino acids (peptide
132-153), 11 amino acids (peptide 143-153), 9 amino acids (peptide 145-153) or 7 amino acids (peptide 145-151), each of which

Site 5

```
                                  145                       151
                                  (Lys)Tyr-Lys-Glu-Leu-Gly-Tyr
```

Peptide 145-153

```
        145                              153
        Lys-Tyr-Lys-Glu-Leu-Gly-Tyr-Gln-Gly
```

Peptide 143-153

```
      143                                    153
      Ala-Ala-Lys-Tyr-Lys-Glu-Leu-Gly-Tyr-Gln-Gly
```

Peptide 135-153

```
  135                                                      153
  Leu-Glu-Leu-Phe-Arg-Lys-Asp-Ile-Ala-Ala-Lys-Tyr-Lys-Glu-Leu-Gly-Tyr-Gln-Gly
```

Peptide 132-153

```
132                                                          153
Asn-Lys-Ala-Leu-Glu-Leu-Phe-Arg-Lys-Asp-Ile-Ala-Ala-Lys-Tyr-Lys-Glu-Leu-Gly-Tyr-Gln-Gly
```

Truncated Peptide 139-153

```
139                                          153
Arg-Lys-Asp-Ile-Ala————Lys-Tyr-Lys-Glu-Leu-Gly————Gln-Gly
```

Figure 9. Structure of the synthetic Mb peptides that were first used to study effect of peptide size on antibody response to immunization by free peptides (site 5, peptides 145-153, 143-153, and 132-153) and to generate specific tolerance to preselected antigenic sites of Mb (peptides 143-153, 135-153, 132-153, and truncated 139-153). The continuous lines in truncated peptide 139-153 indicate the absence of Ala and Tyr residues at positions 144 and 151. The residue in parenthesis is not required as part of the antigenic site in all antisera (1).

contain only one antigenic site (1) when the native protein is
the immunizing antigen, is effective in eliciting antibodies
capable of binding specifically to the native protein (48). In
general, the 22- and 11-residue peptides elicited a higher antibody response than the 9- and 7-residue peptides with the responses to the latter two peptides being essentially of comparable magnitude. The results with peptide 145-151 (site 5 clearly
showed that the response to this 7-residue peptide is improved
by further boosting and the antibody titer can be maintained in
the serum for an extended period (48).

These results were the first demonstration that immunization
with a small free (i.e. not coupled to any carrier) synthetic
antigenic site is effective in eliciting antibodies capable of
binding to the ative protein molecule (48).

Having found that a free synthetic antigenic site of only a
few amino acids will elicit antibody responses, we investigated
(49) whether this is a general phenomenon (i.e. whether immunization with free synthetic peptides representing each of the five
antigenic sites of Mb (Figure 2) could produce antibodies that
bind to native Mb). Also, we have investigated (49) the antigenicity, in their free form, of synthetic peptides representing
surface regions of Mb which are non-antigenic when whole Mb is
used as the immunogen (Figure 10).

The results clearly show (49) that immune sera raised to each
of the synthetic peptides (6 or 7 amino acids in size) contain
antibodies that bind specifically to native Mb (Table I). Thus
immunization with a peptide representing a single antigenic site,
at least when native Mb is the immunizing antigen, is effective
in eliciting antibodies that will bind specifically to native Mb
and exclusively to the peptide used in immunization (Table I).
The antibody responses to these peptides were already of considerable titre within 14 days after the immunization and, with
periodic boosting, persisted throughout the immunization period
up to 324 days. Later bleedings were not tested.

Of intriguing interest was the finding (49) that immunization
with free synthetic peptides 1-6 and 121-127 will produce antibodies that bind to native Mb (Table II). These two peptides
represent surface regions within the Mb molecule that are not
antigenic when intact Mb is the antigen (1). Clearly the lack
of antigenicity of these surface regions within Mb is not caused
by some specific structural features that renders the regions
non-antigenic. The antigenic structure of Mb has shown that the
antigenic sites are all surface regions but not every region of
the surface is an antigenic site (1). The present findings pose
many questions concerning our understanding of the molecular and
cellular factors that contribute to produce an immune response
to proteins and peptides. Knowledge of the antigenic structures
of Mb (1), lysozyme (4), the α- and β-chains of human hemoglobin
(5-7), and the six major antigenic sites of serum albumin (8-11)
have revealed (for review see ref. 35) that the antigenicity of

                                  1   6
Peptide 1-6:   Val-Leu-Ser-Glu-Gly-Glu

                                  121   127
Peptide 121-127:   Gly-Asn-Phe-Gly-Ala-Asp-Ala

Figure 10. Peptides representing two surface regions to which no detectable antibody responses are found when intact Mb is the immunizing antigen (1).

the sites in a protein is largely inherent in their conformational locations (32). Furthermore, other cellular factors, external to the molecule, regulate the immune response. The immune responses to Mb are controlled by genes in the I-region of the major histocompatibility complex (46). More importantly, the responses to the synthetic antigenic sites are each under separate genetic control (47,50).

Our observation that small synthetic peptides are antigenic in their free form has not been confined to Mb peptides. Synthetic peptides of other proteins have also been found to be antigenic in their free form. We have obtained similar results with free synthetic peptides of human hemoglobin (51), bovine serum albumin, ragweed allergen Ra3 (38) and influenza virus hemagglutinin (29,30). So far, 36 different synthetic peptides belonging to these protein systems have evoked, without exception in vivo antibody responses in rabbits and mice, and the anti-peptide antibodies bound to the respective protein. Table III shows an example of the antibody response with time to a synthetic peptide of influenza virus hemagglutinin and the binding of these antibodies to the virus (29).

Other parameters of antibody response to free peptides.

We have studied the effect of several adjuvants on the antibody responses to several of the peptides (52,53). In general, the highest responses were obtained in immunization of peptide with complete Freund's adjuvant. Immunizations without adjuvant (in PBS) or with incomplete Freund's adjuvant usually gave little or no responses.

One important consideration is the titer of the anti-protein antibody elicited by peptide compared with that raised by immunization with the native protein. With a short immunization schedule, the titers of antibodies elicited by free small peptides are low. However, if the size of the immunizing synthetic peptide is increased, the antibody titer rises to levels comparable to the titers obtained following immunization with native protein (48). Also, it was shown recently (29) that antibody titer is steadily increased following immunization with a given small synthetic protein after several boosters reaching a level comparable with the antibody titers of antisera obtained by immunization with intact protein. Thus, in general, the level of antibody response to a free peptide immunogen increases with periodic boosting, usually reaching maximum titer in about 2-3 months.

In the initial phase of the response, the antibodies are usually mostly IgM (κ), accompanied occasionally with IgG1 and IgG2a (54). By periodic boosting (usually 3-6 times), as the titer of antibody increases, a gradual switch to IgG antibodies takes place until in fact the IgG antibodies predominate. Usually, but not always, IgG1 and IgG2b are higher than IgG2a and IgG3.

We have also shown (55) that the genetic control of the antibody response to Mb following immunization with the free synthetic peptides is different from the genetic control obtained ·fol-
lowing immunization with native Mb (47). Table IV gives some
examples of these differences. The reasons for these differences
in the genetic control are, at present, unknown. Such differences may be related to the presence of inter-site influences in
the native protein (56) as compared to the free synthetic peptides. In this context it should be noted that inter-site
influences that regulate the immune response to Mb have been
described and they can be cooperative or suppressive in nature
(56). Furthermore, even though the data so far indicate that the
same five antigenic sites recognized by mouse B-cells are also
recognized by mouse T-cells (47,50), the possibility of the
existence on Mb of additional T-cell recognition sites that are
not recognized by B-cells cannot be ruled out at the present time.
These may also contribute via T-helper or T-suppressor cells to
the regulation of the overall immune response to Mb. Further
experiments are in progress to determine the nature of any additional T-cell recognition sites on the native Mb molecule.
     In another series of studies (57) we have found that there
is an optimum dose for each immunizing free peptide which varied
with the peptide. It was also clear from these studies (57) that
some free peptides are more immunogenic than others of equal size.
For example, site 1 of Mb is more immunogenic than sites 2, 3, 4
or 5. At present the underlying reasons for differences in
immunogenicity of free peptides of equal size are unknown.

Production of monoclonal antibodies with preselected specificities

Monoclonal antibodies produced by the techniques of somatic cell
hybridization (42,58) are now being used in many areas of funda-
mental research and clinical medicine (for reviews, see refs.
59-61). Most of these applications have taken advantage of the
precise binding specificities expressed by monoclonal antibodies
to distinct antigenic determinants. Yet in spite of recent
developments in cell fusion and tissue culture techniques (60,62-
64), as well as hybridoma screening methods (65,66), the production of monoclonal antibodies that express desired submolecular
binding specificities to single antigenic sites remains a time
consuming and often expensive endeavor. Indeed, the preparation
of monoclonal antibodies to specific antigenic sites can be
tedious and elusive.
     Having demonstrated that it is possible to elicit antibodies
with preselected submolecular binding specificities to protein
regions by immunization with free peptides (48,49,29,30,38,51),
it appeared possible to produce monoclonal antibodies with similar predetermined specificities by the use of free synthetic peptides as immunogens. The salient features in the development of

this approach are: (1) the use of a model protein whose antigenic structure is known in detail; (2) immunization with free
synthetic peptides rather than peptide-carrier conjugates; (3)
hybrid selection and maintenance using traditional hybridoma
tissue culture techniques; (4) submolecular binding specificities
determined by, and entirely directed to, the synthetic regions
used for immunization; and (5) an apparent similarity between the
monoclonal antibodies secreted by the subcloned hybrids and the
serum anti-Mb antibodies produced by the spleen cell donor mice.

(a) Monoclonal antibodies against the antigenic sites

   Initially, we investigated (67) whether it would be possible
to produce monoclonal antibodies with predetermined antigen binding specificities from mice that had been immunized with antigenic site 5 of Mb (67). Two monoclonal antibodies with preselected submolecular binding specificities to Mb were obtained
(67) by hybridizing Fa/O mouse myeloma cells with spleen cells
derived from mice which had been immunized with free (not coupled
to any carrier) Mb synthetic peptides 132-153 or 145-151 (antigenic site 5). Both monoclonal antibodies were IgG$_1$ (κ) and
their binding specificities were restricted to determinants
present in Mb and in the peptides used for immunization. The
results suggested that monoclonal antibodies with preselected
submolecular binding specificities can be readily obtained by the
techniques of somatic cell hybridization when the corresponding
free synthetic peptides are used as immunogens (67).
   Subsequently, we confirmed (54) that this finding is not
peculiar to antigenic site 5 of Mb but is in fact a general
phenomenon that can be duplicated for other peptides. The five
synthetic antigenic sites of Mb (Figure 2) were used in their
free form (i.e. not coupled to any carrier) to immunize separate
groups of Balb/cByJ mice. Serum samples obtained from each group
of mice contained antibodies that bound specifically to Mb and
exclusively to the immunizing antigenic site. Monoclonal antibodies to each of the five antigenic sites were subsequently
obtained (54) by hydridizing Fa/O mouse myeloma cells with spleen
cells derived from each group of mice. These monoclonal antibodies were either IgM (κ) or IgG$_1$ (κ). They expressed the
same isotypes as the antigen specific serum antibodies produced
by the mice whose spleen cells were used for hybridization. Each
monoclonal antibody, like the immune serum of the parent animal,
bound specifically to Mb and exclusively to the synthetic peptide
used as an immunogen (Table V). These results suggested that the
hybridoma antibodies expressed submolecular binding specificities
that were the result of peptide immunization rather than hybrid
selection (54). This strongly supported our previous findings
(67) that it is possible to produce monoclonal antibodies with
preselected submolecular binding specificities to continuous
protein sites by the techniques of somatic cell hybridization

Table V. Monoclonal antibodies from immunization with free synthetic antigenic sites of Mb

Monoclonal antibody	Antibody bound (CPM) to Mb and to peptides[a]					
	Site 1	Site 2	Site 3	Site 4	Site 5	Mb
MB1-4-15 (anti-site 1)	4414 ± 167	0	0	0	0	20,288 ± 613
MB2-5-4 (anti-site 2)	0	9353 ± 745	0	0	0	29,667 ± 933
MB3-5-13 (anti-stie 3)	0	0	9735 ± 792	0	0	52,190 ± 2030
MB4-3-22 (anti-site 4)	0	0	0	4357 ± 510	0	17,103 ± 201
MB5-16-1 (anti-site 5)	0	0	0	0	13,392 ± 643	62,763 ± 2010
MB5-14-5 (anti-site 5)	0	0	0	0	27,203 ± 3789	30,570 ± 1410

[a] Values represent means (± S.E.M.) of 4 replicate analyses by direct solid phase RIA and have been corrected for binding to baseline control antigens. Baseline control antigen for peptide-BSA conjugates was peptide 121-127-BSA conjugate. Baseline control antigen for Mb was BSA. No binding was detected against a control protein hen egg white lysozyme. Values not significantly > 0 by Student's T-test ($P < 0.05$) reported as 0. Representative data shown.

Table is from Schmitz et al. (54), by permission.

when the corresponding free synthetic peptides are used as
immunogens.

(b) Production of monoclonal antibodies to regions that are non-
immunogenic in a protein

The finding (54) that it is possible to produce monoclonal
antibodies with preselected submolecular binding specificities
to the five antigenic sites of Mb by immunization with free synthetic sites prompted us to investigate even wider applications.
Studies were undertaken (43) to determine whether monoclonal
antibodies with preselected submolecular binding specificities
to surface regions of a protein that are not immunogenic (when
the intact protein is the immunogen) could be produced when the
corresponding synthetic peptides (6-7 residues) are used in their
free form as immunogens.
    Two synthetic peptides corresponding to surface regions of
Mb that are not antigenic in the native molecule were used (43)
in their free form (i.e. not coupled to a carrier) to immunize
separate groups of Balb/cByJ mice. The synthetic peptides cor-
responded to regions 1-6 and 121-127 (Figure 10). Serum samples
obtained from each group of mice contained antibodies that bound
specifically to Mb and exclusively to the immunizing peptide (43).
Monoclonal antibodies to each of the two surface regions were
subsequently prepared (43). These monoclonal antibodies were IgM
(κ). They expressed the same isotype as the antigen specific
serum antibodies produced by the mice whose spleen cells were
used for hybridization. Solid phase radioimmunoassay studies
also indicated that each monoclonal antibody, like the immune
serum of the parent animals, bound specifically to Mb and exclusively to the synthetic peptide used as an immunogen (43) (Table
VI). Thus, the hybridoma antibodies expressed submolecular binding specificities that were the result of peptide immunization
rather than hybrid selection (43). Clearly, monoclonal antibodies with preselected submolecular binding specificities to
protein surface regions that are not immunogenic when the whole
protein is the immunizing antigen can be produced by the techniques of somatic cell hybridization when the corresponding free
synthetic peptides are used as immunogens (43).
Remarks on antibody production by free small peptides
The fact that free synthetic peptides of Mb, six to seven amino
acids in size, were able to evoke an immune response that allowed
for the production of sera antibodies and of monoclonal antibodies runs somewhat counter to the traditional theories concerning the immunogenicity of small peptides. The aforementioned
recent work in this laboratory (48,49,29,30,38,51), however, has
shown that immunization with small synthetic peptides representing each of the five antigenic sites of Mb, antigenic sites of
hemoglobin, influenza virus hemagglutinin or ragweed allergen can

Table VI. Specificity of monoclonal antibodies from immunization with free peptide representing surface regions that are non-antigenic in whole Mb

Peptide/Protein[b]	Monoclonal Antibodies Bound (CPM)[a]		
	MB16-6-1	MB16-8-21	MB121-2-5
Site 1	0	0	0
Site 2	0	0	0
Site 3	0	0	0
Site 4	0	0	0
Site 5	0	0	0
Peptide 1-6	14,231 ± 861	29,665 ± 1060	0
Peptide 121-127	0	0	7,477 ± 374
Mb	18,094 ± 1662	36,390 ± 1060	15,205 ± 1508

[a] Values represent mean (± S.E.M.) of 3-4 replicate analyses by direct solid phase RIA. Results have been corrected for binding to baseline control antigen BSA. Values not significantly >0 by Student's T-test ($P < 0.05$) reported as 0. Representative data shown.

[b] Peptides were conjugated to BSA before use in the RIA.

Table is from Schmitz et al. (43), by permission.

evoke dose dependent serum antibody responses that bind to the respective protein in various strains of mice. We have also demonstrated that it is possible to produce monoclonal antibodies to the antigenic sites of a protein (67,54) and even to regions that are not immunogenic (43) in the protein when the corresponding synthetic peptides are used as immunogens. The fact that neither region 1-6 or 121-127 is immunogenic in native Mb (1) despite its exposed location, suggests that some constraints must be placed on these regions during the immune response to the whole protein. These constraints, which are not yet fully understood, may in part be related, as already mentioned, to intersite cellular influences (56) (T-helper or T-suppressor) and to Ir-gene control (47,50).

From the incidence of positive growth fusion wells that initially secreted anti-protein antibodies, it was apparent, that the production of hybrid lines by free synthetic peptide immunization is similar to conventional procedures in that it does not require selective enrichment for antigen specific B cells. The binding specificities of the monoclonal antibodies to the antigenic sites and to non-immunogenic regions of Mb were the result of peptide immunization rather than hybrid selection. The isotype of each monoclonal antibody was also the same as the predominant isotype of the site-specific serum antibodies, suggesting that the monoclonals were also an adequate representation of the antibodies produced in the animals.

The ability to produce large quantities of antibodies whose binding specificities are selected before hybridization obviates the time-consuming and expensive requirement to screen large numbers of hybrid cultures for the presence of antibodies that express the desired specificity. The protein antigen can be used exclusively for screening, and no further examination of specificity should ordinarily be needed since specificity is determined by, and is exclusively directed against, the immunizing peptide.

These results suggest that, during immune recognition, in addition to sequence identity, some conformational similarity must also exist between the free synthetic peptides and the corresponding locations of these regions in the native molecule. Although synthetic peptides exist in an equilibrium comprising a multitude of dynamic conformational states, the time-average of which is random, each peptide is able to assume a favorable conformational state that resembles the shape of the corresponding region in the native protein (23). Binding to cell receptors, as in binding to antibody (1,4), may also induce the peptide to assume this favorable state (23), thus shifting the conformational equilibrium to that state which would more closely resemble the shape of the surface region in the whole molecule. This would allow for both the molecular and submolecular binding specificities (43,54) expressed by each of the monoclonal antibodies described above.

The ability to produce antisera and monoclonal antibodies that express predetermined binding specificities to desired protein regions, even to those that are non-immunogenic when the protein is the immunogen, by immunizing with free peptides represents a breakthrough in immunology. It affords valuable reagents that may be employed as powerful probes of the conformation of essentially any surface region of a protein, irrespective of whether that region is immunogenic in the native molecule. With this enormous versatility, the monoclonal antibodies produced will help elucidate the molecular basis of immunity and should assist in the development of sensitive therapeutic and diagnostic reagents that have precise binding capabilities that would otherwise be difficult or impossible to obtain.

Preparation of T-lymphocyte lines and clones with specificities to preselected protein sites.

The antibody response to protein antigens has been extensively studied. As briefly outlined, the complete antigenic structures of several proteins have now been determined by chemical methods and confirmed by synthesis (for reviews, see refs. 1,4,35,44). In contrast, little is known about the molecular parameters involved in the T-lymphocyte responses to protein antigens. The inability to prepare T-cells of preselected specificities to desired protein regions has been responsible, in part, for our poor understanding of the T-cell responses.

The recent advent of the T-cell cloning technique (68,69) has made it possible to obtain T-lymphocyte clones that are monospecific to protein antigenic sites (70). However, the isolation of a clone of a desired specificity is tedious, time-consuming, and often elusive. Determination of the site specificity of the clones is extremely difficult and has been done either with multi-determinant fragments (70) or with proteins having known sequence substitutions. The latter approach, fraught with electrostatic, steric and conformational complications is unsatisfactory for localization of antigenic sites as has already also been demonstrated for its application to regions recognized by antibodies (for review, see refs. 35, 44). Caution should also be exercised in applying this approach to localization of T-cell recognition sites, especially in view of the findings both for Mb (71) and for lysozyme (72) that T-cell recognition can also be dependent on native conformation.

Our finding that the small (6-7 residues) synthetic antigenic sites of Mb stimulated T-cells from peritoneal exudates of Mb-primed mice (47), suggested to us (73) that free synthetic peptides may be used during in vitro passage to enrich for T-cells with a selected specificity. However, lymph node cells usually

give a lower proliferative response with the small synthetic
sites (71). Indeed attempts to maintain Mb-primed lymph node
T-cells with the neat sites (i.e. without additional residues)
were usually unsuccessful. Upon extending the sites (Figure 11)
by an additional 5-6 residues (i.e. a total peptide size of 13
residues), the proliferative response of lymph node cells was
greatly improved (73). Therefore, these extended sites were
used to drive the culture into a T-cell population of a single
desired specificity (73). Lymph node cells from mice primed in
vivo with Mb were periodically passaged in vitro with a synthetic extended site. After several passages, the peptide-
driven long term T-cell cultures responded to the intact protein
and exlusively to the peptide that was used to drive the cells
(73) (Tables VII and VIII). from these cultures, T-cell clones
were prepared (73) that responded only to the driving peptide and
to the whole protein (Table IX).
      It has been cautioned (73) that passage of the T-cell cul-
tures with longer peptides is undesirable since they are more
likely to be multivalent (i.e. carry more than one T-cell recognition site) and as a consequence of increasing length they
become more impure and more difficult to purify. Also, passage
of the cells with peptide fragments obtained from protein cleavage is not advisable because of the high likelihood of contamination with traces of intact protein and/or other fragments.
      The ability to obtain T-cell lines (and henceforth T-cell
clones) with specificity to selected protein regions by employing
free synthetic peptides affords a measure of control that has not
hitherto been possible. It completely removes the element of
chance inherent in the present techniques. Furthermore, it makes
it feasible to obtain T-cell lines or clones having a preselected
specificity to biologically or clinically important antigens.
T-cell lines of a preselected specificity would have numerous
applications in basic investigations to probe the molecular basis
of T-cell specificity and cell-cell interactions in immune recognition. Also, many hitherto untapped therapeutic and diagnostic
applications of T-cells may be realized.

Induction of tolerance to preselected protein antigenic sites by
free synthetic peptides

Recently, as a part of our studies on the T-cell recognition of
Mb, we have reported (74) the ability to induce neonatal tolerance to preselected antigenic regions of the protein by the use
of free synthetic peptides carrying those regions. In these
studies neonatal mice (Balb/cByJ) were either tolerized with Mb
or with synthetic peptides of Mb containing Mb antigenic sites
(e.g. antigenic site 5 of Mb; Figure 11). Tolerization with Mb
and subsequent immunization with Mb gave T-cells that did not
proliferate in vitro to Mb or any of the peptides. T-cells from

Extended site 1 (Pept 10-22):

```
           10                                    22
Val-Leu-His-Val-Trp-Ala-Lys-Val-Glu-Ala-Asp-Val-Ala
```

Extended site 2 (pept 50-62):

```
           50                                    62
Lys-Thr-Glu-Ala-Glu-Met-Lys-Ala-Ser-Glu-Asp-Leu-Lys
```

Extended site 3 (pept 87-100):

```
           87                                        100
Lys-Pro-Leu-Ala-Glu-Ser-His-Ala-Thr-Lys-His-Lys-Ile-[Pro]
```

Extended site 4 (pept 107-120):

```
           107                                       120
Ile-Ser-Glu-Ala-Ile-Ile-His-Val-Leu-His-Ser-Arg-His-[Pro]
```

Extended site 5 (pept 141-153):

```
           141                                   153
Asp-Ile-Ala-Ala-Lys-Tyr-Lys-Glu-Leu-Gly-Tyr-Gln-Gly
```

Figure 11. Extension of the five antigenic sites of Mb. The five antigenic sites (underlined residues) were extended by 6-7 residues each to enhance their T-cell proliferative activity. These peptides were used to prepare T-cell lines and T-cell clones with submolecular specificity to preselected protein sites (73).

Table VII. Responses of lymph node cells and long term T-lymphocyte cultures obtained by in vitro passage with Mb or with free extended site 5

[³H-Thymidine incorporation in Δcpm (and S.I.)[a]]

Challenge Antigen	Lymph node cells		15 passages with Mb		14 passages with Ext. Site 5	
	Opt. Dose[b] (μg/ml)	Δcpm (S.I.)	Opt. Dose[b] (μg/ml)	Δcpm (S.I.)	Opt. Dose[b] (μg/ml)	Δcpm (S.I.)
Mb	10	67,390 (14.7)	100	57,510 (3.7)	300	40,330 (9.9)
Ext. Site 1	50	18,220 (4.7)	2.5	31,060 (2.4)		n.d.
Ext. Site 2	50	23,610 (5.8)	5	27,950 (2.3)	5	4,700 (1.9)
Ext. Site 5	30	31,420 (7.4)	10	35,730 (2.67)	15	102,540 (19.5)
Site 5 (pept 145-151)	30	15,050 (4.1)		n.d.	1.2	15,100 (3.7)

a Values are given relative to unchallenged cells and cells challenged with hen lysozyme. Lymph node cells and T cells passaged with Mb or ext. Site 5 responded to 1 μg/ml Con A: Δcpm 47250, 61660, and 52690, respectively. Whereas, 100 μg/ml PPD or 500 μg/ml LPS elicited responses only in lymph node cells, Δcpm 194,560 and 120,970, respectively. S.I. is Stimulation Index.

b The optimum dose is indicated although studies were done in a range of 1-300 μg/ml.

Table is from Yoshioka et al. (73), by permission.

Table VIII. Proliferative response of an SJL T-cell line
obtained by 4 passages with free extended site 4

Challenge Antigen	[^{3}H]-Thymidine incorporation (Δcpm)[a]		
	2.5 µg/ml	5 µg/ml	10 µg/ml
Mb	92,240	121,760	96,510
Ext. Site 1	0	0	0
Ext. Site 2	0	0	0
Ext. Site 3	0	0	0
Ext. Site 4	73,360	124,760	154,630
Ext. Site 5	0	0	0

[a] The values are given in Δcpm relative to the counts of medium or lysozyme challenged cells. Cells responded to Con A (Δcpm 181, 929) but not to LPS or PPD.

Table is from Yoshioka et al. (73), by permission.

Table IX. Proliferative responses of T-cell clones obtained from SJL and Balb/c T-cell long term cultures that were passaged with <u>free extended site 4 or extended site 5</u>

[³H]-Thymidine incorporated in Δcpm (and S.I.)

Challenge Antigen[d]	SJL T-cell clones		Balb/c T-cell clone[c] (#8C) from line specific to Ext. Site 5
	Clone #4.EIV-1[a] from cell line specific to Ext. Site 4	Clone #5.EV-4[b] from cell line specific to Ext. Site 5	
Mb	183,600 (47.6)	5,560 (5.32)	13,500 (22.8)
Ext. Site 1	0	0	0
Ext. Site 2	0	0	0
Ext. Site 3	0	0	0
Ext. Site 4	294,450 (75.8)	0	0
Ext. Site 5	0	5,500 (5.30)	13,600 (23.0)

a This clone responded to Con A (Δcpm 303,620; S.I. 78.12), but not to PPD, LPS or hen lysozyme (Δcpm 0; S.I., 0.86).

b This clone responded to Con A (Δcpm 37,620; S.I. 62.6), but not to PPD, LPS or hen lysozyme (Δcpm 0; S.I. 0.88).

c Cells responded to Con A (Δcpm 19,025; S.I. 32.1) but not LPS or PPD or hen lysozyme (Δcpm 0; S.I. 0.98).

d Extended sites were tested in the dose range of 1 to 5 μg/ml. Values represent responses at the optimum dose.

Data are from Yoshioka et al. (73), by permission.

mice that were tolerized with a truncated peptide 139-153 (having
deletions at Tyr-151 and Ala-144) and subsequently immunized with
Mb proliferated in vitro to Mb and to peptides 132-153, 135-153
and 143-153. Tolerization with peptides carrying site 5 had no
effect on the recognition of, and the response to other antigenic
sites of native Mb by the T-cells, whereas the response to the
tolerizing peptides was completely removed (74).

Conclusions

These studies have demonstrated for the first time the enormous
effectiveness of peptides, in their free form, as immunogens.
Thus, contrary to a long-held belief, free small synthetic
peptides will in fact induce antibody and T-lymphocyte immune
responses. The ability to induce antibodies can readily be
exploited to prepare monoclonal antibodies of preselected specificities to desired protein regions. Antibodies can even be
prepared against regions that are not antigenic, when the native
protein is used as immunogen, by immunization with the appropriate free synthetic peptide. Free synthetic peptides have also
proved to be powerful reagents for preparation of T-cells of preselected specificity and for inducing specific tolerance to preselected regions of a protein. These immunogenic properties
should afford important and simple tools for basic immunological
investigations and in disease related antigens and invasive
agents (e.g., viruses, bacteria, toxins, allergens, etc.) for
therapeutic and diagnostic purposes.

Acknowledgments

The work reviewed here was supported by grants AM-18920 and
AI-18657 from the National Institutes of Health, U.S. Public
Health Service.

Literature Cited

1. Atassi, M. Z. Immunochemistry 1975, 12, 423-438.
2. Anderer, F. A. Biochim. Biophys. Acta 1963, 71, 246-248.
3. Atassi, M. Z., in "Immunochemistry of Proteins"; Atassi, M.
   Z., Ed.; Plenum Press: New York, 1977; Vol. 2, pp. 77-176.
4. Atassi, M. Z. Immunochemistry 1978, 15, 909-936.
5. Kazim, A. L.; Atassi, M. Z. Biochem. J. 1980, 191, 261-264.
6. Kazim, A. L.; Atassi, M. Z. Biochem. J. 1982, 203, 201-208.
7. Yoshioka, N.; Atassi, M. Z. 5th Int. Congr. Immunol. 1983,
   Abstr. 232, 0023.
8. Atassi, M. Z.; Sakata, S.; Kazim, A. L. Biochem. J. 1979,
   179, 327-331.
9. Sakata, S.; Atassi, M. Z. Biochim. Biophys. Acta 1980, 625,
   159-162.

10. Sakata, S.; Atassi, M. Z. Mol. Immunol. 1980, 17, 139-142.
11. Atassi, M. Z. Biochim. Biophys. Acta 1982, 704, 552-555.
12. Atassi, M. Z., in "Specific Receptors of Antibodies and
    Cells"; Pressman, D.; Tomasi, T. B.; Grossberg, A. L.; Rose,
    N. R., Eds.; S. Karger, Basel, 1972; pp. 118-136.
13. Atassi, M. Z., in "Immunochemistry of Proteins"; Atassi, M.
    Z., Ed.; Plenum Press: New York, 1977; Vol. 1, pp. 1-161.
14. Atassi, M. Z.; Lee, C.-L.; Pai, R.-C. Biochim. Biophys. Acta
    1976, 427, 745-751.
15. Lee, C.-L.; Atassi, M. Z. Biochem. J. 1976, 159, 89-93.
16. Atassi, M. Z; Smith, J. A. Immunochemistry 1978, 15, 609-610.
17. Lee, C.-L.; Atassi, M. Z. Biochim. Biophys. Acta 1977, 495,
    354-368.
18. Lee, C.-L.; Atassi, M. Z. Biochem. J. 1977, 167, 571-581.
19. Atassi, M. Z.; Lee, C.-L. Biochem. J. 1978, 171, 419-427.
20. Atassi, M. Z. Biochem. J. 1967, 103, 29-35.
21. Andres, S. F.; Atassi, M. Z. Biochemistry 1970, 9, 2268-2275.
22. Twining, S. S.; Lehmann, H.; Atassi, M. Z. Mol. Immunol.
    1981, 18, 473-479.
23. Atassi, M. Z.; Saplin, B. J. Biochemistry 1968, 7, 688-698.
24. Twining, S. S.; Atassi, M. Z. J. Biol. Chem. 1978, 253,
    5259-5262.
25. Kazim, A. L.; Atassi, M.Z. Biochem. J. 1980, 187, 661-666.
26. Amzel, L. M.; Poljak, R. J.; Saul, F.; Varga, J. M.;
    Richards, F. F. Proc. Natl. Acad. Sci. U.S.A. 1974, 71,
    1427-1430.
27. Padlan, E. A.; Davies, D. R.; Rudikoff, S.; Porter, M.
    Immunochemistry 1976, 13, 945-949.
28. Atassi, M. Z. Mol. Immunol. 1981, 18, 1021-1025.
29. Atassi, M. Z.; Webster, R. G. Proc. Natl. Acad. Sci. U.S.A.
    1983, 80, 840-844.
30. Atassi, M. Z.; Webster, R. G., unpublished data.
31. Kazim, A. L.; Atassi, M. Z. Biochem. J. 1977, 167, 275-278.
32. Atassi, M. Z.; Kazim, A. L, in "Immunobiology of Proteins
    and Peptides"; Atassi, M. Z.; Stavitsky, A. B., Eds.; Plenum
    Press: New York, 1978; Vol. 1, pp. 19-40.
33. Yoshida, T.; Atassi, M. Z. Immunol. Commun. 1984, in press.
34. Twining, S. S.; Lehmann, H.; Atassi, M. Z. Biochem. J. 1980,
    191, 681-697.
35. Atassi, M. Z. Mol. Cell. Biochem. 1980, 32, 21-44.
36. Hopp, T. P.; Woods, K. R. Proc. Natl. Acad. Sci. U.S.A.
    1981, 78, 3824-3828.
37. Chou, P. Y.; Fasman, G. D. Biochemistry 1974, 13, 222-224.
38. Atassi, H.; Atassi, M. Z., unpublished data.
39. Atassi, M. Z.; Habeeb, A. F. S. A., in "Immunochemistry of
    Proteins"; Atassi, M. Z., Ed.; Plenum Press: New York,
    1977; Vol. 2, pp. 177-264.
40. Takagaki, Y.; Hirayama, A., Fujio, H; Amano, T. Biochemistry
    1980, 19, 2498-2505.

41. Dean, J.; Schechter, A. N. J. Biol. Chem. 1979, 254, 9185-9193.
42. Kohler, G.; Milstein, C. Nature 1975, 256, 495-497.
43. Schmitz, H. E.; Atassi, H.; Atassi, M. Z. Immunol. Commun. 1983, 12, 161-175.
44. Atassi, M. Z., in "Molecular Immunology"; Atassi, M. Z.; van Oss, C. J.; Absolom, D., Eds.; Marcel Dekker: New York, 1973; pp. 15-52.
45. Weir, D. M., in "Handbook of Experimental Immunology"; Blackwell Scientific Publications: Oxford, 1973; Vol. 3, 2nd edition, pp. A2.10-A2.11.
46. Okuda, K.; Christadoss, P.; Twining, S.; Atassi, M. Z.; David, C. S. J. Immunol. 1978, 121, 866-868.
47. Okuda, K.; Twining, S.; David, C. S.; Atassi, M. Z. J. Immunol. 1979, 123, 182-188.
48. Young, C. R.; Atassi, M. Z. Immun. Commun. 1982, 11, 9-16.
49. Young, C. R.; Schmitz, H. E. Atassi, M. Z. Mol. Immunol. 1983, 20, 567-570.
50. Twining, S. S.; David, C. S.; Atassi, M. Z. Mol. Immunol. 1981, 18, 447-450.
51. McCormick, D.; Atassi, M. Z., unpublished data.
52. Young, C. R.; Atassi, M. Z., unpublished data.
53. Atassi, M. Z.; Young, M. Z. Immunology Today 1984, in press.
54. Schmitz, H. E.; Atassi, H.; Atassi, M. Z. Mol. Immunol. 1983, 20, 719-726.
55. Young, C. R.; Schmitz, H. E.; Atassi, M. Z. J. Immunogen. 1983, in press.
56. Atassi, M. Z.; Yokota, S.; Twining, S. S.; Lehmann, H.; David, C. S. Mol. Immunol. 1981, 18, 945-948.
57. Young, C. R.; Schmitz, H. E.; Atassi, M. Z. Immunol. Commun. 1983, in press.
58. Kohler, G.; Milstein, C. Eur. J. Immun. 1976, 6, 511-519.
59. Scharff, M. D.; Roberts, S.; Thammana, P. J. Infect. Dis. 1981, 143, 346-351.
60. Kaplan, H. S.; Olsson, L.; Raubitschek, K., in "Monoclonal Antibodies in Clinical Medicine"; McMichael, A. J.; Fabre, J. W., Eds.; Academic Press: London, 1982; pp. 17-35.
61. Milstein, C., in "Monoclonal Antibodies in Clinical Medicine"; McMichael, A. J.; Fabre, J. W., Eds.; Academic Press: New York, 1982; pp. 3-16.
62. Fazekas de St. Groth, S.; Scheidegger, D. J. Immun. Meth. 1980, 35, 1-21.
63. Davis, J. M.; Pennington, J. E.; Kubler, A.-M.; Conscience, J.-F. J. Immun. Meth. 1982, 50, 161-171.
64. Murakami, H.; Masui, H.; Sato, G. H.; Sueoka, N.; Chow, T. P.; Kanosueoka, T. Proc. Natl. Acad. Sci. U.S.A. 1982, 79, 1158-1162.
65. Buchanan, D.; Kamarck, J.; Ruddle, N. H. J. Immun. Meth. 1981, 42, 179-185.

66. Yolken, R. H.; Leister, F. J. J. Immun. Meth. 1981, 43, 209-218.
67. Schmitz, H. E.; Atassi, H.; Atassi, M. Z. Mol. Immunol. 1982, 19, 1699-1702.
68. Fathman, C. G.; Hengartner, H. Nature, 1978, 272, 617-618.
69. Sredni, B.; Tse, H. Y.; Chen, C.; Schwartz, R. H. J. Immunol. 1980, 126, 341-347.
70. Infante, A. J.; Atassi, M. Z.; Fathman, C. G. J. Exp. Med. 1981, 154, 1342-1356.
71. Young, C. R.; Atassi, M. Z. Adv. Exp. Med. Biol. 1982, 150, 73-93.
72. Bixler, G. S.; Atassi, M. Z. J. Immunogen. 1983, in press.
73. Yoshioka, M.; Bixler, G. S.; Atassi, M. Z. Mol. Immunol. 1983, 20, 1133-1137.
74. Young, C. R.; Atassi, M. Z. J. Immunogen. 1983, 10, 161-169.
75. Atassi, M. Z.; Lee, C.-L. Biochem. J. 1978, 171, 429-434.

RECEIVED January 15, 1984

Studies on New Microbial Secondary Metabolites with Potential Usefulness

Antibiotics, Enzyme Inhibitors, and Immunomodifiers

HAMAO UMEZAWA

Institute of Microbial Chemistry, 3-14-23 Kamiosaki, Shinagawa-ku, Tokyo 141, Japan

I have been studying antibiotics since 1944. By 1951, penicillin, streptomycin, chloramphenicol, and tetracyclines were introduced into the clinical use and chemotheraphy of bacterial and rickettsia diseases were almost completely established. Thus antibiotic research was expanded to include antitumor antibiotics since about 1953. In about 1957, resistant strains appeared in hospital patients and the study of antibacterial antibiotics for the development of effective agent against resistant strains was started. By these studies many B-lactam antibiotics and aminogylcoside antibiotics were studied and their derivatives and analogues were developed for the treatment of resistant infections. By 1965, organic chemistry had developed sufficiently to permit determination of structure of natural products very rapidly. This permitted optimization of the search for enzyme inhibitors, out of which the discovery of many compounds which have various pharmacological activities resulted. Enzyme inhibition research has expanded also to low molecular weight immunomodifiers which are useful in the treatment of cancer. Thus in these developments in antibiotic research, which might be called the second era, I could contribute to the opening of these research areas.

In this paper, I will review the studies which have pioneered new research areas and recent studies on the new microbial secondary metabolites with potential usefulness.

Studies on Antimicrobial Antibiotics:
Kanamycin and Derivatives of Aminoglycoside Antibiotics

In 1957, strains resistant to all chemotherapeutic agents at that time appeared in hospital patients. At that time we discovered kanamycin (83) and this antibiotic was highly regarded for its effect against resistant strains. The occurrence of these resistant strains stimulated the study of B-lactam antibiotics and this study is still contributing to the development of new effective agents against resistant strains. For instance, during three years from January 1981 to January 1983, 19 new B-lactams had been introduced into the clinical use in Japan.

In 1965, Staphylococci and gram-negative organisms resis-

0097-6156/84/0251-0073$09.00/0
© 1984 American Chemical Society

tant to kanamycin also appeared in hospital patients. I elucidated the enzymatic mechanism of resistance to aminoglycoside
antibiotics in 1967 (78): resistant strains produced phospho-
transferase (3'-O-phosphotransferase), which transferred the terminal phosphate of ATP to the 3'-hydroxyl group of kanamycin,
neomycin, and paromomycin; 3'-deoxykanamycin A and 3', 4'-dideo-
xykanamycin B inhibited the growth of resistant strains (Fig. 1)
(60). Following this study, 2"-O-phosphotransferase, 4' and 2"-
O-adenylyltransferases, 3-, 2'- and 6'-N-acetyltransferases were
also found to be involved in the mechanism of resistance (60,63).

Thus, I opened up a new research area where structure of
derivatives effective against resistant strains are predicted by
mechanism of resistance and such derivatives are synthesized.

At present, neither phospho- nor adenylyltransferase, which
transfer the phosphate or adenylyl group of ATP to 5, 2', 4" and
6"-hydroxyl groups has yet appeared in resistant strains. However, these enzymes may appear in future resistant strains.
Therefore, I was interested in the antibacterially active structures which had the least number of hydroxyl groups. We synthesized deoxyderivatives of kanamycins A and B. This study revealed that the amino groups play a predominant role in the antibacterial action of kanamycins, while the hydroxyl groups do not.
5,2',3',4',4",6"-Hexadeoxykanamycin A has almost the same antibacterial activity as kanamycin A (73), and heptadeoxykanamycin,
which has no hydroxyl group, still has a good antibacterial
activity. (73).

Also, by screening, fortimicin, sporaricin, istamycin, and
dactimicin, all of which contain only one hydroxyl group, have
been found by 4 Japanese research groups (63).

It has been known that there are cross-resistance relationships between aminoglycosides and peptide antibiotics such as
viomycin among resistant strains which have been made resistant
by passage through media containing these antibiotics. This can
easily be understood in terms of the predominant role of amino
groups in the antibacterial action of aminoglycosides. Negamycin
(18,36), a peptide antibiotic which we discovered inhibits protein synthesis on bacterial ribosomes and causes miscoding as do
aminoglycoside antibiotics. It has only one hydroxyl group. We
have found that deoxynegamycin has almost the same activity as
negamycin (Fig. 2) (59).

Besides these studies on antibacterial antibiotics and the
derivatives with usefulness, we have discovered about 85 antimicrobial antibiotics and elucidated structures of about 40 of them.
Among these antibiotics, there is kasugamycin (Fig. 3) (77,40,41)
which had been used to prevent the most dreadful rice plant diseases.

Parallel to the study of structure-activity relationships in
aminoglycoside antibiotics, the development study of new amino-
gylcosides effective against resistant infections or with potential agricultural usefulness will continue.

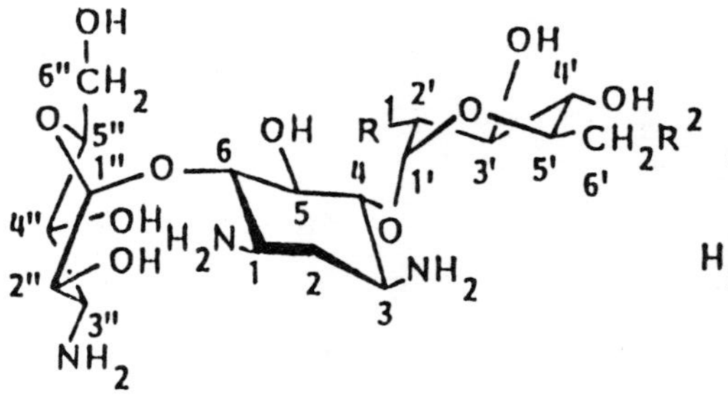

kanamycin A: $R^1 = OH$, $R^2 = NH_2$

kanamycin B: $R^1 = NH_2$, $R^2 = NH_2$

kanamycin C: $R^1 = NH_2$, $R^2 = OH$

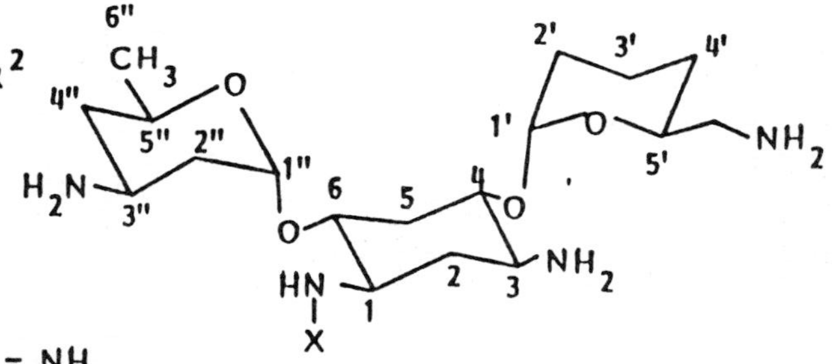

1-N-X-Heptadeoxykanamycin

Figure 1. Kanamycins and 1-N-X-heptadeoxykanamycin, which has strong antibacterial activity and the least number of hydroxyl groups.

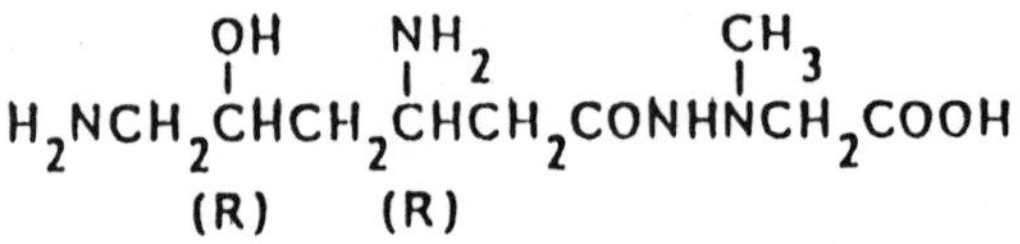

Figure 2.   Negamycin.

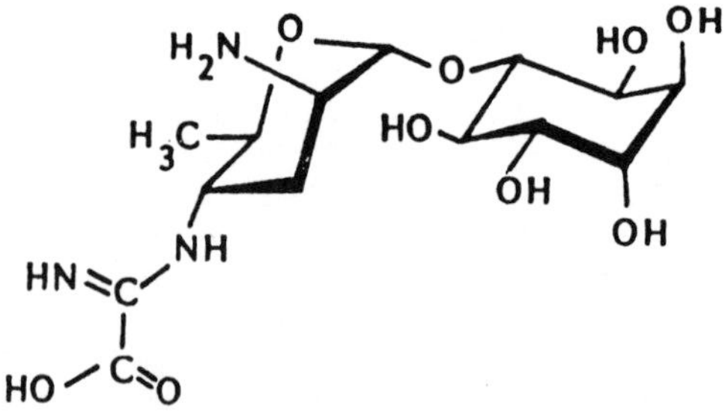

Figure 3.   Kasugamycin.

Studies on Antitumor Antibiotics, Their
Derivatives and Analogs

Here again I should like to backtrack to 1951. At that time
resistant organisms except for streptomycin-resistant tubercle
bacilli had not yet appeared and the chemotherapy of bacterial
diseases seemed to be almost completed. Therefore, I endeavored
to extend antibiotic research to a new area and initiated the
screening of antitumor antibiotics. I reported the discovery of
two microbial products, substance No. 289 and sarkomycin (67).
This was the first report of the successful screening of antibiotics for antitumor activity. Antibiotic research was thus expanded to also cover antitumor research. The term antitumor antibiotics was coined to include those compounds that are produced
by microorganisms and inhibit the growth of tumor cells and tumors.
Since that time, I have been continuing the study of new antitumor
antibiotics. Up to now with my collaborators I discovered about
65 antitumor antibiotics and elucidated structures of about 50 of
them. Among them, bleomycin which we discovered in 1966 (76,79)
has been used in the treatment of Hodgkin's lymphoma, tumors of
the testis, and carcinomas of the skin, head, neck, and cervix.
In 1972, we elucidated the structure of bleomycin except for the
side-chain part of the pyrimidoblamyl moiety (53), and in 1978,
we determined the structure of bleomycin conclusively, as is
shown in Fig. 4 (52). One of the amino acids contained in bleomycin has a pyrimidine ring; we named this amino acid "pyrimidoblamic acid". During the study of biosynthesis, demethylpyrimi-
doblamylhistidinylalanine was obtained and its copper complex was
crystallized. Based on the x-ray analysis of this crystal (10),
we proposed the structure of bleomycin in Fig. 4. We also confirmed this structure by ^{15}N-nmr (25).

In 1980, in collaboration with Professor Ohno, Faculty of
Pharmaceutical Sciences, the University of Tokyo, we were successful in the chemical synthesis of pyrimidoblamic acid (84). This
was one of the most important parts of the total synthesis of
bleomycin. Soon thereafter, Dr. Takita et al. (55) in my institute were successful in the synthesis of the entire peptide part
of bleomycin A2 1981 and then in the total synthesis of bleomycin
A2 in the same year (56,54). Before this, we chemically converted bleomycin A2 to bleomycin demethyl A2 and established synthetic processes for preparing bleomycinic acid from bleomycin demethyl A2 and for preparing various bleomycins from bleomycinic acid
(62). Thus, the structures of bleomycins shown in Fig. 4 were
conclusively established. After our synthesis, Hecht et al.also
reported on the synthesis of the deglycobleomycin demethyl A2 (3)
and the synthesis of bleomycin demethyl A2 (1).

Fujii et al., the Research Institute of Nihon Kayaku Co. who
collaborated with our bleomycin study, isolated 8 peptides from
culture filtrates of a bleomycin-producing strain. They were suggested by the structures to be biosynthetic intermediates of bleo-

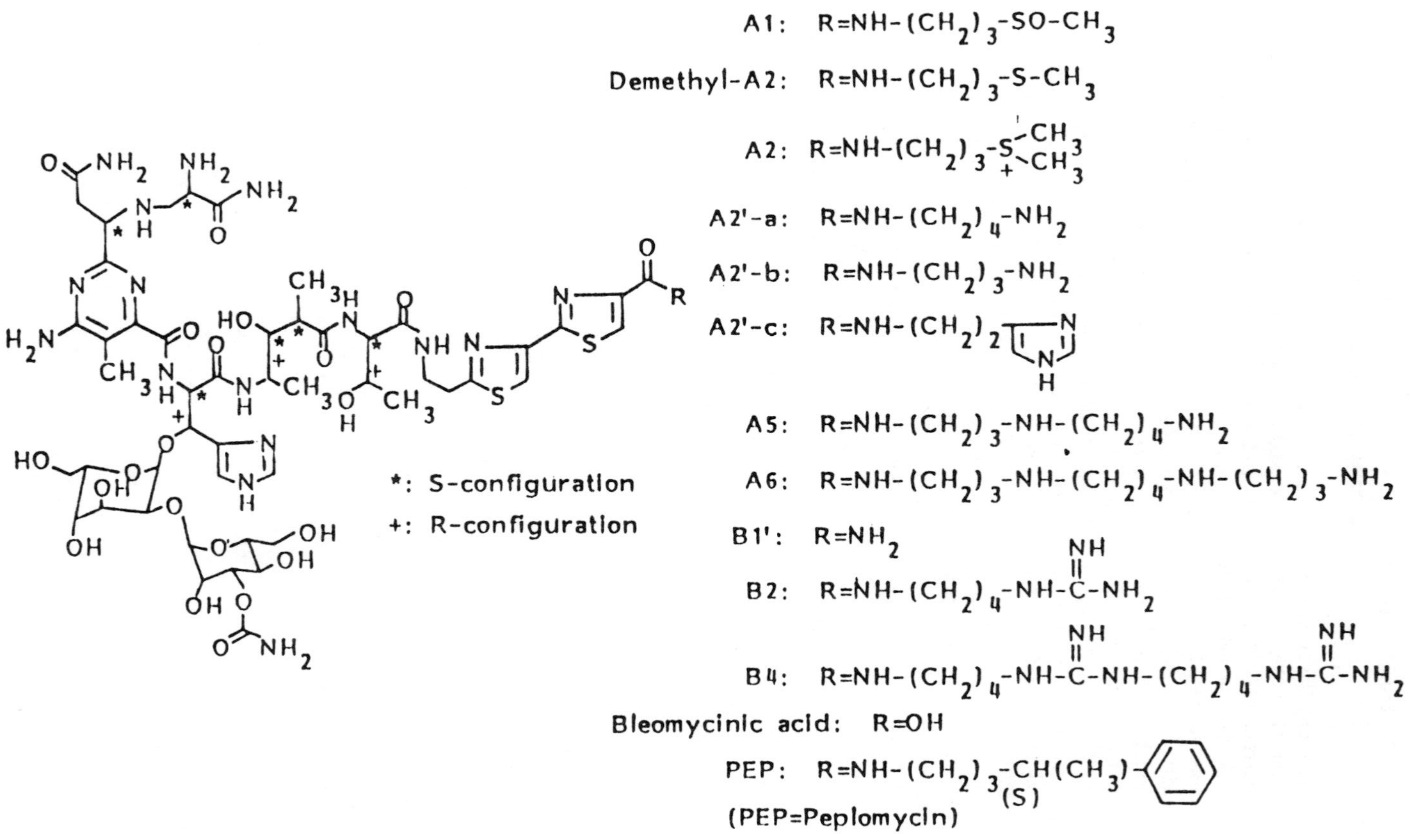

A1:   R=NH-(CH$_2$)$_3$-SO-CH$_3$

Demethyl-A2:   R=NH-(CH$_2$)$_3$-S-CH$_3$

A2:   R=NH-(CH$_2$)$_3$-S$^+$$\overset{-CH_3}{\underset{CH_3}{\diagdown}}$

A2'-a: R=NH-(CH$_2$)$_4$-NH$_2$

A2'-b: R=NH-(CH$_2$)$_3$-NH$_2$

A2'-c: R=NH-(CH$_2$)$_2$-$\langle$N$\rangle$NH

A5:   R=NH-(CH$_2$)$_3$-NH-(CH$_2$)$_4$-NH$_2$

A6:   R=NH-(CH$_2$)$_3$-NH-(CH$_2$)$_4$-NH-(CH$_2$)$_3$-NH$_2$

B1':   R=NH$_2$

B2:   R=NH-(CH$_2$)$_4$-NH-C-NH$_2$
                          ‖
                          NH

B4:   R=NH-(CH$_2$)$_4$-NH-C-NH-(CH$_2$)$_4$-NH-C-NH$_2$
                          ‖   ‖
                          NH   NH

Bleomycinic acid: R=OH

PEP: R=NH-(CH$_2$)$_3$-CH(CH$_3$)
                          (S)
(PEP=Peplomycin)

*: S-configuration
+: R-configuration

Figure 4.   Bleomycins.

mycin. On the basis of the structures of these peptides, the following pathway may be suggested for the biosynthesis of the peptide part of bleomycin:

demethylpyrimidoblamylhistidine (abbreviated as demethylPMB-His) ——→ demethylPMB-His-Ala ——→ demethylPMB-His-4-amino-2-hydroxy-4-methylpentanoic (abbreviated ad demethylPMB-His-AHP) ——→ demethyl-PMB-His-AHP-Thr ——→ PMB-His-AHP-Thr ——→ PMB-His-AHP-Thr-2'-(2-aminoethyl)-2,4' -bithiazole-4-carboxylic acid (abbreviated as PMB-His-AHP-Thr-BTC) ——→ PMB-B-hydroxy-histidine-AHP-Thr-BTC (abbreviated as PMB-B-OH-His-AHP-Thr-BTC) ——→ PMB-B-OH-His-AHP-Thr-BTC-(3-aminopropyl) dimethylsulfonium (the peptide part of bleomycin A2).

The methyl group of pyrimidoblamyl moiety (PMB) and the 2-methyl group of the 4-amino-3-hydroxy-2-methylpentanoyl moiety (AHP) were confirmed to be derived from the methyl group of methionine. The study of the incorporation of labeled amino acids into the pyrimidoblamyl moiety has suggested that the main molecular part of this amino acid is synthesized from L-serine and L-asparagine, and that the methyl group is derived from L-methionine. Labeled 2'-(2-aminoethyl)-2,4'-bithiazole-4-carboxylic acid is not incorporated into this amino acid moiety of bleomycin. This amino acid moiety is produced from B-aminopropionate and 2 molecules of cysteine, suggesting the cyclization of the (3-aminopropionyl) cyteinylcyteine moiety for the formation of the bithiazole-4-carboxylic acid moiety.

The biosynthetic pathway described above indicates the possible involvement of multifunctional enzyme complexes in the biosynthesis of the peptide part of bleomycin. The peptide part of bleomycin has no cytotoxicity. Probably, in the final step of the biosynthesis, the disaccharide part is transferred to the B-hydroxyl group of the B-hydroxylhistidyl moiety and the bleomycin thus synthesized is rapidly released extracellularly.

Bleomycin binds strongly with Cu^{2+}, and an equimolar bleomycin-Cu^{2+} complex is thus formed. We determined the structure of this complex as is shown in Fig. 5 (51,82). As is shown in Fig. 5, the secondary amide between the pyrimidoblamyl and B-hydroxyhistidyl moieties is deprotonated. This deprotonation is shown by the results of the crystal analysis of demethylpyrimidoblamyl-histidylalanine (25) and by the behavior of the bleomycin copper complex during electrophoresis and chromatography. The quenching of the fluorescence of bleomycin by DNA, first found by Horowitz et al. (7), indicates the binding of the bithiazole moiety of both copper-free and copper-bleomycin complexes to the guanine moiety of DNA (16). The positive charge of the terminal amine facilitates the binding of bleomycin to DNA (16).

In the presence of ferrous ions and oxygen, copper-free bleomycin causes a double-strand scission of DNA. The bleomycin-Cu^{2+} complex binds to DNA, but does not cause strand scission.

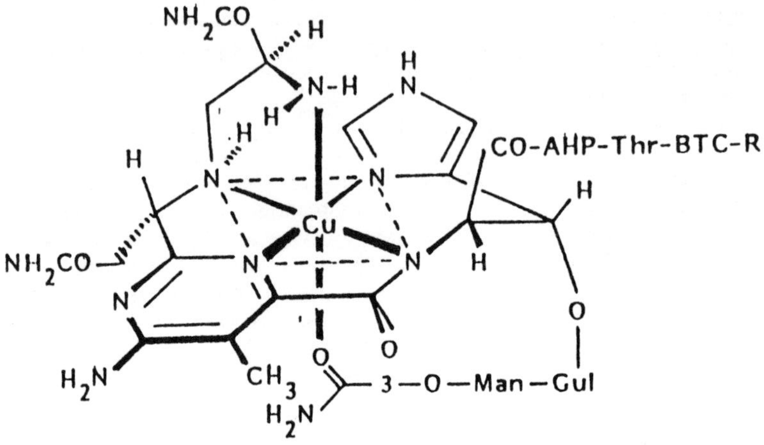

AHP = 4-amino-3-hydroxy-2-methylpentanoyl

Thr = threonyl

BTC = 2'-(2-aminoethyl)-2,4'-bithiazole-4-carboxyl

R = terminal amine

Man-Gul = 2-O-(α-D-mannopyranosyl)-α-L-gulopyranosyl

Figure 5.   Bleomycin-Cu2+-complex.

Although it has not yet been proven, we have proposed a structure for the bleomycin-iron-O_2 complex in which Fe^{2+} replaces Cu^2 in Fig. 5 (51,82). Oppenheimer et al. once proposed a structure different from ours for the bleomycin-Fe^{2+}-CO complex. On the basis of pmr analysis, the same authors (32, 31) later reported that the steric relationship between the a-methin proton of the a-aminocarboxamide part of the pyrimidoblamyl moiety and the adjacent methylene protons is different from that in the demethylpyrimidoblamylhistidylalanine-Cu^{2+} complex crystals (shown by x-ray analysis) (10) and deglycobleomycin-Fe^{2+}-CO complex. This result does not really contradict the structure which we previously proposed (51), for CPK-model study shows that both gauche-trans and gauche-gauche conformers between the methin and methylene protons can exist in the 5-membered chelate-ring constructed as follows:

$$Fe^{2+} \longrightarrow NH_2 \longrightarrow CH(CONH_2) \longrightarrow CH_2 \longrightarrow NH(CH\text{---})\longrightarrow$$
$$(Fe^{2+})$$

The active species of the bleomycin-iron-O_2 complex involved in the reaction with DNA has been suggested to be the bleomycin-Fe^{3+}-O_2^{2-} complex (22,6)   The products of DNA fragmentation caused by the bleomycin-iron-O_2 complex were isolated by Grollman and Takeshita (9). On the basis of these reaction products, the following scheme can be proposed for the DNA-fragmentation reaction caused by bleomycin: bleomycin-Fe^{3+}-O_2^{2-} binding to DNA abstracts the hydrogen radical from the 4-carbon of the 2-deoxyribose moiety, leaving a radical at the 4-C position; this radical then reacts with molecular oxygen; as the result of this reaction, the 4-carbon is oxygenated, and the ring cleavage of the deoxyribose moiety is followed by cleavages of the phosphate and ester bonds in various ways.

Bleomycin intercalates between bases of double-stranded DNA(34). In this connection, it is interesting that phleomycin which has the dihydrobithiazole moiety, does not intercalate with DNA (33). It causes more single-strand scission than double-strand scission (30).

Injected bleomycin binds with Cu^{2+} in the blood. After penetrating into cells, the Cu^{2+} of the bleomycin copper complex is reduced to Cu^+ by reducing agents such as cysteine. In the cells the Cu^+ is then tranferred to a cellular protein which can bind selectively to Cu^+ (62,45). The copper-free bleomycin thus formed undergoes reaction with bleomycin hydrolase, which hydrolyzes the a-aminocarboxamide bond of the pyrimidoblamyl moiety of bleomycin (62,72). This enzyme is widely distributed in human and animal cells. Copper-free bleomycin, which escapes this enzymic action, reaches the nuclei, binds, and reacts with DNA as has been described above. Our knowledge of the mechanism of the action has been utilized for designing derivatives or analogs with improved therapeutic activities.

We have established fermentation and chemical methods for the preparation of artificial bleomycins which contain various terminal amines. With the addition of many kinds of amines to the fermentation medium, various bleomycins containing the added amines are produced while the production of other bleomycins is suppressed (62). We found acyl agmatine hydrolase in Fusarium sp., which hydrolyzes the terminal peptide bond of bleomycin B2, thus yielding bleomycinic acid (62,81). Bleomycinic acid can also be obtained by the reaction of cyanogen bromide with bleomycin demethyl A2 (50). Various bleomycins are synthesized from bleomycinic acid. By testing the toxicity of various bleomycins, the degree of renal and pulmonary toxicity was found to be dependent on the terminal amine. Moreover, it has been shown by the clinical study that peplomycin (Fig. 6), a semi-synthetic bleomycin (23), is more effective than the present bleomycin against carcinomas sensitive to bleomycin treatment, and has a lower pulmonary toxicity, and a wider anticancer spectrum. Peplomycin has also been confirmed to be effective against prostatic carcinoma.

As has already been described, bleomycin hydrolase hydrolyzes the carboxamide of the a-aminocarboxamide bond of the pyrimidoblamyl moiety, and the product of this hydrolysis can be used as the starting material for the modification of the a-aminocarboxamide moiety. Two examples of such derivatives, PEP-PEP and DBP-PEP, are shown in Fig. 6. Both are resistant to bleomycin hydrolase and have a low pulmonary toxicity. Their therapeutic index against Ehrlich carcinoma is as high as that of bleomycin. Bleomycin analogues and derivatives of this type which may be more effective and useful in cancer treatment than bleomycin will undoubtedly be developed in the future.

After we were successful in the total synthesis of bleomycin in 1981, as we reported last year, we improved the method of the synthesis (35). We synthesized bleomycin analogues containing the 4-aminobutanoyl, (3S)-4-amino-3-hydroxybutanoyl or (3S,4R)-4-amino-3-hydroxypentanoyl moiety instead of the (2S,3S,4R)-4-amino-3-hydroxy-2-methylpentanoyl moiety of bleomycin A2. Then, only the last analogue had the same degree of the activity as bleomycin in inhibiting the growth of B. subtilis and causing strand scission of DNA. Thus, the 5-methyl group of the 4-amino-3-hydroxy-2-methyl-pentanoyl moiety was shown to play a role in the reaction with DNA. Probably the hydroxyl group is also involved in the reaction. The functional groups for the action of bleomycin can be elucidated by the synthesis of new analogues, and further improved analogues will be developed for cancer treatment.

Adriamycin, discovered by Dr. Arcamone, is one of the most effective cancer chemotherapeutic agents. Thus, many researchers have been continuing the study of anthracyclines. For instance, the 4'-epi-adriamycin and 4-demethoxydaunomycin.

Although many anthracycline antibotics have been isolated since the discovery and structure determination of early anthracyclines in the decade of 1950, the screening for red- or yellow-pigment antitumor antibiotics still leads to the finding of new

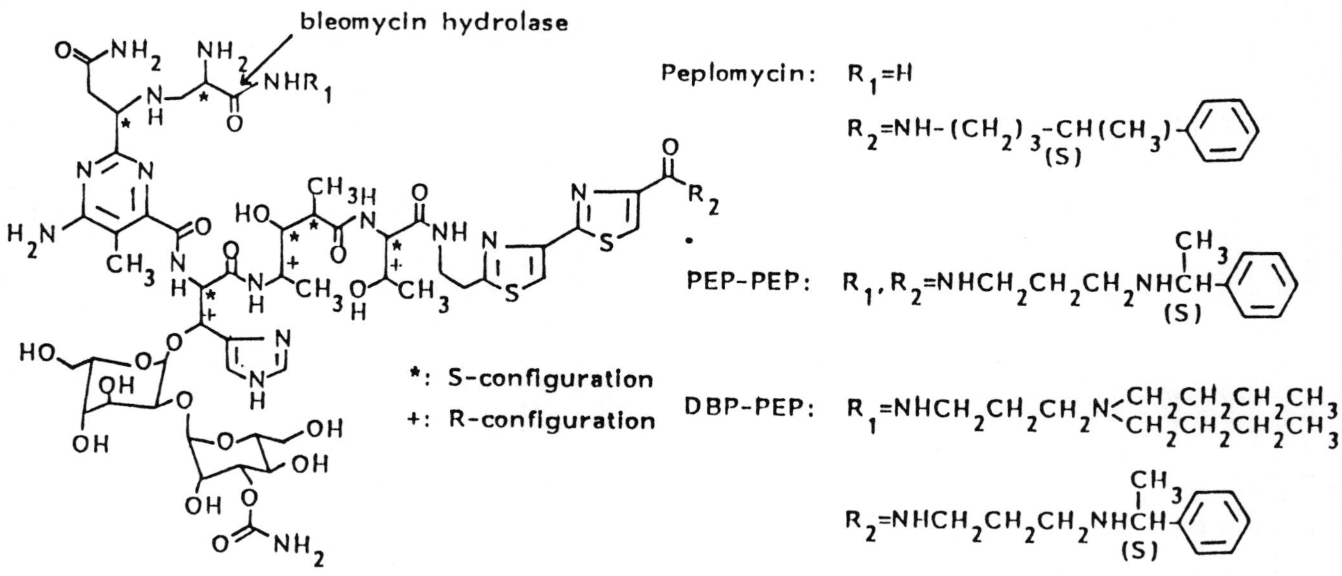

Figure 6.   Artificial bleomycins: Peplomycin, PEP-PEP, and DBP-PEP.

types of anthracyclines. Very recently we found decilorubicin (Fig.7) containing two molecules of a nitro-sugar which we named "decilonitrose" (11). Recently we also found three ditrisarubicins A, B and C, each consisting of B-rhodomycinone and trisaccharides at both the 7-C-OH and 11-C-OH positions (Fig. 8) (58).

A new anthracycline, aclacinomycin A (Fig. 9) which we discovered in 1976 (28), has been proved by clinical study to be indispensable in the treatment of leukemia. It exhibits a therapeutic effect against leukemia and lymphoma, even against cases resistant to treatment with daunomycin and adriamycin. Dantchev et al. (8) proved that aclacinomycin A has markedly a lower cardiac toxicity in hamsters than does adriamycin. This low cardiac toxicity has also been confirmed by clinical study.

We studied the biosynthesis of anthracyclines and obtained various mutants which produce neither red nor yellow pigments and which convert aglycones to anthracyclines. In addition, we found a mutant which produced 2-hydroxyaklavinone (aklavinone is the aglycone of aclacinomycin). By adding 2-hydroxyaklavinone to the culture medium and culturing a pigmentless mutant of an aclacinomycin-producing strain, we obtained 2-hydroxyaclacinomycins A and B (29). This is the first finding of a 2-hydroxy analog of anthracyclines. 2-Hydroxyaclacinomycins A and B have higher therapeutic indices against L1210 leukemia than does aclacinomycin A.

We have also discovered baumycins (Fig. 10) in culture filtrates of daunomycin-producing strains (47). Baumycin Al showed a strong action against L1210 in our laboratories. Therefore, we started the synthesis of 4'-O-acetal derivatives of adriamycin and daunomycin. Among about the fifty derivatives thus synthesized, one of the 4'-O-tetrahydropyranyladriamycins (Fig. 10) showed a stronger effect against L1210 than adriamycin and daunomycin (80). This effective anomer is abbreviated as THP. THP has a similar or a slightly greater degree of antitumor activity than that of adriamycin against various experimental mouse tumors. Dantchev et al. (8) proved that THP has a significantly lower cardiac toxicity than adriamycin in hamsters. This low cardiac toxicity has also been observed by clinical study. Such side effects as hair loss, nausea, and vomiting which often occur during adriamycin treatment are very slight in the case of THP. THP has shown a strong therapeutic effect against lymphomas, lymphatic leukemia, tumors of the ovary, uterus, head, and neck, etc.

THP, adriamycin, and their metabolites can be determined by liquid chromatography using a flourescence detector. The results of the determination of intracellular amounts of THP and adriamycin have indicated that THP is much more rapidly taken up by cancer cells than is adriamycin (20). There is a cross-resistance between adriamycin and THP, but it is not complete; for instance, the 50% inhibition concentrations of adriamycin against two resistant cell lines of P388 were 60-70 times higher than that against the parental sensitive cell line, and the 50% inhibition concentrations of THP against the resistant cell lines were 13 times higher than that against the sensitive cell line.

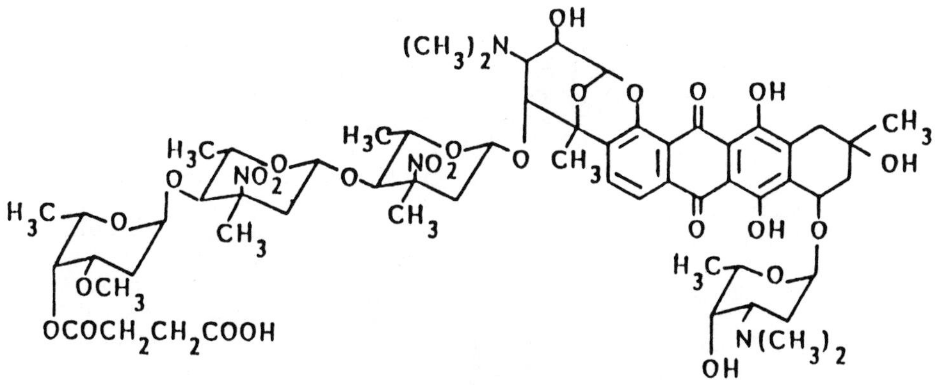

Figure 7. Decilorubicin.

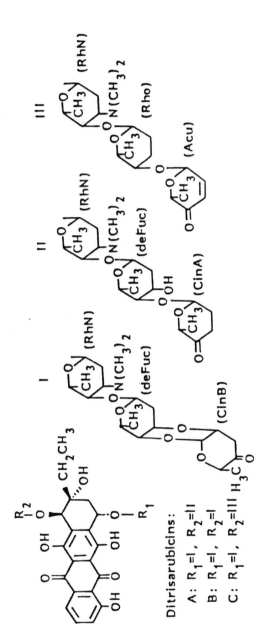

Figure 8. Ditrisarubicins.

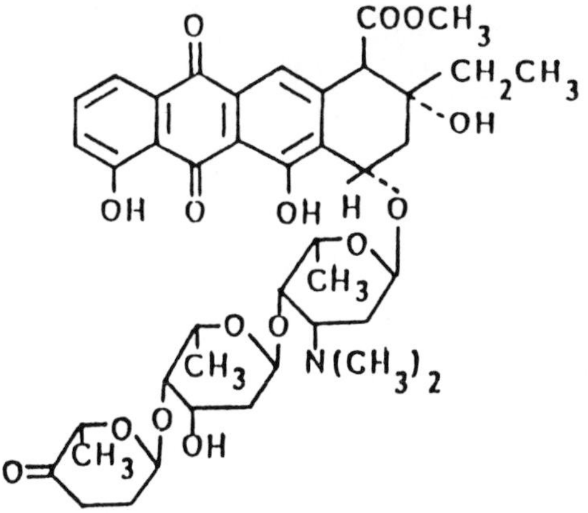

Figure 9. Aclacinomycin.

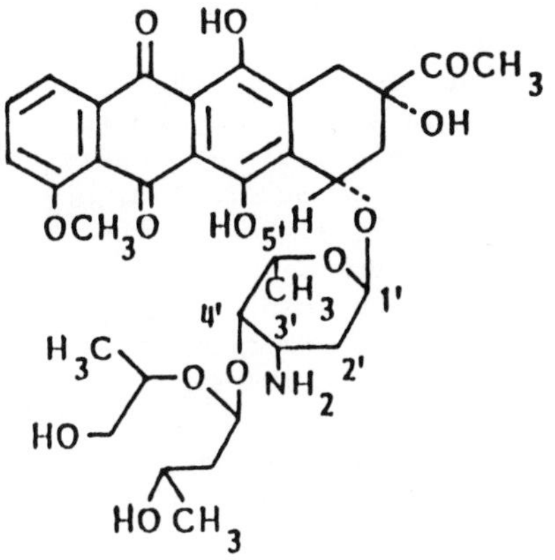

Baumycin A1 was found in a
daunomycin-producing strain

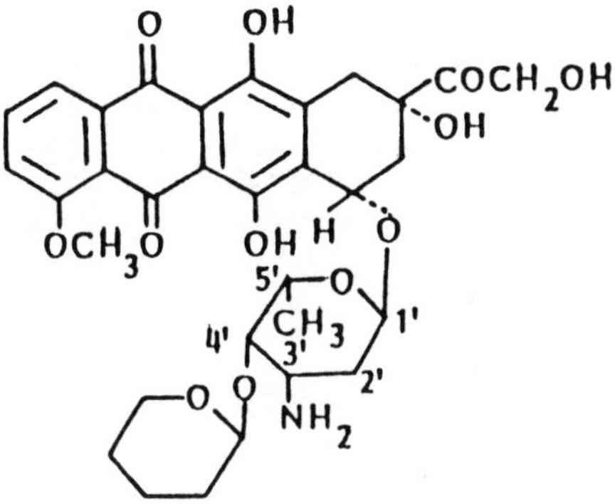

Figure 10. Baumycin A1 and 4'-0-tetrahydropypyranyl-
adriamycin (THP, theprubicin).

As has been described above, it seems that the continuation of the present study will lead to the development of new anthracyclines which have a much lower toxicity and a stronger therapeutic effect than the anthracyclines used clinically at present. Moreover, the screening study for anthracyclines effective against resistant cell lines may lead to the discovery of interesting new compounds with potential usefulness.

Thirty years have passed since I reported the first successful screening for antitumor antibiotics. Even at present, by applying various screening methods, new types of antitumor antibiotics can be discovered.

In 1981, we discovered a completely new type of antitumor antibiotic (75,17). This was produced by a strain of bacteria which we classified as Bacillus laterosporus. On the basis of its structure (Fig. 11), we named this antibiotic "spergualin".

Spergualin strongly inhibits L1210 leukemia. About on half of the mice treated with 3.13 or 12.5 mg/kg daily for 10 days survived, and the surviving mice rejected a second inoculation of the same tumor. Spergualin does not inhibit DNA, RNA, and protein synthesis, but its mechanism of action has not yet been determined. Spergualin is an interesting new antitumor compound with a strong antitumor effect against L1210 mouse leukemia, a low chronic toxicity, and an undetermined action mechanism. We have synthesized spergualin and its analogs. Spergualin (Fig. 11) contains two hydroxyl groups. We have prepared 15-deoxyspergualin and 11,15-dideoxyspergualin. All acted to prolong the survival period of mice with L1210 mouse leukemia: 15-deoxyspergualin has the strongest activity, while the dideoxyspergualin has a slighly weaker activity than spergualin. In other spermidine-containing antibiotics such as bleomycin, edeines A and B, laterosporamine, BA-1808, glysperins A, B, and C, and glycinnamoylspermidine, the amino group of the 3-aminopropyl moiety of spermidine links to the residual part of the molecule. However, in the case of spergualin the amino group of the 4-aminobutyl moiety of spermidine links to the carboxyl group of the residual portion of the molecule. We synthesized spergualin analogues containing various amines instead of the spermidine. The analogue in which the amino group of the 3-aminopropyl moiety of spermidine is involved in the linkage to the residual part of the molecule has a much weaker activity in inhibiting the growth of L1210 cells in vitro and has no activity in inhibiting L1210 in vivo (66). The removal of the amidino group of the guanidine moiety of spergualin eliminates the effect in vivo. Analogue studies of spergualin thus indicate a predominant role of the amino and guanidine groups in the antitumor action and suggests the importance of the distances between the amine nitrogen atoms.

Glyo II found by the study of inhibitors of glyoxalase and exhibited antitumor effect. Glyo II reacts with SH-compounds as follows (48):

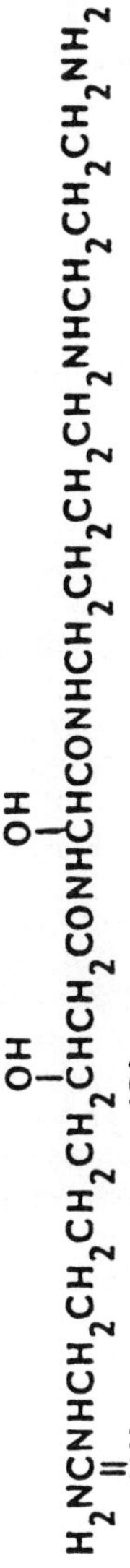

$$\underset{\substack{\|\\ NH}}{H_2NCNHCH_2CH_2CH_2CH_2} \underset{\substack{|\\ OH}}{CHCH_2} CONHCH_2 \underset{\substack{|\\ OH}}{CHCONHCH_2CH_2CH_2CH_2} NHCH_2CH_2CH_2NH_2$$

(S)

Figure 11. Spergualin.

$$\text{(structure)} + RSH \longrightarrow \text{(structure)} + CH_3CH=CHCOOH$$

The cytotoxic action of Glyo II was thus elucidated by its reaction with RSH.

In the last 20 years, microbial culture filtrates have been screened for the activity to inhibit L1210 mouse leukemia, P388 leukemia, sarcoma 180, Ehrlich carcinoma, etc., and the antitumor antibiotics which exhibit therapeutic effect against leukemia, lymphoma, breast cancer tumor of the ovary, uterus, testis, head, neck and skin have been developed. However, antitumor compounds which exhibit a strong therapeutic effect against cancer of the stomach and lung have not yet been discovered. Therefore, the antibiotics that exhibit the cytotoxic action through interesting mechanisms may be interesting.

Low Molecular Weight Enzyme Inhibitors - Microbial
Secondary Metabolites with Various Pharmacological Activity

By 1965, NMR and x-ray crystallography had been introduced into natural product chemistry, and it became possible to elucidate the structures of microbial products very quickly. Moreover, at about this time, an understanding of the biochemistry of various diseases began to make rapid progress.

Therefore, with my collaborators I initiated the screening of culture filtrates for low molecular weight enzyme inhibitors. We reported the first paper in 1969, and have since discovered about 50 inhibitors (65).

Trypsin hydrolyzes peptide bonds at the carboxyl side of arginine and lysine; chymotrypsin, at the carboxyl side of phenylalanine, and pancreas elastase, at the carboxyl side of alanine. Those of inhibitors (Fig. 12) which we discovered, that is, leupeptin and antipain inhibiting trypsin, chymostatin inhibiting chymotrypsin and elastatinal inhibiting elastase, had the argininal, phenylalaninal or alaninal group respectively (65,61). The C-terminal aldehyde structure for the inhibition of serine and thiol proteases was first found in these inhibitors. Pepstatin inhibiting pepsin, cathepsin D, and renin, and phosphoramidon inhibiting metallo-proteinases, also have interesting structures, as is shown in Fig. 12. In determining the structures of enzyme inhibitors and antibiotics, we became interested in why so many

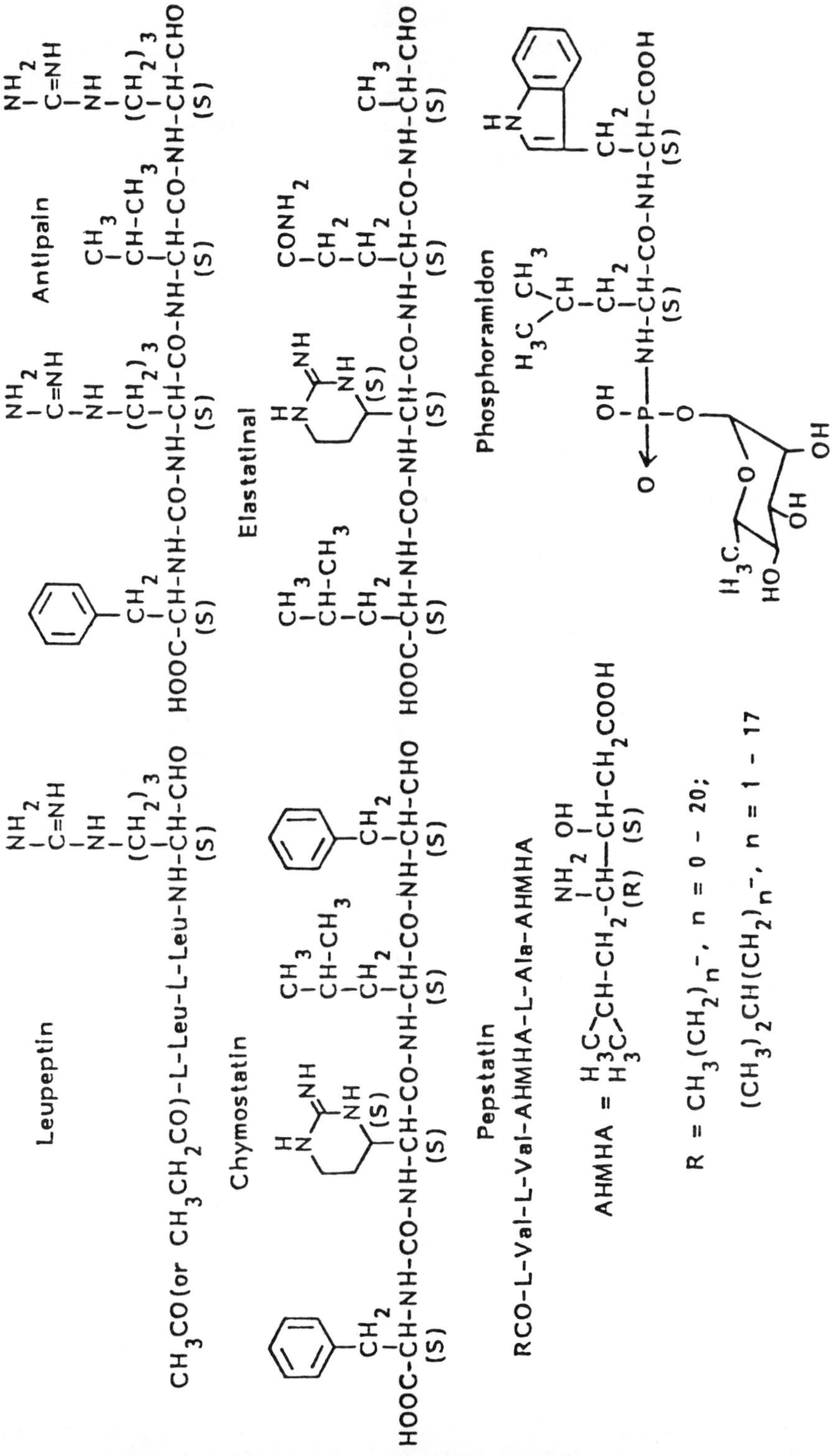

Figure 12. Protease inhibitors.

compounds with various structures are produced by microorganisms;
therefore, we studied the biosynthesis of leupeptin. In this study,
we were successful in the isolation of all three enzymes (43,44,
42) involved in leupeptin biosynthesis, that is, leucine acetyl-
transferase, leupeptin acid synthetase, and leupeptin acid reductase. These enzymes were extracted from <u>Streptomyces</u> <u>roseus</u> MA
839-A1 producing leupeptin.   Leupeptin acid (acetylleucylleucy-
larginine)is synthesized by leupeptin-acid synthetase, which requires ATP. The reaction sequence for this multifunctional enzyme can be shown as follows:

$$\text{acetyl-Leu + L-Leu} \xrightarrow{\text{ATP}} \text{acetyl-L-Leu-L-Leu + L-Arg}$$

$$\xrightarrow{\text{ATP}} \text{acetyl-L-Leu-L-Leu-L-Arg}$$

Leupeptin acid is reduced to leupeptin by leupeptin acid reductase which requires ATP and NADPH. This enzyme is located in cell
membranes.

Leupeptin-acid reductase is inhibited by leupeptin, but not
by elastatinal (42). This specific inhibition indicates that
leupeptin acid which has no antiprotease activity is produced
within cells; on the other hand, the leupeptin produced from leupeptin acid is not accumulated in cells, but is rapidly released
extracellularly.

Compounds like leupeptin acid, which are the precursors of
secondary metabolites, should not have cytotoxicity, and in many
cases, the enzyme involved in the last step of the biosynthesis
may be inhibited by the last product as in the case of leupeptin
acid reductase. It is also possible that multifunctional enzyme
complexes may be involved in the synthesis of many secondary metabolites.

As has been described in a recent review of low-molecular-
weight enzyme inhibitors of microbial origin (65), hypotensive
compounds, compounds useful in the treatment of diabetes or obe-
sity, and compounds useful in the treatment of hypercholestremia
have been discovered by the screening for inhibitors of catecho-
lamine-synthesizing enzymes, amylase, or 3-hydroxy-3-methylglu-
taryl coenzyme A reductase respectively.

Low Molecular Weight Immunomodifiers

I extended the study of enzyme inhibitors to the study of
low molecular weight immunomodifiers. We searched for inhibitors
of enzymes on cell surfaces, that is, microbial product which can
bind to surfaces or membranes of animals and we could identify
immunomodifiers.

We discovered three antitumor antibiotics produced by
<u>Coriolus</u> <u>consor</u> in 1969 (49), we named them coriolins A, B, and C
and determined their structures (Fig. 13) (46). We also prepared
diketocoriolin B, which was a derivative of coriolin B. This
mushroom is called "saruno-koshikake" in Japanese, and an extract

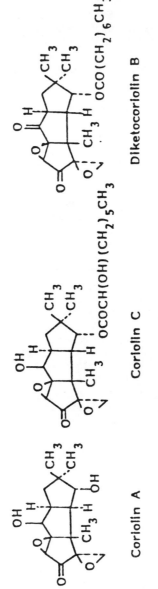

Corlolin A

Corlolin C

Dlketocorlolln B

Figure 13. Coriolins produced by <u>Coriolus consors</u> (saruno-<u>koshikaka</u> in Japanese) and diketocoriolin B.

from it has long been used as a folk medicine for cancer. In 1972, we found that the administration of a very small dose of coriolins A and C and diketocoriolin B to mice increased the number of spleen cells producing an antibody (12). We also found that coriolins and diketocoriolin B inhibit Na^+-K^+-ATPase (21). This enzyme is located in cell membranes of all kinds of animal cells. I first thought, therefore, that the binding of diketocoriolin B to membranes of the cells involved in antibody formation resulted in an increase in the number of antibody-forming cells. Later, we confirmed that diketocoriolin B acts directly on the antibody-producing B lymphocytes (15). I assumed that the screening for compounds which bind to cell membranes or surfaces would result in the discovery of immunity-modifying compounds. In order to find low molecular weight microbial products which can bind to cells, we searched for inhibitors of enzymes on cell surfaces or membranes. In this study we found that all aminopeptidases which hydrolyze N-terminal peptide bonds are located on cell surfaces (2). These enzymes are not released extracellularly. We also found that alkaline phosphatases and esterases are also located on cell surfaces. Searching for inhibitors of these enzymes, we discovered bestatin (70,39,26,74), inhibiting aminopeptidase B ($Ki+6x10^{-8}M$) and leucine aminopeptidase ($Ki=2x10^{-8}M$); amastatin (4), inhibiting aminopeptidase A ($Ki=1.5x10^{-7}M$) and leucine aminopeptidase ($Ki=1.5x10^{-6}M$); forphenicine (5,24), inhibiting chicken intestine alkaline phosphatase; and esterastin (68,19) ($Ki=2x10^{-10}M$) and ebelactones A and B (71,85) ($Ki=9.2x10^{-8}M$ for A; $Ki=5x10^{-10}M$ for B) inhibiting esterase. Their structures are shown in Fig. 14.

Recently, we found the arphamenines. Arphamenines A and B, which we discovered recently in culture filtrates of Chromobacterium violaceum are specific inhibitors of aminopeptidase B. As is shown in Fig. 15, by structural study arphamenines A and B were elucidated to be the methylene analogues of L-arginyl-L-phenylalanine or L-arginyl-L-tryosine respectively. Arphamenines A and B (Fig. 15) (69,27) inhibit aminopeptidase B very strongly (Ki of of A=$2.5x10^{-9}M$ and Ki of B=$8x10^{-10}M$). Arphamenines do not, however, inhibit aminopeptidase A and leucine aminopeptidase.

A low dose (1-100 µg/mouse) of bestatin enhanced delayed-type hypersensitivity (DTH) to sheep red blood cells, while a high dose of it (1 mg/mouse) increased the number of antibody-forming cells in the spleen. Amastatin increased the number of antibody-forming cells. Forphenicine (1-100 µg/mouse) enhanced DTH and also increased the number of antibody-forming cells when given at a dose of 10-1,000 µg/mouse. Ebelactone A enhanced DTH (71). However, esterastin suppressed DTH and reduced the number of antibody-forming cells. Arphamenine A enhanced DTH.

We have also synthesized bestatin and its stereoisomers (38). Bestatin and 3 isomers which had the S-configuration at the 2-C position of the 3-amino-2-hydroxy-4-phenylbutyryl moiety have been found to act strongly to inhibit aminopeptidase B. Conforming

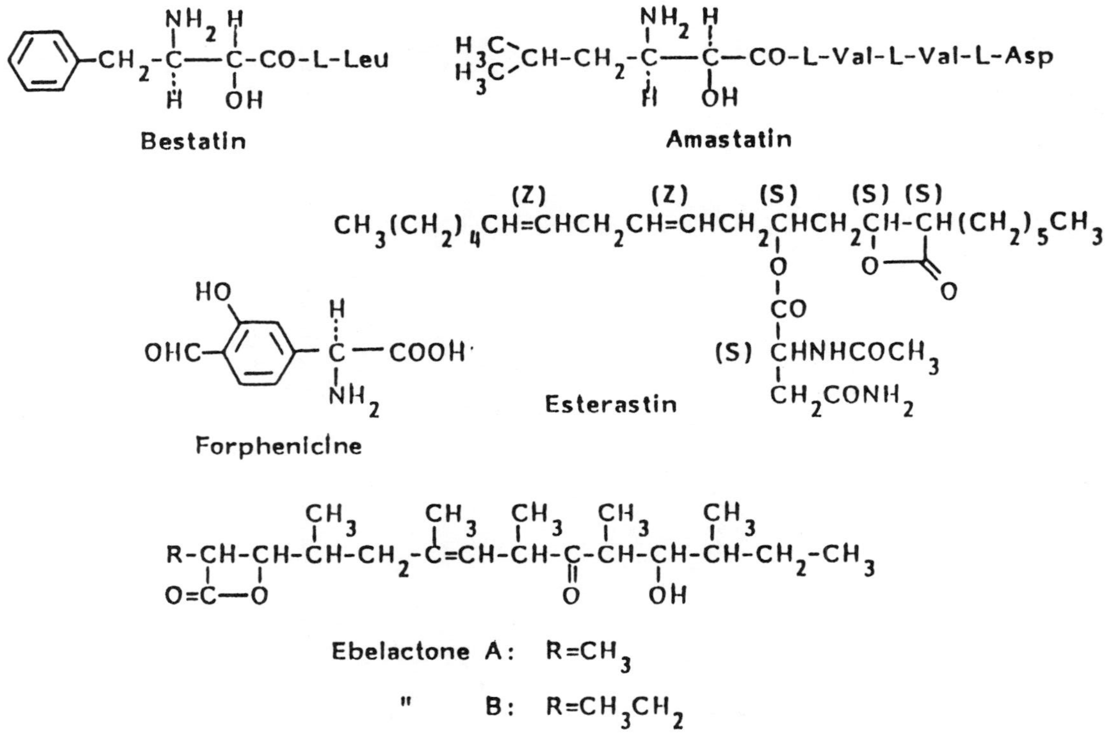

Figure 14. Bestatin, amastatin, forphenicine, esterastin, and ebelactones.

with this activity, all of them acted strongly to enhance delayed-type hypersensitivity. Amastatin, like bestatin, also has the 3-amino-2-hydroxy-propionyl moiety. The stereoisomers which had the S-configuration at the 2-C position of this moiety acted to inhibit aminopeptidase A, but the isomer of the R at the 2-C position had very weak activity or none at all (57).

The type of inhibition of chicken intestine alkaline phosphatase by forphenicine was not competitive, but uncompetitive with the substrate. Its derivative, forphenicinol, which contains a hydroxymethyl group instead of the formyl group in the forphenicine molecule, did not inhibit alkaline phosphatase but, it did bind to cells. Forphenicinol enhanced delayed-type hypersensitivity (13,14) and the phagocytic activity of macrophages.

Among these low-molecular-weight immuno-modifiers, bestatin, forphenicine, forphenicinol, and arphamenines A and B have been tested for antitumor effects against mouse tumors. All showed antitumor action against some mouse tumor strains in vivo and enhanced the antitumor effect of adriamycin, bleomycin, mitomycin, etc. They all have very low toxicity. Of these low-molecular-weight immunomodifiers, bestatin has been studied in greatest detail. Experimental results from testing the effects of bestatin on the mouse-immune system have been presented in a monograph on bestatin (64).

Bestatin has been studied clinically during the last 6 years. Daily oral administration of 30 or 60 mg to cancer patients restored the lowered immunity indices in such patients (64). Clinical randomization tests for the therapeutic effects of bestatin have been conducted. For instance, the survival period of patients with melanoma after the macroscopic elimination of tumors by surgery and chemotherapy has been significantly prolonged by bestatin administration (30 mg, daily, orally) compared with the cases of controls without such bestatin treatment.

As well known, suppressor cells which suppress the immune resistance to cancer have increased in cancer patients, and it is necessary to prepare compounds which can inhibit the generation or action of suppressor cells. We, therefore, have initiated a search for microbial products that inhibit the generation or action of suppressor cells.

It is reasonable to assume that there might exist cytotoxic antibiotics which inhibit the generation or the action of suppressor cells more strongly than that of other immune cells. In fact, anticancer drugs, such as cyclophosphamide, 6-mercaptopurine, aclacinomycin, and bleomycin, etc. have been confirmed to inhibit the generation of suppressor cells.

We discovered completely new nucleoside-like antitumor antibiotic containing a new heteroaromatic ring and named it oxanosine (37) (Fig. 16). We found a dynamic structural change of oxanosine with base and acid as shown in Fig. 16. On the basis of this finding, oxanosine was synthesized (86). This antibiotic produced a significant prolongation of the survival period in mice

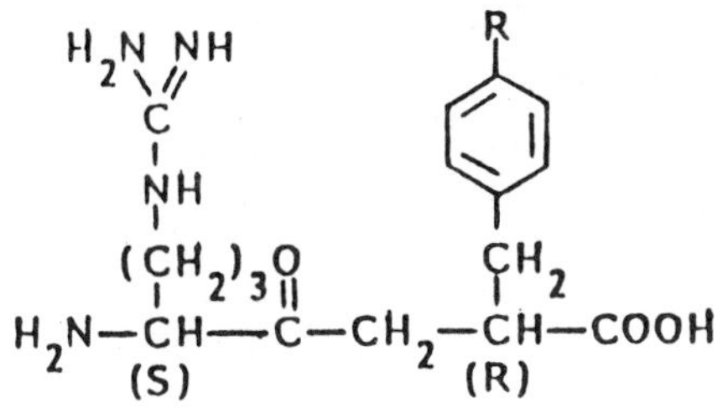

Figure 15.   Arphamenines A (R=H) and B (R=OH).

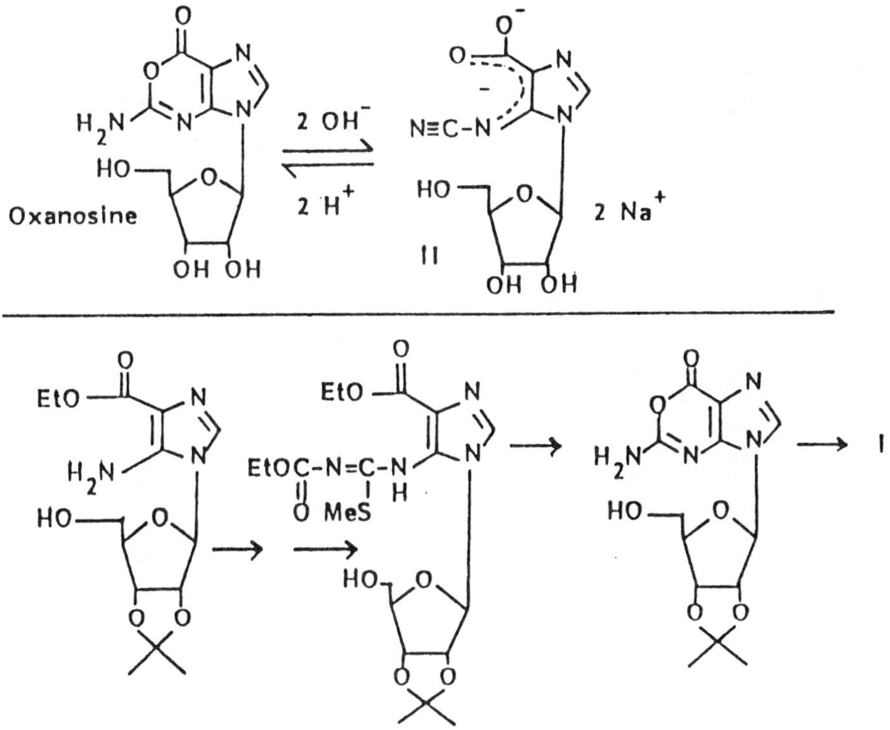

Figure 16.   Oxanosine, its dynamic structure change and synthesis.

with L1210 tumor. The suppressor cells are produced in the spleen of mice with IMC carinoma; the transfer of these suppressor cells to mice eliminates the immune resistance to IMC carcinoma in the latter. If the mice with IMC carcinoma are treated with oxanosine (50-400 mg/kg), then the suppressor activity of the transferred spleen cells is markedly reduced or eliminated. Moreover, one (50 mg/kg) or two injections 6 or 7 days after the inoculation of tumor cells inhibited the growth of IMC carcinoma, although the injections 1 or 3 days after the inoculation of IMC carcinoma cells (10^6) did not produce any antitumor effect. Thus, oxanosine was shown to inhibit the generation or action of suppressor cells. Encouraged by these effects of oxanosine, we have been continuing the study of oxanosine derivatives and its analogues, such as 2'-deoxyoxanosine.

It is also possible to find compounds inhibiting the generation of suppressor cells among low-molecular-weight immunomodifiers. We have confirmed that bestatin, forphenicinol, and arphamenines A and B inhibit the generation and action of suppressor cells which suppress delayed-type hypersensitivity. The effect of bestatin, forphenicinol, arphamenine inhibiting suppressor cells which suppress the cancer immunity is suggested by their effect in inhibiting IMC carcinoma when given 6 and 7 days after the inoculation of the tumor cells; the treatment on 3 or 4 days after the inoculation of tumor cells is not effective. The antitumor effect of the arphamenines has been suggested to be due to their effect of inhibiting the generation of suppressor cells.

Conclusion

I have been successful in expanding the research area of microbial secondary metabolites, isolating new types of compounds which have biological and pharmacological activities with my collaborators. We determined their structures, and synthesized them and their derivatives and analogues. Studies of their derivatives and analogues have also led to the development of more effective antibacterial and antitumor compounds than the parental antibiotics. These studies have also made a great contribution to the understanding of the structure-activity relationships. The study of microbial secondary metabolites and their chemistry has made a great contribution to the progress of medicinal chemistry, and I believe further that the chemistry of the microbial products has been brought to the forefront of life science of today. I also believe that in the near future, methods to produce new microbial products will be established.

Literature Cited

(1) Aoyagi, T., Katano, K., Suguna, H., Primeau, J., Chang,L.-H., Hecht, S. M., J. Am. Chem. Soc. 104, 5537 (1982).

(2) Aoyagi, T., Suda, H., Nagai, M., Ogawa, K., Suzuki, J., Takeuchi, T., Umezawa, H., Biochim. Biophys. Acta 452, 131 (1976).

(3) Aoyagi, Y., Suguna, H., Murugesan, N., Ehrenfeld, G. M., Chang, L.-H., Ohgi, T., Shekhani, M. S., Kirkup, M. P., Hecht, S. M., J. Am. Chem. Soc. 104, 5237 (1982).

(4) Aoyagi, T., Tobe, H., Kojima, F., Hamada, M., Takeuchi, T., Umezawa, H., J. Antibiotics (Japan) 31, 636 (1978).

(5) Aoyagi, T., Yamamoto, T., Kojiri, K., Kojima, F., Hamada, M., Takeuchi, T., Umezawa, H., J. Antibiotics (Japan) 31, 244 (1978).

(6) Burger, R. M., Peisach, J., Horwitz, S. B., J. Biol. Chem. 256, 11636 (1981).

(7) Chien, M., Grollman, A. P., Horwitz, S. B., Biochem. 16, 3641 (1977).

(8) Dantchev, D., Paintrand, M., Hayat, M., Bourut, C., Mathe, G., J. Antibiotics (Japan) 32, 1085 (1979).

(9) Giloni, L., Takeshita, M., Johnson, F., Iden, C., Grollman, P., J. Biol. Chem. 256, 8608 (1981).

(10) Iitaka, Y., Nakamura, Y., Nakatani, T., Muraoka, Y., Fujii, A., Takita, T., Umezawa, H., J. Antibiotics (Japan) 31, 1070 (1978).

(11) Ishii, K., Kondo, S., Nishimura, Y., Hamada, M., Takeuchi, T., Umezawa, H., J. Antibiotics (Japan) 36, 451 (1983).

(12) Ishizuka, M., Iinuma, H., Takeuchi, T., Umezawa, H., J. Antibiotics (Japan) 25, 320 (1972).

(13) Ishizuka, M., Ishizeki, S., Masuda, T., Momose, A., Aoyagi, T., Takeuchi, T., Umezawa, H., J. Antibiotics (Japan) 35, 1042 (1982).

(14) Ishizuka, M., Masuda, T., Kanbayashi, N., Watanabe, Y., Matsuzaki, M., Sawazaki, Y., Ohkura, A., Takeuchi, T., Umezawa, H., J. Antibiotics (Japan) 35, 1049 (1982).

(15) Ishizuka, M., Takeuchi, T., Umezawa, H., J. Antibiotics (Japan) 34, 95 (1981).

(16) Kasai, H., Naganawa, H., Takita, T., Umezawa, H., J. Antibiotics (Japan) 31, 1316 (1978).

(17) Kondo, S., Iwasawa, H., Ikeda, D., Umeda, Y., Ikeda, Y., Iinuma, H., Umezawa, H., J. Antibiotics (Japan) 34, 1625 (1981).

(18) Kondo, S., Shibahara, S., Takahashi, S., Maeda, K., Umezawa, H., Ohno, M., J. Am. Chem. Soc. 93, 6305 (1971).

(19) Kondo, S., Uotani, K., Miyamoto, M., Hazato, T., Naganawa, H., Aoyagi, T., Umezawa, H., J. Antibiotics (Japan) 31, 797 (1978).

(20) Kunimoto, S., Miura, K., Takahashi, Y., Takeuchi, T., Umezawa, H., J. Antibiotics (Japan) 36, 312 (1983).

(21) Kunimoto, T., Hori, M., Umezawa, H., Biochim. Biophys. Acta 298, 513 (1973).

(22) Kuramochi, H., Takahashi, K., Takita, T., Umezawa, H., J. Antibiotics (Japan) 34, 576 (1981).

(23) Matsuda, A., Yoshioka, O., Takahashi, K., Yamashita, T., Ebihara, K., Ekimoto, H., Abe, F., Hashimoto, Y., Umezawa, H., "Bleomycin: Current Status and New Developments", p. 311, Academic Press, 1978.

(24) Morishima, H., Yoshizawa, J., Ushijima, R., Takeuchi, T., Umezawa, H., J. Antibiotics (Japan) 35, 1500 (1982).

(25) Naganawa, H., Takita, T., Umezawa, H., Hull, W. E., J. Antibiotics (Japan) 32, 539 (1979).

(26) Nakamura, H., Suda, H., Takita, T., Aoyagi, T., Umezawa, H., Iitaka, Y., J. Antibiotics (Japan) 29, 102 (1976).

(27) Ohuchi, S., Suda, H., Naganawa, H., Takita, T., Aoyagi, T., Umezawa, H., Nakamura, H., Iitaka, Y., J. Antibiotics (Japan) 36, 1576 (1983).

(28) Oki, T., Matsuzawa, Y., Yoshimoto, A., Numata, K., Kitamura, I., Hori, S., Takamatsu, A., Umezawa, H., Ishizuka, M., Naganawa, H., Suda, H., Hamada, M., Takeuchi, T., J. Antibiotics (Japan) 28, 830 (1975).

(29) Oki, T., Yoshimoto, A., Matsuzawa, Y., Takeuchi, T., Umezawa, H., J. Antibiotics (Japan) 34, 916 (1981).

(30) Okubo, H., Abe, Y., Hori, M., Asakura, H., Umezawa, H., J. Antibiotics (Japan) 34, 1213 (1981).

(31) Oppenheimer, N. J., Chang, C., Chang, L.H., Ehrenfeld, G., Rodriguez, L.O., Hecht, S. M., J. Biol. Chem. 257, 1606 (1982).

(32) Oppenheimer, N. J., Rodriguez, L. O., Hecht, S. M., Biochem. 18. 3439 (1979).

(33) Povirk, L. F., Biochem. 20, 665 (1981).

(34) Povirk, L. F., Hogan, M., Dattagupta, N., Biochem. 18, 96 (1979).

(35) Saito, S., Umezawa, Y., Yoshioka, T., Muraoka, Y., Takita, T., Umezawa, H., J. Antibiotics (Japan) 36, 92 (1983).

(36) Shibahara, S., Kondo, S., Maeda, K., Umezawa, H., Ohno, M., J. Am. Chem. Soc. 94, 4353 (1972).

(37) Shimada, N., Yagisawa, N., Naganawa, H., Takita, T., Hamada, M., Takeuchi, T., Umezawa, H., J. Antibiotics (Japan) 34, 1216 (1981).

(38) Suda, H., Aoyagi, T., Takeuchi, T., Umezawa, H., Archiv. Biochem. Biophys. 177, 196 (1976).

(39) Suda, H., Takita, T., Aoyagi, T., Umezawa, H., J. Antibiotics (Japan) 29, 100 (1976).

(40) Suhara, Y., Maeda, K., Umezawa, H., Ohno, M., Tetrahedron Letters 1966, 1239; Advances in Chemistry Series 74", p. 15 American Chemical Society, 1968.

(41) Suhara, Y., Sasaki, F., Maeda, K., Umezawa, H., J. Am. Chem. Soc. 90, 6559 (1968); Suhara, Y., Sasaki, F., Koyama, G., Maeda, K., Umezawa, H., Ohno, M., J. Am. Chem. Soc. 94, 6501 (1972).

(42) Suzukake, K., Hori, M., Hayashi, H., Umezawa, H., "Peptide Antibiotics - Biosynthesis and Functions", p. 325, Walter de Gruyte and Co., 1982.

(43) Suzukake, K., Hori, M., Tamemasa, O., Umezawa, H., Biochim. Biophys. Acta 661, 175 (1981).

(44) Suzukake, K., Takada, M., Hori, M., Umezawa, H., J. Antibio tics (Japan) 33, 1172 (1980).

(45) Takahashi, K., Yoshioka, O., Matsuda, A., Umezawa, H., J. Antibiotics (Japan) 30, 861 (1977).

(46) Takahashi, S., Naganawa, H., Iinuma, H., Takita, T., Maeda, K., Umezawa, H., Tetrahedron Letters 1971, 1955.

(47) Takahashi, Y., Naganawa, H., Takeuchi, T., Umezawa, H., J. Antibiotics (Japan) 30, 622 (1977).

(48) Takeuchi, T., Chimura, H., Hamada, M., Umezawa, H., Yoshioka, O., Oguchi, N., Takahashi, Y., Matsuda, A., J. Antibiotics (Japan) 28, 737 (1975).

(49) Takeuchi, T., Iinuma, H., Iwanaga, J., Takahashi, S. Takita, T., Umezawa, H., J. Antibiotics (Japan) 22, 215 (1969).

(50) Takita, T., Fukuoka, T., Umezawa, H., J. Antibiotics (Japan) 26, 252 (1973).

(51) Takita, T., Muraoka, Y., Nakatani, T., Fujii, A., Iitaka, Y., Umezawa, H., J. Antibiotics (Japan) 31, 1073 (1978).

(52) Takita, T., Muraoka, Y., Nakatani, T., Fujii, A., Umezawa, Y., Naganawa, H., Umezawa, H., J. Antibiotics (Japan) 31, 801 (1978).

(53) Takita, T., Muraoka, Y., Yoshioka, T., Fujii, A., Maeda, K., Umezawa, H., J. Antibiotics (Japan) 25, 755 (1972).

(54) Takita, T., Umezawa, Y., Saito, S., Morishima, H., Tsuchiya, T., Miyake, T., Umezawa, H., Muraoka, Y., Suzuki, M., Otsuka, M., Ohno, M., Tetrahedron Letters 23, 521 (1982).

(55) Takita, T., Umezawa, Y., Saito, S., Morishima, H., Umezawa, H., Muraoka, Y., Suzuki, M., Otsuka, M., Kobayashi, S., Ohno, M., Tetrahedron Letters 22 671 (1981).

(56) Takita, T., Umezawa, Y., Saito, S., Morishima, H., Umezawa, H., Muraoka, Y., Suzuki, M., Otsuka, M., Kobayashi, S., Ohno, M., Tsuchiya, T., Miyake, T., Umezawa, S., "Peptides: Synthesis-Structure-Function", p. 29 Proceedings of the 7th American Peptide Symposium, 1981.

(57) Tobe, H., Morishima H., Aoyagi, T., Umezawa, H., Ishiki, K., Nakamura, K., Yoshioka, T., Shimauchi, Y., Inui, T., Agric. Biol. Chem. 46, 1865 (1982).

(58) Uchida, T., Imoto, M., Masuda, T., Immura, K., Hatori, Y., Sawa, T., Naganawa, H., Hamada, M., Takeuchi, T., Umezawa, H., J. Antibiotics (Japan) 36, 1080 (1983).

(59) Uehara, Y., Hori, M., Kondo, S., Hamada, M., Umezawa, H., J. Antibiotics (Japan) 29, 937 (1976).

(60) Umezawa, H., "Advances in Carbohydrate Chemistry and Bio-chemistry", p. 183, Academic Press, 1974.

(61) Umezawa, H., "Methods in Enzymology", P. 678, Academic
     Press, 1976.
(62) Umezawa, H., "GANN Monograph on Cancer Research", p. 3,
     University of Tokyo Press, 1976.
(63) Umezawa, H., Jap. J. Antibiotics (Japan) 32 (Suppl.), S1
     (1979).
(64) Umezawa, H., "Small Molecular Immunomodifiers of Microbial
     Orgin - Fundamental and Clinical Studies of Bestatin",
     Japan Scientific Societies Press/Pergamon Press, 1981.
(65) Umezawa, H., "Annual Review of Microbiology", p. 75, Annual
     Reviews Inc., 1982.
(66) Umezawa, H., "Advances in Polyamine Research", Vol. 4,
     Raven Press (1983) in press.
(67) Umezawa, H., Proc. Royal. Soc. Lond. B217, 357 (1983).
(68) Umezawa, H., Aoyagi, T., Hazato, T., Uotani, K., Kojima, F.,
     Hamada, M., Takeuchi, T., J. Antibiotics (Japan) 31, 639
     (1978).
(69) Umezawa, H., Aoyagi, T., Ohuchi, S., Okuyama, A., Suda, H.,
     Takita, T., Hamada, M., Takeuchi, T., J. Antibiotics (Japan)
     36, 1572 (1983).
(70) Umezawa, H., Aoyagi, T., Suda, H., Hamada, M., Takeuchi, T.,
     J. Antibiotics (Japan) 29, 97 (1976).
(71) Umezawa, H., Aoyagi, T., Uotani, K., Hamada, M., Takeuchi,
     T., Takahashi, S., J. Antibiotics (Japan) 33, 1594 (1980).
(72) Umezawa, H., Hori, S., Sawa, T., Yoshioka, T., Takita, T.,
     Takeuchi, T., J. Antibiotics (Japan) 27, 419 (1974).
(73) Umezawa, H., Iwasawa, H., Ikeda, D., Kondo, S., J. Anti-
     biotics (Japan) 36, 1087 (1983).
(74) Umezawa, H., Ishizuka, M., Aoyagi, T., Takeuchi, T., J.
     Antibiotics (Japan) 29, 857 (1976).
(75) Umezawa, H., Kondo, S., Iinuma, H., Kunimoto, S., Ikeda, Y.,
     Iwasawa, H., Ikeda, D., Takeuchi, T., J. Antibiotics (Japan)
     34, 1622 (1981).
(76) Umezawa, H., Maeda, K., Takeuchi, T., Okami, Y., J. Antibio-
     tics (Japan) Ser. A-19, 200 (1966).
(77) Umezawa, H., Okami, Y., Hashimoto, T., Suhara, Y., Hamada,
     M., Takeuchi, T., J. Antibiotics (Japan) Ser. A-18, 101
     (1965).
(78) Umezawa, H., Okanishi, M., Kondo, S., Hamana, K., Utahara,
     R., Maeda, K., Mitsuhashi, S., Science 159, 1559 (1967).
(79) Umezawa, H., Suhara, Y., Takita, T., Maeda, K., J. Antiobio-
     tics (Japan) Ser. A-19, 210 (1966).
(80) Umezawa, H., Takahashi, T., Kinoshita, M., Naganawa, H.,
     Masuda, T., Ishizuka, M., Tatsuta, K., Takeuchi, T.,
     J. Antibiotics (Japan) 32 1082 (1979).
(81) Umezawa, H., Takahashi, Y., Fujii, A., Saino, T., Shirai,T.,
     Takita, T., J. Antibiotics (Japan) 26, 117 (1973).
(82) Umezawa, H., Takita, T., Structure and Bonding 40, 73 (1980).
(83) Umezawa, H., Ueda, M., Maeda, K., Yagishita, K., Kondo, S.,
     Okami, Y., Utahara, R., Osato, Y., Nitta, K., Takeuchi, T.,
     J. Antibiotics (Japan) Ser. A-10, 181 (1957).

(84) Umezawa, Y., Morishima, H., Saito, S., Takita, T., Umezawa, H., Kobayashi, S., Otsuka, M., Narita, M., Ohno, M., J. Am. Chem. Soc. 102, 6630 (1980).
(85) Uotani, K., Naganawa, H., Kondo, S., Aoyagi, T., Umezawa, H., J. Antibiotics (Japan) 35, 1495 (1982).
(86) Yagisawa, N., Takita, T., Umezawa, H., Tetrahedron Letters 24, 931 (1983).

RECEIVED January 6, 1984

Conformation of Nucleic Acids and Their Interactions with Drugs

ANDREW H.-J. WANG

Department of Biology, Massachusetts Institute of Technology, Cambridge, MA 02139

The recent availability of synthetic oligonucleotides of defined sequence has ushered in a new era in our understanding of the nucleic acids. We can now crystallize fragments of nucleic acids and analyze their structure by single crystal X-ray diffraction analysis, which often produces data at atomic or near-atomic resolution. Examples will be discussed of both right-handed and left-handed double helical structures as well as structures containing both RNA and DNA. It is important to note the contributions of nucleotide conformation in these different examples. In addition, the structure of several drug-nucleic acid complexes will be described. It shows in great detail the manner in which these drug molecules have both intercalating components, which bind to the minor groove of B-DNA, as well as hydrogen bonding components which anchor the drug to DNA through its interaction with base pairs on either side of the intercalative site. Analysis at this level makes it possible to contemplate the rational design of molecules such as daunomycin as well as triostin A so that they would interact more strongly as well as more specifically with particular nucleic acid sequences.

Most of our knowledge of the detailed three-dimensional conformation of nucleic acids came from x-ray diffraction studies. The earlier studies of natural and synthetic DNA polymers were carried out on fibers (1). However, fiber diffraction studies have intrinsic limitations as their x-ray diffraction patterns provided only a limited amount of experimental information. In general, it is impossible to solve the molecular structure of a

0097-6156/84/0251-0105$09.00/0
© 1984 American Chemical Society

macromolecule from a fiber diffraction pattern without making many
assumptions as to the nature of the structure or using model
building.
    The availability of chemically synthesized oligonucleotides
of defined sequences has changed the nature of nucleic acid
structural studies from fiber to single crystal x-ray analysis.
Unlike fibers, single crystals have the advantage that they
usually diffract to quite high resolution, sometimes up to atomic
resolution (less than 1 A resolution). Furthermore, there is a
large amount of diffraction data available from single crystals
and it is not necessary to assume any models for the structural
analysis. Recently, a wealth of information has been accumulated
through these studies. A variety of DNA conformations has now
been shown to exist (2), including some molecules that were found
to have more than one conformation in their polynucleotide
backbone. The fine details of the B-DNA structure started to
appear from the recent work of Dickerson and his colleages on a
DNA dodecamer fragment d(CGCGAATTCGCG) (3-4). In this report, I
review some of the recent work dealing with DNA structures from
chemically synthesized oligonucleotides and their interactions
with drugs.

Right-handed DNA Conformation

DNA is known to adopt a number of right-handed double-helical
structures. Two different diffraction patterns could be produced
from DNA fibers depending upon the relative-humidity of the local
environments (5). If the fibers were allowed to expose to air
with 75% relative humidity, they produced an A-type diffraction
pattern, and if the fibers remained hydrated, a B-type diffraction
pattern was obtained. The familiar Watson and Crick double
helical DNA model was derived using the B-type diffraction pattern
(6). The relative ease with which these two forms can
interconvert shows that DNA is conformationally active and clearly
polymorphic. It is generally assumed that B-DNA exists in
biological systems, though the evidence for this is not very
strong.
    There are several differences between A- and B-DNA, for
example, the tilting of the base pairs relative to helical axis,
the displacement of the base pairs away from the helix as well as
the pucker of the furanose ring. The latter is illustrated in
Figure 1, which shows the five-member ring of the deoxyribose
sugar drawn so that the plane defined by the atoms C1', O1', C4'
is horizontal. The two other ring atoms, C2' and C3', can be
oriented in two different classes of positions. Those in which
the C2' atom is above the horizontal plane are called C2' endo,
whereas if atom C3' is above that it is called C3' endo. The
major effect of these differences in sugar pucker is that they
alter the separation between the phosphate groups attached to the
sugar by over 1 Å. In the C3' endo conformation the phosphate

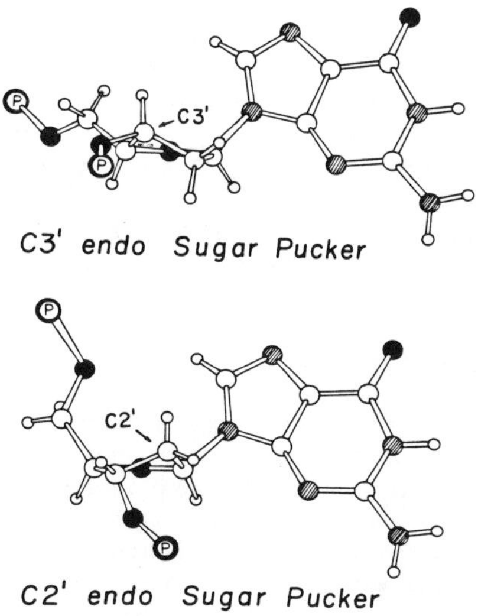

C3' endo Sugar Pucker

C2' endo Sugar Pucker

Figure 1: A diagram illustrating the two major families of furanose ring pucker in ribonucleotides and deoxynucleotides. The C1',O1',C4' atoms are drawn in a horizontal plane. Atoms above that plane are in the <u>endo</u> conformation. Note that in the C2' <u>endo</u> conformation the phosphate groups are further apart than in the C3' <u>endo</u> conformation.

groups are closer together while in the C2' __endo__ conformation they are further apart. This results in the introduction of an elastic element in the backbone of polynucleotides. These differences in distance are widely used in naturally occurring nucleic acid structures. For example, in the three-dimensional structure of yeast phenylalanine transfer RNA a majority of the 76 nucleotides are in the C3' __endo__ conformation. However, eight of them are in the C2' __endo__ conformation (7) and they occur in specific positions such as where the polynucleotide chain has to be extended to acommodate or surround an intercalating base. They also occur when the polynucleotide chain is stretched out.

A Modified A-DNA Conformation

Although DNA structures are often described as being either A-DNA or B-DNA, it is important to recognize that these represent only idealized models of molecules and the actual conformation which a particular molecule adopts reflects to varying extents an individual sequence. Generally only one of the lowest energy conformations for that sequence is observed in the crystal. The deviations from ideality may be considerable, as for example, if we consider the structure of the octamer d(GpGpCpCpGpGpCpC) (8). Although this molecule is predominantly in the A-DNA form, it actually has a central segment containing the two different families of sugar pucker so that the molecule has an interesting mixture of A-DNA and B-DNA features. Fig. 2 illustrates some of the features of this structure in comparison to A- and B-DNA. It was found that the molecules in the crystal underwent a small temperature dependent conformational change so that two different structures were solved at $-8°$ and $-18°C$. Fig. 2 shows side views of the van der Waals diagrams of the molecule. The center two drawings show the conformations obtained at the two different temperatures, while on the left and the right respectively are idealized models of A-DNA and B-DNA constructed using the same sequence.

A-DNA and B-DNA are different in several ways. In B-DNA the bases occupy the center of the molecule and they are almost perpendicular to the axis. In A-DNA the base pairs are removed from the central axis of the molecule and they have a considerable tilt in the opposite direction. In B-DNA the rise per residue along the axis is 3.34 Å, which is the thickness of the unsaturated purine-pyrimidine base pair. Due to the tilting of the bases in A-DNA the rise per residue is 2.56 Å along the axis. The diameter of the A-DNA molecule is slightly larger. In A-DNA the minor groove is flat and wide while the major groove is deep and extends through the central axis of the molecule. The tilt of the base pairs brings the phosphate groups closer together on opposite strands across the major groove of A-DNA than they are in B-DNA. Fig. 2 shows the differences by the arrow at the right of the figure, which measures the vertical distance along the helix

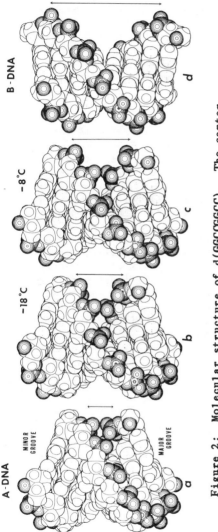

Figure 2: Molecular structure of d(GGCCGGCC). The center diagrams b and c show the form of the octamer which is observed experimentally at −18°C and at −8°C. Models of pure A-DNA (a) and B-DNA (b) are shown on either side for comparison. The upper diagrams are van der Waal's drawings of the four different DNA structures. The helix axis is vertical and a horizontal two-fold axis is located in the plane of the paper. The arrows to the right of each structure represent the vertical distance between the terminal phosphates of the two chains. The phosphorous and oxygen atoms have a heavier shading than the other atoms. The tilt to the bases from the horizontal is 19° in A-DNA and −7° in B-DNA, while base pairs in b and c are tilted approximately 14° and 12° respectively.

axis between the phosphate groups at either end of the molecule. This distance is much smaller in A-DNA than in B-DNA. Thus, in the two octamer structures we find that they have a conformation which is intermediate between A and B.

The reason that the octamer structure is not a pure A-DNA is mainly due to the alternating sugar pucker of successive residues. The numbering of the self complementary octamer structure goes from G1 to C8 down one strand and then G1* to C8* along the other strand. Thus residues G1 and G2 are paired to C8* and C7* of the opposite strands. All four of these residues have conformations close to A-DNA. However, the central segment of four base pairs, C3 through G6, consists of residues which have alternating ring puckers, i.e., alternatively near C2' endo, C3' endo, C2' endo, C3' endo. These differences in ring puckers are also reflected in differences in the twist angle between adjacent base pairs. This is the angle between the line C1'-C1' of one base pair with the next base pair. The variations in twist angle vary from 45° in C3pC4 step to 16° in C4pG5 step, and these are to be compared with a constant twist angle of 33° which is found in the idealized A-DNA structure and 36° found in B-DNA.

It is not certain whether this alternating A-DNA conformation is found in a particular sequence. It is interesting that the octamer d(CCCCGGGG) crystallizes in virtually the identical lattice as the octamer d(GGCCGGCC) (8). Furthermore, examination of sample diffraction patterns from crystals of that octamer show that it is virtually identical to that of the octamer with the sequence d(GGCCGGCC). These two octamers both have the sequence CCGG in their central four base pairs. Two other molecules, d(iodoCCGG) (9) and d(GGTATACC) (10-11), also have a somewhat similar A-DNA conformation as observed here. Thus it is possible that this alternating A conformation may be favored by a sequence involving two pyrimidines followed by two purines or it may be favored by the sequence CCGG.

Conformation of a DNA-RNA Hybrid

During DNA replication a single strand of DNA is used as a template for assembling complementary deoxynucleotides. For one of the two strands of the double helix, DNA replication takes an unusual form in which segments of DNA are assembled, Okazaki fragments (12), which are later joined to form an intact final strand. The synthesis of DNA Okazaki fragments is primed at the 5' end by a small number of ribonucleotides which initiate the synthesis. Synthesis is then continued by covalently joined deoxynucleotides. In an attempt to learn something of the structure of this initiating complex and more generally learn something about DNA-RNA hybrid molecules, the structure of an oligonucleotide, r(GCG)d(TATACGC) ,was solved which contains three ribonucleotides at the 5' end connected covalently to seven deoxynucleotides (13). This molecule is self-complementary and

forms two DNA-RNA hybrid segments with three base pairs
surrounding a central region of four base pairs of double helical
DNA. All three parts of the molecule adopt a conformation which
is close to that seen in A-DNA or in the 11-fold RNA double helix.
Fig. 3 shows side views of the hybrid molecule. In these
diagrams the ribo components are shaded and the 2' hydroxyl groups
are black. These three different views 90° apart illustrate the
typical A-DNA geometry of the complex. The major groove is deep
and narrow and the minor groove is broad and shallow. The base
pairs have an average twist angle of 33° with a small variation
among the residues. The base pairs have a rise along the axis of
2.6 Å and in this helix there are 10.9 residues per turn. The
base pairs are considerably removed from the axis of the molecule
and are tilted approximately -20° from the axis of the molecule.
It is interesting that the hybrid molecule has a fairly regular
geometry even though it contains both RNA and DNA. The molecule
has an almost perfect A-type geometry with all of the ribose and
deoxyribose sugars in the C3' endo conformation. There are no
structural discontinuities between the hybrid helix and the DNA
helix itself. While a slight discontinuity associated with the
structure of the central four base pairs containing the sequence
d(TATA) is observed. In contrast to the six hybrid G-C base pairs
at either end which have rather normal hydrogen bond distances,
the four AT base pairs have somewhat longer NH---O hydrogen bond
lengths. In addition, there are some discontinuities in the
orientation of the helix axis in the d(TpA) segments. The results
from a high resolution NMR study are consistent with the structure
observed here (14).

These discontinuities in the TATA region may be an expression
of structural features which are an inherent part of the TATA
sequence possibly associated with stacking modifications. This
might be of biological interest, since the base sequence TATA is
one of the common signals which is used in the initiation of
transcription by RNA polymerase.

Lattice Interactions

The manner in which these A-DNA octamer and RNA-DNA hybrid decamer
fragments form a lattice is quite interesting. The flat, shallow
minor groove is used as one of the component building blocks for
organizing the molecules into a lattice. In particular, the
planar C-G base pair at the end of the molecule is found to stack
on the flat surface in the minor groove of an adjacent molecule in
a manner which is shown in Fig. 4. In the stereodiagram 4A, the
octamer itself is drawn as open circles but the terminal two base
pairs of adjacent molecules are drawn with shaded atoms. It
clearly shows the manner in which the adjacent molecules use the
flat surface of the minor groove to stabilize, through van der
Waals forces, the interactions between adjacent molecules to build
up a lattice.

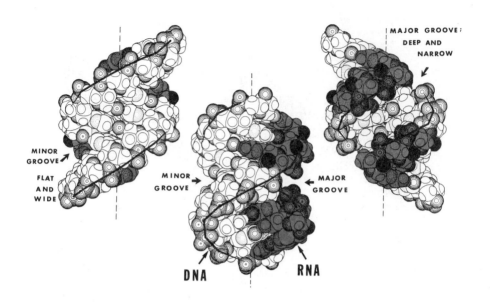

Figure 3: A space-filling drawing of the DNA-RNA hybrid
   r(GCG)d(TATACGC). The molecule is shown in three different
   orientations 90° apart from each other about the dashed
   vertical axis. At the left we are looking into the broad,
   flat minor groove of the molecule. Phosphate groups on
   opposite strands are 8.6 Å apart across the minor groove.
   The heavy black lines are drawn from phosphate to phosphate
   to show the flow of the polynucleotide chains. The
   ribonucleotides are shaded and the ribose 2' oxygen atoms are
   black. The center figure, rotated 90°, shows both the minor
   groove on the upper part of the molecule and the major groove
   at the lower right. The shaded ribonucleotide backbone
   segments are close to each other on either side of the major
   groove. The bases are tilted 19° from the vertical axis. In
   the center view the tilt reverses itself in going from the
   upper part to the lower part of the molecule. The view on
   the right is rotated 90° from the center of the molecule and
   we are looking down into the deep and narrow major groove of
   the molecule. The phosphate groups are 4.7 Å away from each
   other across this groove. Oxygen atoms are solid circles;
   nitrogen atoms are stippled; phosphorous atoms have spiked
   circles.

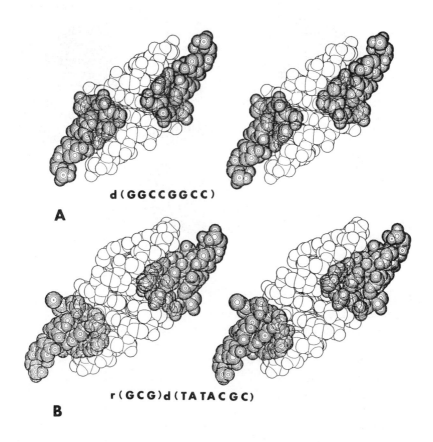

d(GGCCGGCC)

A

r(GCG)d(TATACGC)

B

Figure 4:   Stereo diagrams illustrating the interaction between
molecules in the crystal lattices of (A) the octamer
d(GGCCGGCC) and (B) the decamer hybrid r(GCG)d(TATACGC). In
both cases, a complete molecule is shown with unshaded atoms.
The shaded atoms represent the base pairs at the end of
adjoining molecules. Two or three base pairs from the
adjoining molecules are shown with shaded atoms in order to
illustrate the packing of the terminal planar base pairs on
the flat minor groove surface of the unshaded molecule in the
center.

Likewise, the packing of the hybrid A-DNA segments in the crystal lattice uses the same type of molecular interactions as those which were found in the organization of the octamer lattice described above. Fig. 4B shows a stereodiagram of this similar stacking interactions. The hybrid decamer is shown with unshaded atoms and three base pairs of the neighboring stacking molecules adjoining it are shown with shaded atoms. It can be seen that the packing motif is one in which the terminal planar purine-pyrimidine base pair stacks on the flat surface of the minor groove A-type double helix in the same way as seen for the octamer stacking in Fig. 4A. This stacking motif appears to be used in several other crystal structures (9-11).

Attention has been drawn to the fact that the size and shape of the purine-pyrimidine base pair in this case is rather similar to the size and shape of the benzo[a]pyrene nucleus, which is a powerful carcinogen (8). That carcinogen is known to bind covalently to the N2 position of guanine (15). In the present lattice the planar purine-pyrimidine base pair rests in a position close to the guanine N2. Thus, this mode of interaction may also be a model for the interaction of planar carcinogen molecules with DNA.

Furthermore, many planar intercalating drugs are known to have "outside" binding affinity to nucleic acids. For example, proflavin has been shown to bind to a specific site in the yeast phenylalanine tRNA molecule in a non-intercalative manner (16). It is interesting to note that both grooves in B-DNA structure are quite deep and the width as well as the shape of these grooves are not well suited for such type of interaction involving large planar molecules.

In the octamer d(GGCCGGCC) and the DNA-RNA hybrid, both of them are found in an A-DNA conformation and this can be explained using two different mechanisms. For the pure deoxy octamer it was speculated that it may be the sequence of stacking of two adjacent deoxyguanosine residues which favors an A structure. In the DNA-RNA hybrid it is clearly the influence of the ribonucleotide which favors the C3' endo conformation which forces the entire molecule to adopt an A conformation. It should be recognized that the A conformation and B conformation are always in dynamic equilibrium and the actual conformation in a crystal structure is one of the most stable energy states. Due to the fact that the crystal is carrying out a sampling operation, it is possible that other conformations in equilibrium with this may be represented in solution to a significant extent, for example, in the case of the Z-DNA structure described below. The strength of single crystal X-ray analyses is that they provide firm information about molecular conformation. The limitation is that it focuses on one conformation and does not provide information about the other conformations which are in equilibrium with it in solution. It is important to consider this point in thinking about the conformation of nucleic acids in biological systems.

Left-Handed Z-DNA

B-DNA to A-DNA conformational transition is a small change in comparison to the molecular rearrangement which occurs when DNA adopts the left-handed Z-DNA conformation. This left-handed structure was discovered in an atomic resolution X-ray diffraction analysis of a single crystal of a hexanucleoside pentaphosphate with the sequence $(dC-dG)_3$ (17-18) and subsequently with $(dC-dG)_2$ (19-20). Figure 5 shows a van der Waal's drawing of the Z-DNA in comparison to the more familiar right-handed B-DNA. The left-handed double helix has the phosphate groups arranged in a zig-zag array hence the name Z-DNA. The structure is favored by sequences which have an alternation of purines and pyrimidines. The reason for this is seen in Fig. 6 which shows the conformation of deoxyguanosine as found in Z-DNA and B-DNA. In Z-DNA, the deoxyguanosine residues have the C3' _endo_ pucker, while the deoxycytidine residues have C2' _endo_ pucker. Further, the guanine residues adopt the _syn_ while the cytosines have an _anti_ conformation. This is in contrast to B-DNA where all residues have the _anti_ conformation. The asymmetric unit in Z-DNA thus is a dinucleotide in contrast to the mononucleotide found in B-DNA. The Z-DNA helix has 12 base pairs per turn of the helix with a pitch of 44.6 Å, whereas in right-handed DNA it has 10 base pairs per turn occupying a distance of 34 Å. The diameter of the Z-DNA helix is only 18 Å compared to the somewhat thicker 20 Å found in B-DNA as can be seen in Figure 7.

In the crystal lattice, the hexamer Z-DNA fragments are stacked upon each other in such a manner that they make a structure in which the base pairs have a stacking which runs continuously through the crystal parallel to the _c_ axis, and around it the sugar-phosphate chains form a continuum except that they are interrupted by the absence of a phosphate group every six residues. The structure has enough regularity so that it is visualized in the form of a continuous helix. The Z-DNA helix is shown in Figure 5 in which the helical groove is shaded and the heavy black line which forms a zig-zag array around the groove shows the position of the phosphate groups along the serrated edge of the chain. There is only one groove in Z-DNA compared to two in B-DNA. The Watson-Crick base pairs which form the outer convex surface of the molecule in Z-DNA correspond to the major groove of the B-DNA helix.

Topologically, one cannot go from B-DNA to Z-DNA by simply turning the helix around the other way. In addition to the rotation of the helix in the opposite direction, the base pairs must "flip over," as they have an orientation relative to the backbone opposite to that which is found in B-DNA. Thus, the transition from B-DNA to Z-DNA is a rather complex process involving many structural rearrangements.

The transition from B-DNA to Z-DNA was first observed in solution by the near inversion of the circular dichroism of

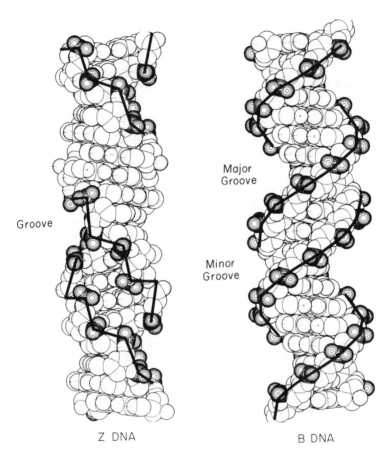

Figure 5: Van der Waals side views of Z-DNA and B-DNA. The zig-zag path of the sugar-phosphate backbone is shown by the heavy lines. The groove in Z-DNA is deep, extending to the axis of the double helix. This is in contrast to B-DNA which has two grooves.

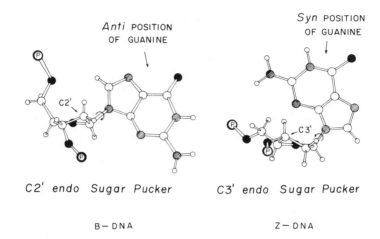

C2′ endo Sugar Pucker   C3′ endo Sugar Pucker

B—DNA   Z—DNA

Figure 6: A diagram illustrating the conformation of
deoxyguanosine in Z—DNA and B—DNA. In Z—DNA the guanosine
residues have the C3′ endo sugar pucker and the guanine base
is found in the syn conformation. Both of these are
different from the conformation found in B—DNA. However, the
deoxycytidine residues of Z—DNA have the C2′ endo sugar
pucker and the anti position of cytidine.

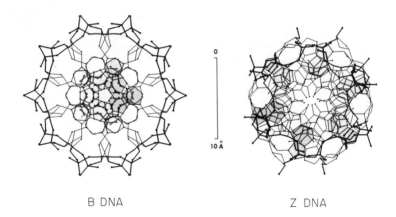

B DNA   Z DNA

Figure 7: End views of B—DNA and Z—DNA are shown in which the
guanine residues of one strand have been shaded. The Z—DNA
figure represents a view down the complete c axis of the
crystal structure encompassing the hexamers. The approximate
6—fold symmetry is apparent in the figure. The B—DNA figure
represents one full turn of helix. It can be seen that Z—DNA
is a slimmer helix than B—DNA.

poly(dG-dC) when the salt concentration (NaCl) in the solution was raised to 4M (21). We have shown that the high salt form of poly(dG-dC) in solution is indeed Z-DNA using the identity of the Raman spectra from poly(dG-dC) in high salt solution and from the crystals of d(C-G)$_3$ (22). In solution there is an equilibrium between Z-DNA and B-DNA. The equilibrium constant is determined by many factors, such as base sequence and the nature of the ions in the solution. It is interesting that the crystals of Z-DNA were grown from a solution containing a low concentration of cations so that the major species in the solution was B-DNA (17-18). However, the crystals which nucleated were Z-DNA and as these crystals grew the equilibrium shifted until finally all of the material had converted to Z-DNA in the crystal lattice.

Methylation of Cytosine Stabilizes Z-DNA

One of the principal modifications of the nucleic acids, especially in the higher eukaryotes, is methylation of cytosine on the 5 position where that cytosine precedes a guanine. Extensive studies have been carried out which have shown that methylation of DNA is generally associated with gene regulation (23-24). It is interesting to note that CG sequences play an important role in the Z conformation. Accordingly, it is reasonable to ask whether methylation might modify the distribution between B-DNA and Z-DNA. Behe and Felsenfeld have demonstrated that poly(dG-m^{5}dC) could convert to Z-DNA by adding very small amount of magnesium ion (0.6 mM) (25). In order to convert poly(dG-dC) to Z-DNA, it is required to have 760 mM magnesium ion. This is a decrease of three orders of magnitude in the amount of magnesium ions needed to stabilize Z-DNA when the polymer is methylated.

We have recently solved the structure of a hexamer, (m^{5}dC-dG)$_3$ (26). Figure 8 compares these two helices. The overall form of the methylated Z-DNA molecule is similar to that seen in the unmethylated molecule. This result is reasonable in view of the fact that antibodies raised against non-methylated Z-DNA can also recognize Z-DNA formed by the methylated polymer (27). However, there have been some subtle changes in the geometry of the molecule, principally associated with the fact that the methyl group is very close to the carbon atoms C1' and C2' of the adjacent guanosine residue. This has made a small change in the helix twist angle of Z-DNA. The methylated polymer has a twist angle for CpG which is $-13°$ compared to an average value of $-9°$ for the unmethylated polymer. There is a similar change averaging 4° for the sequence GpC. The net effect of these changes is that the methyl groups on the surface of the molecule are brought closer together from 5.2 Å to 4.6 Å in the methylated polymer than they would be if they were attached to the unmethylated polymer without such a change. The results from a recent 500MHz proton NMR study of the Z-DNA form of d(m^{5}C-G)$_3$ in methanolic solution are in complete agreement with the structural features observed in the crystal (28).

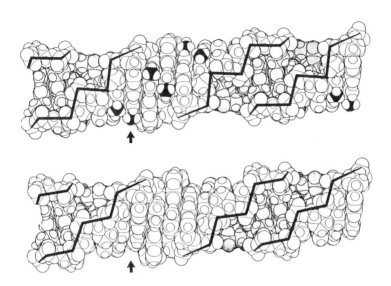

Figure 8: Two van der Waals drawings showing structure of Z-DNA
in both its (A) unmethylated and (B) methylated forms as
determined in single crystal structures of (dC-dG)$_3$ and
(m^{5}dC-dG)$_3$ respectively. The groove in the molecule is shown
by the shading. The black zig-zag line goes from phosphate
group to phosphate group to show the arrangement of the sugar
phosphate backbone. In the methylated polymer (B), the
methyl groups on the C5 position of cytosine are drawn in
black. The arrow illustrates that a depression found in the
unmethylated polymer (A) is filled by methyl groups in (B).
The methyl group indicated by the arrow is in close contact
with the imidazole ring of guanosine above it and the C1 and
C2' carbon atoms of the sugar ring.

The stabilization of Z-DNA by methylation is due to two factors. One of these is that the methyl group fills a vacancy or depression on the surface of Z-DNA. This is shown in Figure 8, in which the arrow near the unmethylated polymer (A) points to a depression at the side of the molecule, whereas in the methylated polymer (B) that depression is filled by the methyl group. The methyl group is in van der Waal's contact with the imidazole ring of guanine immediately above it in Figure 8B, and also with the C1' and C2' carbon atoms of the same guanosine. In effect, these produce small hydrophobic patch on the surface of the molecule. This is in contrast to the situation in B-DNA where the evenly distributed methyl groups project out into the solvent from the major groove of the double helix. The effect of methylation is thus two-fold: one, to destabilize B-DNA by interposing a hydrophobic group into the water; and secondly, to stabilize Z-DNA by hydrophobic interactions. This provides a structural rationale for why methylation of DNA might favor the formation of small segments of Z-DNA.

Adenine-Thymine Base Pairs in Z-DNA

Segments of DNA in negatively supercoiled plasmids have been shown to form Z-DNA through the use of Z-DNA specific antibodies, and they contain AT base pairs (29-30). However, AT base pairs are known to be less stable than CG base pairs, as for example AT containing DNA segments convert to Z-DNA much less readily. We have addressed the problem by solving the structure of Z-DNA with AT base pairs (31). Two of the molecules are hexamers with the general self-complementary sequence d(CGTACG) in which the cytosine residues have either methyl groups or bromine atoms on their 5 positions. Another molecule which has been crystallized in Z-DNA structure is an unmodified octamer, d(CGCATGCG) (32).

The structures of both the 5-methyl and 5-bromo derivatives of d(CGTACG) are similar to each other and likewise similar to the structure of $(dC-dG)_3$ as well as $(m^5dC-dG)_3$. They form a double helix with six base pairs and stack together to form an essentially continuous Z-DNA double helix running along the c axis of the unit cell. The crystal of the methylated hexamer diffracts to a resolution of 1.2 Å, and the brominated derivative to 1.5 Å. Both crystals form an isomorphous lattice with that of the $(dC-dG)_3$. Thus it is not surprising that the gross form of Z-DNA is the same whether it is made of CG base pairs or AT base pairs.

The overall helical parameters are quite similar, and there are only small changes in the base stacking geometry and small differences in the hydrogen bond distances of the base pairs. This is not totally unexpected, as both the monoclonal as well as polyclonal antibodies against Z-DNA containing only CG base pairs also react with high specificity against negatively supercoiled plasmids containing CA sequences (29-30).

During the refinement of the crystal structure of d(m^5CGTAm^{5}CG), a large number of solvent molecules were located. The majority of these peaks are water molecules, although five of the peaks have been identified as cations due to the coordination geometry associated with them.

From the analysis of the hydration organization of these Z–DNA crystal structures, two different types of water molecules are generally found in the groove of Z–DNA. The water molecule of the first kind bridges the amino group on position 2 of guanine and a phosphate oxygen of the same deoxyguanosine nucleotide. This bridging water molecule is in a position such that it can stabilize the _syn_ conformation of guanine. Second type of water molecule fits in the groove where it lies near halfway between oxygen O2 of pyrimidine residues in successive base pairs. In the case of the structure of both the unmethylated hexamer (dC–dG)$_3$ (17) and the methylated hexamer (m^5dC–dG)$_3$, (26), both of these water molecules are found occupying the helical groove of the Z–DNA. Thus there are two water molecules hydrogen bonded to electronegative nitrogen and oxygen atoms at the bottom of the Z–DNA helical groove per base pair.

The situation is quite different in the case of the AT base pairs, as no ordered water molecules can be seen in the groove hydrogen bonded to the AT base pairs. First, as the adenine residue does not have an N2 amino group, the bridging water molecule is absent. Second, the water molecule which is hydrogen bonded directly or through another water molecule onto the pyrimidine O2 atoms along the bottom of the groove does not appear in the electron density map either.

A visualization of the hydration around the Z–DNA molecule is shown in the stereodiagram of Figure 9 with a van der Waals model of d(m^5CGTAm^{5}CG) (31) together with solvent molecules (stippled spheres). The convex outer portion of the molecule is heavily covered with a sheath of water molecules which are binding to most of the electronegative atoms in the molecule. There are small patches of hydrophobic residues which do not have water molecules covering them. Figure 9 also shows that the helical groove of Z–DNA is filled with water molecules except at the position occupied by the two base pairs. At the bottom of the helical groove, the base pairs themselves can be visualized devoid of ordered hydration structure, even though there are water molecules at the outer part of the groove which are hydrogen bonded to the negatively charged phosphates. Two of these (at positions marked x) have been removed in Figure 9 in order to visualize the disordered hydration at the bottom of the groove. While the geometry of the Z–DNA molecule is not altered to a significant extent through the introduction of AT base paris, hydration in the helical groove is modified considerably.

It is known that AT base pairs in B–DNA are somewhat less stable than CG base pairs. In Z–DNA, they are probably considerably less stable, not only due to the absense of a third

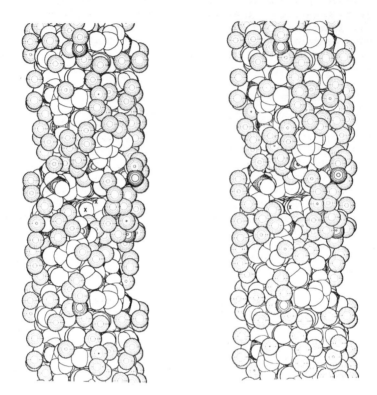

Figure 9: A stereodiagram of a van der Waals model of the hexamer
d(m⁵CGTAm⁵CG) showing the first shell hydration. Only
solvent molecules are included for which the temperature
factor is lower than 45 $\mathring{A}^2$. Water molecules are represented
as spheres with stippled circles, magnesium metal ions are
drawn as spheres with concentric circles, while phosphorus
atoms are drawn with circles with cross striations. The
helical groove is generally filled with ordered water
molecules except in one region where the two AT base pairs
lie. In order to visualize this section of the groove, two
water molecules were removed which are bound to the phosphate
groups near the periphery of the molecule.

hydrogen bond between the bases, but also due to the lack of ordered hydration structure in the helical groove. In addition, the reactivity and accessibility of various sites of the AT vs GC base pairs might be another factors which can influence the the relative stability of B- vs Z-DNA structures. Since the Z-DNA sequences contain information, it is likely that these differences in stability will be used in nature for various biological processes.

Z-DNA in Biological Systems

The structural studies on Z-DNA suggest that there exists a stable alternative conformation of DNA in the left-handed form which may exist in vivo. Several studies have provided evidence for the existence of Z-DNA in biological system(27,29-30,33-34). Through the use of antibodies specific to Z-DNA, it has been shown that segments of DNA in negatively supercoiled plasmids as well as SV40 virus can exist in Z-DNA conformation. Furthermore, form V DNA contains significant portions of left-handed Z-DNA as judged by Raman and CD spectroscopy. Recently, it has been estimated that in E. coli there exists about 1% potential Z-DNA forming sequences (34). Proteins that bind to Z-DNA specifically have also been partially purified from Drosophilla (35). Thus there is an increasing amount of information being accumulated with regard to the possible biological significance of the left-handed Z-DNA. What is not clear at the present time is the size of the smallest Z-DNA which might exist in the middle of B-DNA. Is it possible that a small d(m^{5}CpG) dinucleotide could actually form Z-DNA in the middle of a B-DNA strand? Further structural studies in which the B-Z interface is trapped in a crystal lattice might provide some insights toward a better understanding of the processes which stabilize this conformational change.

The Double Helix Changes Conformation Upon Intercalation

The interactions between a planar molecule with the somewhat hydrophobic surface of the relatively flat and shallow minor groove of A-DNA have been discussed above. But the more frequently encountered conformational changes in double helical nucleic acids due to the binding of a planar molecule are those involving intercalation of the planar molecule between the base pairs. It does this by changing the sugar-phosphate backbone conformation in a significant way. Intercalation has two important effects: it separates the adjacent base pairs from 3.4 Å to 6.8 Å. This is due to the planarity of the intercalator which has the unsaturated pi system of 3.4 Å thick. In addition, it unwinds the double helix.

A number of structures have been solved involving intecalators, mostly with RNA and DNA dinucleoside monophosphate fragments. Fig. 10 shows an example of the structure of a ribose

CpG together with the intercalator acridine orange solved at atomic resolution (36). It can be seen tha the 3' end of the double helical RNA fragment has adopted the C2' endo conformation while the 5' end maintains the normal C3' endo conformation. A large number of intercalator structures of this type have been solved and they have been summaried elsewhere. Sobell and his colleages pointed out that the intercalation is associated with a modification of the pucker of the ribonucleotide chain on the 3' end of the intercalator (37-38). Although intercalation is generally associated with the conformations similar to those seen in Fig. 10, a number of alternative conformations have been found with more complex intercalators.

For "simple" intercalators, it is possible to make a simplified generalization about the way double helical DNA and RNA accommodate intercalator. This can be accomplished by elongating DNA or RNA molecules to accept an intercalator by adopting a similar C3'-endo(3',5')C2'-endo mixed sugar pucker conformation. These conformational changes provide a reasonable explanation for the nearest neighbor exclusion effect. If a DNA or RNA double helix is saturated with an intercalator, the most that can be accommodated is one intercalator per two base pairs. The reason for this is probably due to the necessity for mixed sugar pucker on either side of the intercalator. However, for more complex intercalators the situation is not so strightforward as will be described below.

Interaction between Daunomycin and DNA

Daunomycin was the first antibiotic to be used in the treatment of leukemia in human(39-40). Daunomycin (Fig. 11) and the closely related adriamycin (14-hydroxydaunomycin) are both widely used in the treatment of human tumors. Even though these substances are closely related to each other, they have quite distinct biological activities. Daunomycin is used in the treatment of leukemias, whereas adriamycin is used in the treatment of solid tumors. These agents are believed to act by inhibiting both DNA replication and transcription.

Numerous studies have been reported concerning the interactions of these molecules with DNA. These antibiotics are known to intercalate through the planar part of the anthracycline chromophore into DNA molecule, usually at a saturation level of one daunomycin per three base pairs. Although models has been suggested about the manner in which these molecules interact with DNA, no definitive conclusion could be arrived. In particular, it was not clear why different modifications of ring A have profound effect on the biological activities of the molecule. Ring A has both equatorial and axial substituents, among them an amino sugar daunosamine. The great importance of these drugs has prompted the syntheses of over 500 derivatives in an attempt to improve their biological activities.

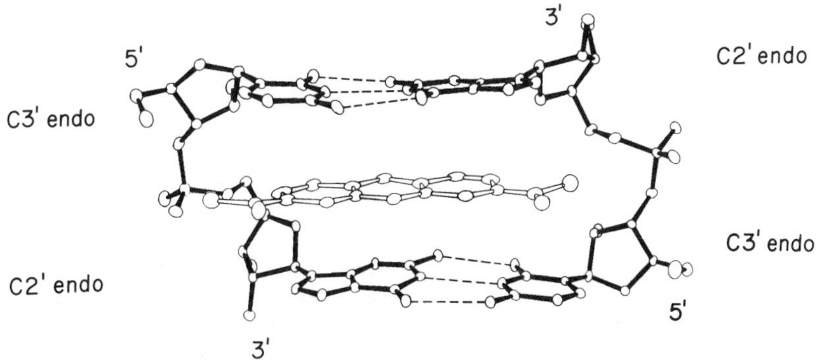

Figure 10: The structure of the CpG—acridine orange intercalator complex. The C2' _endo_ sugar conformation at the 3' end of the RNA chain surrounding the intercalator is indicated. This mixed sugar pucker conformation is associated with an extension of the polynucleotide chain.

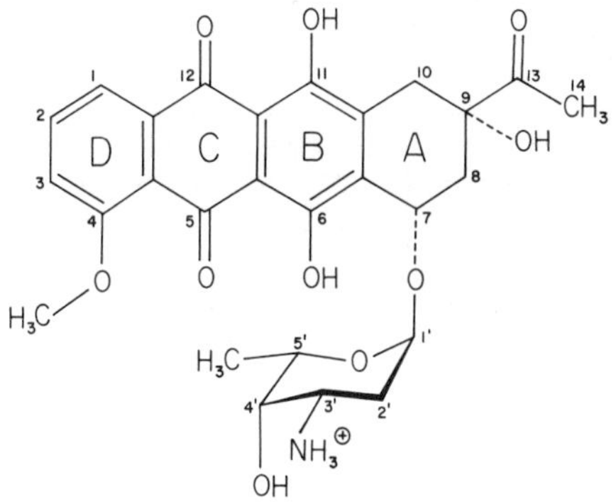

Figure 11: Molecular formula of daunomycin.

In order to understand how these drugs interact with DNA, daunomycin was co-crystallized with a DNA fragment, d(CGTACG). The self-complementary DNA hexamer forms a 1:1 complex with daunomycin in a tetragonal lattice (41). Originally, the crystal structure was solved by molecular replacement method and refined to an R-factor of 20% to 1.5 Å resolution. Recently we have collected the diffraction data to 1.2 Å resolution under low temperature and refined the structure to an R-factor of 17% (unpublished results). The structure contains a double helix of modified B-DNA six base pairs long with two daunomycins intercalating between the dCpG steps. There is a crystallographic two fold axis passing through the center of the duplex. Figure 12 illustrates the structure of this complex with van der Waals diagrams. It can be seen that the DNA forming a right-handed double helix with the CpG at either end separated to allow the intercalation of the planar anthracycline chromophore. The two fold axis is horizontal in the plane of the paper in the middle of the molecule in Figure 12(a-c). In Figure 12b the chromophore is drawn and in the upper part the non-planar ring A can be seen with the 9-hydroxy pointing down towards the middle of the molecules. At the bottom of the Figure 12b ring D can be seen protruding into the major groove of the double helix with its methoxy group at the left. In Figure 12c the amino sugar is added to the chromophore and it can be seen at the top that it fits into the minor groove of the helix. It should be noted that the geometry of the daunomycin is nicely suited to intercalate into right-handed double helix, since the manner in which the amino sugar comes off the chromophore has a right-handed chirality. In Figure 12d the molecule has been rotated 90° so that we are looking down the two fold axis. This shows the extent to which the amino sugars of the two daunomycin molecules fill the minor groove of the double helix with the positively charged amino group in the middle of the minor groove well separated from two negatively charged phosphate groups on either side. The daunomycin molecule covers almost three base pairs, thereby accounting for stoichiometry of DNA fully saturated with daunomycin.

Figure 13 shows a view looking down the helix axis with the two dCpG accomodating the intercalated daunomycin molecules. It can be seen that the elongated chromophore skewers the base pair with ring D protruding well into the major groove of the helix and ring A in the minor groove. It is worth noting that the base pair G2-C5* is displaced in the direction of the major groove relative to the base pair C1-G6*. This nearly 1 Å displacement is only one of the distortions associated with binding of the drug. There is also an unwinding of the helix. Interestingly, this unwinding does not take place in the base pairs which surround the intercalator but instead one base pair further away. The total unwinding angle per daunomycin molecule in the structure is 8°, which is very close to the 11° which has been reported in solution. Several studies have been carried out on the

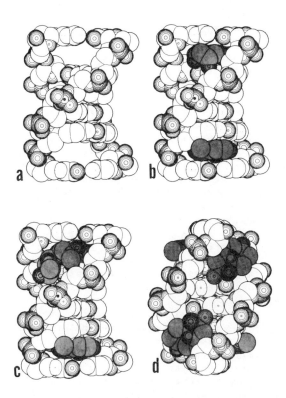

<u>Figure 12</u>: Van der Waals drawings of the daunomycin-d(CGTACG) complex. In a–c, the two fold axis is horizontal and in the plane of the paper. (a) DNA hexamer by itself. (b). DNA and aglycone without acetyl group on C9. (c). DNA and complete daunomycin. (d). The complex is viewed into the minor groove.

interactions of daunomycin with DNA in solution (42–44). The results from these stdies are in consistent with the detailed geometry observed in this crystal structure, for example the skewering orientation of the chromophore relative to the surrounding base pairs and the amino sugar being located in the minor groove.

Specificity of Drugs through Anchoring Function

The interaction between daunomycin and the double helix is shown diagramatically in Figure 14 viewing at a slight angle to the base pairs. It can be seen that there are hydrogen bonds which link substiuents of half saturated ring A with the adjacent base pairs. This hydroxyl group on O9 forms a strong hydrogen bond (2.6 Å) to the N3 atom of guanine G2. The hydroxyl group further receives a hydrogen bond (2.9 Å) from the N2 amino group of the same guanine. In addition, a water molecule (W) is found which forms a hydrogen bonded bridge between the O13 of the acetyl group and O2 of the cytosine residue on the opposite side of the amino sugar above the intercalation site. A octahedrally coordinated sodium ion is also found to locate in the major groove directly bridging the drug and the molecule (unpublished results). This sodium ion strongly coordinates to the N7 of the G6* residue and to the O4 as well as O5 atoms of the daunomycin molecule. In addition, there are two bridging water molecules which connect the sodium ion to the O6 of G6* and to the phosphate group of the same G6*. This sodium ion then provides a further stabilization and specificity from the major groove side.

This demonstrates that the interaction of daunomycin with the DNA double helix not only has base stacking components associated with the intercalation and the electostatic interactions associted with the positively charged daunomycin and the negatively charged DNA, but it also has some specific hydrogen bonds which provide an "anchoring function" holding the antibiotic to the double helix. This can be achieved through direct hydrogen bonds, metal ion coordination or through tightly bonded bridging water molecule. In the present case, although good hydrogen bonds seem to be formed with the CG pair, they do not have high specificity. For example, if an adenine were present instead of guanine 2, the O9 hdroxyl could still form a hydrogen bond to N3 of the adenine. Likewise, the water molecule (W) could form a hydrogen bond with bases other than cytosine, since all four bases have an electronegative atom very close to the position of the O2 of cytosine 1. However, the sodium ion which is coordinated to N7 of G6* indicates that a purine is prefered at that site. Thus the specificity is obtained through the use of a combination of different types of interactions described above.

The specificity of the interactions of the anchoring funtion implys that it plays an important role in the binding of daunomycin to minor groove and major groove of the double helix.

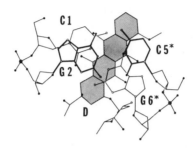

Figure 13: View of the intercalator perpendicular to the base
plane. The daunomycin (D) ring system is shaded. Note that
the center of the G2–C5* base pair has moved toward the major
groove relative to the C1–G6* pair.

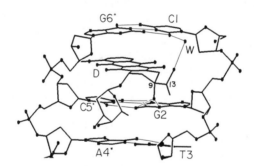

Figure 14: Diagram of the daunomycin-d(CGTACG) complex showing
the intermolecular interactions which include intercalation
and hydrogen bonds. Note that there are two hydrogen bonds
between O9 of daunomycin and N2 and N3 of G2.

These might explained some of the reasons for the requirement for certain substituents on ring A or electronegative atoms on ring C. For example, an inversion of the two groups on C9 position of daunomycin results in a complete loss of activity.

It is interesting to consider adriamycin which has an extra hydroxyl group on the 14 position of daunomycin. We have solved the structure of a complex between 4'-deoxyadriamycin and the same DNA hexamer to an R-factor of 16% at 1.5 Å resolution (unpublished results). It was found that the 14 hydroxyl group form a hydrogen bond to a water molecule which in turn brdiges to the phosphate group of T3 residue. This difference in the hydrogen bonding is associted with significances in the biological spectrum of these antibiotics as they are effective against different types of tumors. The basis for this differentiation is not clear, but this type of structural studies provide a detailed view of the interaction between the antibiotic and the ultimate target DNA molecule. It provides a framework in developing rational drug design, in particular for the further modifications of daunomycin and adriamycin to obtain a second generation antibiotic with high activities and low toxicities.

Triostin A can Bis-intercalate into DNA

Triostin A is a member of several families of natural occuring bis-intercalating antibiotics which have recently received a great deal of attention (45). Triostins and the closely related echinomycin belong to the quinoxaline family of antibiotics which contains a cyclic octadepsipeptide ring with a sulfur-containing cross-bridge and two 2-carboxquinoxaline chromophores. Triostin A has a two fold symmetry axis which relates the two halves of the molecule with a disulfide crosslinking the backbone of the cyclic depsipeptide ring. Both echinomycin and triostin A are potent antitumor antibiotics.

Although numerous models of the interactions between the quinoxaline antibiotics and DNA have been proposed, no definitive conclusion about the precise manner of the interactions could be made (46). Recently, the crystal structure of a synthetic analog of triostin A, des-N-tetramethyltriostin A (TANDEM) (47), has been determined. A naturally occuring quinoline-containing antibiotic, luzopeptin, has been purified and characterized and its three dimensional structure determined (48).

In order to understand the interactions between these bis-intercalating drugs and DNA more fully, we have crystallized several complexes of them and undertaken the structure determination by x-ray diffraction technique. One of the crystal forms diffracts to 1.6 Å resolution with a space group of F222. The crystal structure was determined by the multiple isomorphous replacement method using three different heavy atom derivatives. The structure was refined to an R-factor of 19% and there were moderate number of solvent molecules clearly visible. The crystal is found to contain one triostin A molecule and one DNA hexamer d(CGTACG) in the asymmetric unit of the unit cell (unpublished results). The geometry of the complex is a highly distorted double helix with some unusual features in it. The triostin A molecule is found to use the two quinoxaline rings to sandwich two d(GpC) base pairs at either end of the molecule. There is a crystallographic two-fold axis relating the two segments of the complex. Fig. 15 shows the van der Waals diagrams of the complex from two orientations. It can be seen that in Fig. 15(a-b) the diad axis is perpendicular to the paper. The cyclic depsipeptide ring of the triostin A molecule occupys the minor groove of the DNA molecule while one quinoxaline ring intercalates between the d(GpT) step and the other one covers the outside beyond the terminal CG base pair. In this complex, the triostin A adopts the conformation in which the quinoxaline rings and the valyl side chains are on one side of the peptide ring, while the disulfide bridge protrudes out on the other side. Figure 15(c-d) shows the view 180° away looking into the major groove.

There are several type of interactions which are responsible for the conformation observed in this complex. First, the amide nitrogen of the un-methylated glycine residues forms a hydrogen bond to N3 atom of the guanine residue. This might explain the reason why there are always two unmethylated glycines in this type of antibiotics including triostins, echinomycins, as well as luzopeptin. This is also true for other type of DNA interacting peptide antibiotics. For example, in actinomycin D there are two equivalent D-valine residues which have un-methylated amide nitrogens. These two amide groups are also involved in a similar type of hydrogen bonding interactions with N3 atoms of guanine (49-50). Second, the alanyl side chains are in van der Waals contacts with the sugar residues of the DNA frament. These contacts appears to be important in holding the sugar moieties further apart and causing the adjacent sandwiched bases to be inclined by nearly 20°. In a sense, there is a loss of stacking energy due to the separation of the bases. However, this is undoubtly compensated by the extra stacking from the insertion of the qunioxaline ring between base pairs. If this alanyl residue were to be replaced by a bulkier residue such as valyl residue, this would generate an even more unfavorable contacts.

Another surprising feature observed in this structure is that the central two TA base pairs have adopted a non-Watson-Crick base pairing(51). The adenine residue has turned to a _syn_ conformation and pairs to thymine in a Hoogsteen geometry. The reason for this is not totally clear. It could be due to the enhanced stacking between quinoxaline and adenine base, or it could be that this is a mechanism to relieve the energy stored in this highly constrained conformation. This is believed to be the first case in which a Hoogsteen base pair is seen in a stretch of DNA double helix. This could have important consequence in thinking about sequence-dependent conformation in biological system.

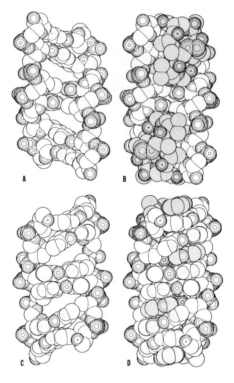

Figure 15: Van der Waals diagrams of the triostin A and d(CGTACG)
    complex. In A–B, the molecular two fold axis is
    perpendicular to the paper and we are looking into the minor
    groove. It can be seen that the double helix is highly
    distorted and the sugar–phosphate backbone no longer follows
    a smoothed curved path. In C–D, the molecule is rotated 180°
    about the vertical axis. (A,C). DNA hexamer by itself.
    (B,D). DNA and triostin A.

Conclusion

Recent structural studies on right- and left-handed fragments of DNA have considerably broadened our perspective about the conformational vitality of DNA (52-53). The high prevalence of A-DNA structures existing in crystalline lattices suggests that these structures may also exist in biological systems and may be stabilized by particular sequences or by interactions with proteins. In the same way, the discovery of Z-DNA in a crystal structure has led to its discovery in biological systems. We now have an entirely different image of DNA than was available a few years ago. The molecule may now be appropriately regarded as one which is in dynamic equilibrium among a number of different conformations. The detailed conformation assumed by the molecule is one which will be influenced by nucleotide sequence, ions in the surrounding medium, the particular proteins that bind to the molecule, and the degree of negative supercoiling stress that the molecule feels. All of these factors will be important in defining a highly dynamic system in which a number of different conformations are found.

There might be other conformations of DNA yet to be found. The answer to this is unclear at present. Although DNA has been studied extensively for over three decades, only recently have we become aware of the fact that the molecule is dynamically active, and this awareness may lead to even further discoveries in the future.

Acknowledgments: This research was supported by grants from the National Institutes of Health, the American Cancer Society, and the National Science Foundation to A. Rich and A. H.-J. W. Additional support from the National Aeronautics and Space Administration to A. R. is also acknowledged. I would like to thank Dr. A. Rich for his generous support and advice. The assistance and contribution from Drs. Gary Quigley, Satoshi Fujii, Toshio Hakoshima, Giovanni Ughetto and Juli Feigon is highly appreciated.

Literature Cited

1. Leslie, A. G. W.; Arnott, S.; Chanddrasekaran R.; Ratliff, R. L. J. Mol. Biol. 1980, 143, 49-60.
2. Wang, A. H.-J.; Fujii, S.; van Boom, J. H.; Rich, A. Cold Spring Harbor Sym. Quan. Biol. 1983, 47, 33-44.
3. Wing, R. M.; Drew, H. R.; Takano, T.; Broka, C.; Tanaka, S.; Itakura, K.; Dickerson, R. E. Nature 1980, 287, 755-757
4. Dickerson, R. E.; Drew, H. R. J. Mol. Biol. 1981, 149, 761-786.
5. Franklin, R. E.; Gosling, R. Nature 1953, 171, 740-1.
6. Watson, J. D.; Crick, F. H. C. Nature 1953, 171, 737.
7. Quigley, G. J.; Rich. A. Science 1976, 194, 796-807.
8. Wang, A. H.-J.; Fujii, S.; van Boom J. H.; Rich, A. Proc. Nat. Acad. Sci. USA 1982, 79: 3968-3972.
9. Conner, B. N.; Takano, T.; Tanaka, S.; Itakura, K.; Dickerson, R. E. Nature 1982, 295, 294-301.
10. Shakked, Z.; Rabinovich, D.; Cruse, W. B. T.; Egert, E.; Kennard, O.; Sala, G.; Salisbury S. A.; Viswamitra, M. A. Proc. Roy. Soc. (London) 1981, B213, 479-485.
11. Shakked, Z.; Rabinovich, D.; Kennard, O.; Cruse, W. B. T.; Salisbury S. A.; Viswamitra, M. A. J. Mol. Biol. 1983, (In press).
12. Ogawa, T.; Okazaki, T. Ann. Rev. Biochem. 1980, 49: 421-434.
13. Wang, A. H.-J.; Fujii, S.; van Boom, J. H.; van der Marel, G. A.; van Boeckel, S. A. A.; Rich, A. Nature 1982, 299, 601-4.
14. Mellema, J.-R.; Haasnoot, C. A. G.; van der Marel, G. A.; van Boeckel, C. A. A.; Wille, G.; van Boom J. H.; Altona, C. Nucleic Acids Res. 1983, 11, 5717-38.
15. Jeffrey, A. M.; Jennette, K. W.; Blobstein, S. H.; Weinstein, I. B.; Beland, F. A.; Harvey, R. G.; Kasai, H.; Miura, I.; Nakanishi, K. J. Amer. Chem. Soc. 1976, 98, 5714-15.
16. Sundaralingam, M.; Liebman, M. N. Acta Cryst. 1978, A34, s54.
17. Wang, A. H.-J.; Quigley, G. J.; Kolpak, F. J.; Crawford, J. L.; van Boom, J. H.; van der Marel G.; Rich, A. Nature 1979, 282, 680-686.
18. Wang, A. H.-J.; Quigley, G. J.; Kolpak, F. J.; van der Marel, G.; van Boom, J. H.; Rich, A. Science 1981, 211, 171-178.
19. Crawford, J. L.; Kolpak, F. J.; Wang, A. H.-J.; Quigley, G. J.; van Boom, J. H.; van der Marel, G.; Rich, A. Proc. Nat. Acad. Sci. USA 1980, 77, 4106-4110.
20. Drew, H. R.; Takano, T.; Tanaka, S.; Itakura, K,; Dickerson, R. E. Nature 1980, 286, 567-572.
21. Pohl, F. M.; Jovin, T. M. J. Mol. Biol. 1972, 67, 375-396.
22. Thamann, T. J.; Lord, R. C.; Wang, A. H.-J.; Rich, A. Nucleic Acids Res. 1981, 9, 5443-57.

23. Razin, A.; Riggs, A. D. <u>Science</u> 1980, <u>210</u>, 604-612.
24. Ehrlich, M.; Wang. R. Y.-H. <u>Science</u> 1981, <u>212</u>, 1350-6.
25. Behe, M.; Felsenfeld, G. <u>Proc. Nat. Acad. Sci. USA</u> 1981,<u>78</u>: 1619-1624.
26. Fujii, S.;. Wang, A. H.-J.; van der Marel G.; van Boom, J. H.; Rich, A. <u>Nucleic Acids Res.</u> 1982, <u>10</u>, 7879-7892.
27. Nordheim, A.; Pardue, M. L.; Lafer, E. M.; Moller, A.; Stollar, B. D.; Rich, A. <u>Nature</u> 1981, <u>294</u>, 417-421.
28. Feigon, J.; Wang, A. H.-J.; van der Marel, G.; van Boom, J. H.; Rich, A. 1983, (Submitted for publication).
29. Nordheim, A.; Rich, A. <u>Proc. Natl. Acad. Sci. USA</u> 1983, <u>80</u>, 1821-5.
30. Nordheim, A.; Rich, A. <u>Nature</u> 1983, <u>303</u>, 674-9.
31. Wang, A. H.-J.; Hakoshima, T.; van der Marel, G.; van Boom, J. H.; Rich, A. 1983, (Submitted for publication).
32. Fujii, S.;. Wang, A. H.-J.; Quigley, G. J.; Westerink, H.; van der Marel, G.; van Boom, J. H.; Rich, A. 1983, (Submitted for publication).
33. Lipps, H. J.; Nordheim, A.; Lafer, E. M.; Ammermann, D.; Stollar, B. D.; Rich. A. <u>Cell</u> 1982, <u>32</u>, 435-441.
34. Thomae, R.; Beck, S.; Pohl, F. M. <u>Proc. Natl. Acad. Sci.</u> 1983, <u>80</u>, 5550-3.
35. Nordheim, A.; Tesser, P.; Azorin, F.; Kwon, Y. H.; Muller, A.; Rich, A. <u>Proc. Natl. Acad. Sci. USA</u> 1982, <u>79</u>, 7729-33.
36. Wang, A. H.-J.; Quigley, G. J.; Rich, A. <u>Nuclic Acids Res.</u> 1979, <u>6</u>, 3879-3890.
37. Tsai, C.-C.; Jain, S. C.; Sobell, H. M. <u>J. Mol. Biol.</u> 1977, <u>114</u>: 301-320.
38. Jain, S. C.; Tsai, C.-C.; Sobell, H. M. <u>J. Mol. Biol.</u> 1977, <u>114</u>, 317-329.
39. Henry, D. W. <u>Cancer Treat. Rep.</u> 1979, <u>63</u>, 845-854.
40. Neidle, S. <u>Prog. Med. Chem.</u> 1979, <u>16</u>, 151-220.
41. Quigley, G. J.; Wang, A. H.-J.; Ughetto, G.; van der Marel, G.; van Boom, J. H.; Rich. A. <u>Proc. Nat. Acad. Sci. USA</u> 1980, <u>77</u>, 7204-9.
42. Phillips, D.; Roberts, G. C. K. <u>Biochemistry</u> 1980, <u>19</u>, 4795-4801.
43. Patel, D. J.; Kozlowski, S. A.; Rice, J. A. <u>Proc. Natl. Acad. Sci. USA</u> 1981, <u>78</u>, 3333-7.
44. Chaires, J. B.; Dattagupta, N.; Crothers, D. M. <u>Biochemistry</u> 1982, <u>21</u>, 3933-40.
45. Waring, M. J.; Wakelin, L. P. G. <u>Nature</u> 1974, <u>252</u>, 653-7.
46. Viswamitra, M. A.; Kennard, O.; Cruse, W. B. T.; Egert, E.; Sheldrick, G. M.; Jones, P. G.; Waring, M. J.; Wakelin, L. P. G.; Olsen, R. K. <u>Nature</u> 1981, <u>289</u>, 817-9.
47. Hossain, M. B.; van der Helm, D.; Olsen, R. K.; Jones, P. G.; Sheldrick, G. M.; Egert, E.; Kennard, O.; Waring, M. J.; Viswamitra, M. A. <u>J. Amer. Chem. Soc.</u> 1982, <u>104</u>, 3401-8.

48. Arnold, E.; Clardy, J. J. Amer. Chem. Soc. 1981, 103,
     1243-4.
49. Sobell, H. M.; Jain, S. C.; Sakore, T. D.; Nordman, C.E.
     Nature New Biol. 1971, 231, 200-2.
50. Takusagawa, F.; Dabrow, M.; Neidle, S.; Berman, H. M.
     Nature, 1982, 296, 466-8.
51. Voet, D.; Rich, A. Progr. Nucl. Acid Res. Mol. Biol.
     1970, 10, 183-265.
52. Rich, A. Cold Spring Harbor Sym. Quan. Biol. 1983, 47,
     1-12.
53. Wells, R. D.; Goodman, T. C.; Hillen, W.; Horn, G. T.;
     Klein, R. D.; Larson, J. E.; Muller, U. R.; Neuendorf, S.
     K.; Panayotatos N.; Stirdivant, S. M. Progr. Nucl. Acid
     Res. Mol. Biol. 1980, 24, 167-267.

RECEIVED November 20, 1983

Substrate Analog Inhibitors of Highly Specific Proteases

JAMES BURTON

Massachusetts General Hospital and Harvard Medical School, Boston, MA 02114

Highly specific proteolytic enzymes cleave a single peptide bond in a naturally occurring substrate. These proteases appear to be integral parts of many biologic processes and may be contrasted with less specific proteases isolated from the gastrointestinal tract. Peptides modeled on the amino acid sequence around the cleavage site of the substrate frequently inhibit the enzyme and provide a starting point for the development of therapeutically relevant drugs which can block a single biologic process. The development of inhibitors for renin, kallikrein, and IgA_1 protease demonstrates the applicability of the substrate analog approach to drug design.

Proteolytic enzymes which split a single peptide bond in a specific amino acid sequence are integral parts of many biologic processes (1). These **highly specific proteases** may be contrasted with the less specific, but more intensively studied, enzymes from the gastrointestinal tract which cleave peptide bonds linking many types of amino acids. Examples of highly specific proteases (Table I) are: renin which cleaves angiotensinogen to initiate generation of the pressor agent angiotensin II (2); the kallikreins which produce either the hypotensive peptides kallidin or bradykinin from kininogen (3); IgA_1 protease which inactivates human secretory immunoglobulin by cleavage of a peptide bond in the hinge region (4); various members of the complement and clotting cascades (5,6); and proteases important in the maturation of viruses (7). Hypertension, shock, infection by both bacteria and viruses, clotting disorders, and immune system dyscrasias could be treated by selective inhibition of the highly specific proteases which are components of these disorders.

Highly specific proteases appear to cleave substrates by the same mechanisms used by more general proteases. Serine proteases, metaloproteases, and aspartyl proteases with greatly restricted specificity have been identified. Specificity appears to reside in the architecture of the active site rather than in functional groups which hydrolyze the peptide bond.

0097-6156/84/0251-0137$06.00/0
© 1984 American Chemical Society

Table I.   Action of Some Highly Specific Proteases

Protease	Substrate	Sequence Cleaved	Action
Renin	Angiotensinogen	DRVYIHPFHLVIH-	Produce Angiotensin I
Kallikrein	Kininogen	-SLMKRPPGFSPFRSSR-	Produce Kallidin
IgA₁ Protease	Secretory IgA1	-TPPTPSPS- -TPPTPSPS-	Inactivate Secretory IgA₁

Highly specific proteases may bind peptides which are homologous with the amino acid sequence of the naturally occurring substrate around the cleavage site. These peptides, which are termed **substrate analog inhibitors** (8), competitively block highly specific proteases. Presumably the substrate analog inhibitors can assume the conformation necessary to fit into in the enzyme active site. These synthetic analogs of the naturally occurring substrate may be contrasted with other proteins and peptides which usually do not bind to highly specific proteases.

The use of substrate analogs has led to the rapid development of inhibitors for several highly specific proteases. Research from this laboratory on the development of renin inhibitors, kallikrein inhibitors, and inhibitors of IgA₁ protease is outlined below.

Renin

Renin (E.C.3.4.99.19) is an aspartyl protease which cleaves angiotensinogen to generate angiotensin I (Table II). After discovery that the N-terminal tetradecapeptide from angiotensinogen was a substrate for renin, L. Skeggs and associates (9) completed a systematic study of the effect of substrate length on the rate of cleavage (V_{MAX}) and concentration of peptide needed to saturate the enzyme (K_M). Enzyme specificity (Table III) does not change appreciably on removal of either the first six amino acid residues from the N-terminus or the seryl residue from the C-terminus of the tetradecapeptide. Removal of the histidyl or tyrosyl residue from the resulting octapeptide His-Pro-Phe-His-Leu-Leu-Val-Tyr however, greatly reduces the rate of cleavage. The

---

Table II.   Sequences in the Renin-Angiotensin System

Angiotensinogen

Asp-Arg-Val-Tyr-Ile-His-Pro-Phe-His-Leu-Val-Ile-His-

Renin

Angiotensin I

Asp-Arg-Val-Tyr-Ile-His-Pro-Phe-His-Leu

Converting Enzyme

Angiotensin II

Asp-Arg-Val-Tyr-Ile-His-Pro-Phe

---

octapeptide is the minimal sequence efficiently cleaved by renin.
Poulsen et al. showed that this octapeptide competitively inhibits renin, reducing the rate at which angiotensin I is produced
(10).

Systematic modification of the octapeptide sequence from angiotensinogen (Figure 1) was undertaken to incorporate desirable
properties into the peptide. Addition of a prolyl residue to the
N-terminus improved solubility at physiologic pH, replacement of
the leucyl-leucine sequence with phenylalanyl residues improved
inhibitory properties by forty-fold, and addition of a lysyl residue to the C-terminus increased solubility and extended half-
life in vivo. These modifications yielded the Renin Inhibitory
Peptide (RIP) which effectively blocks renin both in primates
(11) and man (12).

High affinity substrate analog renin inhibitors have been reported from several laboratories. These were obtained by incorporating elements of a transition state inhibitor into the substrate analog sequence at the cleavage site. Szelke et al. (13)
replaced the peptide bond (-CONH-) between the amino acid residues comprising the cleavage site of various substrate analogs
with a hydroxyethyl group (-CHOH-CH$_2$) to increase affinity several orders of magnitude. Boger and co-workers (14) used the naturally occurring statine residue, which also incorporates a hydroxyethyl group, as a replacement for two amino acid residues in related sequences. Both analogs have a tetrahedral carbon atom at
the putative cleavage site and presumably function as transition
state analogs. In both cases the substrate sequence optimizes
interaction between the transition state analog and the enzyme
active site. Incorporation of the transition state element into

Table III   Cleavage of Synthetic Angiotensinogen Analogs

Asp-Arg-Val-Tyr-Ile-His-Pro-Phe-His-Leu-Leu-Val-Tyr-Ser

K_m (μm)	V_{max} (nmol min^{-1} Gu^{-1})	Specificity
3.7	10.2	2.77
28.0	8.9	0.31
26.1	9.8	0.38
30.7	10.9	0.36
46.8	11.7	0.25
53.6	0.55	0.0102
54.9	7.6	0.16
Not Cleaved		

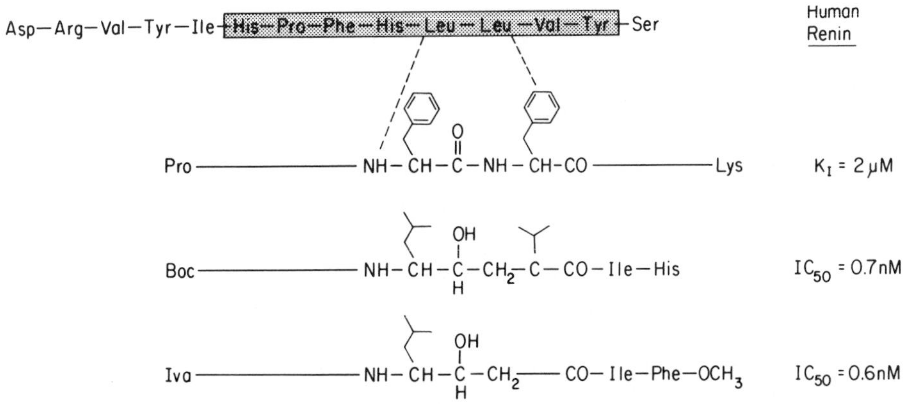

Figure 1.   Amino acid sequences of renin inhibitors based on the amino acid sequence of angiotensinogen.   Details of the synthesis and assay are given in references 11, 13, and 14.

a peptide not normally bound by renin will not yield effective inhibitors. Pepstatin A, which contains statine and is an extremely potent inhibitor of non-selective aspartyl proteases such as pepsin, is several orders of magnitude less effective as a renin inhibitor (15).

Research from this laboratory is now focused on developing orally active renin inhibitors. Initial research demonstrated that intact nona-peptides could cross jejunum. (16, 17). Previously only di- and tri- peptides had been shown to do this (18). Current work is focused on reducing the size, increasing the lipophilicity, and enhancing resistance to proteolytic degradation to optimize absorption of the substrate analog inhibitor from the gastrointestinal tract.

Kallikrein

Kallikrein is a serine protease which cleaves kininogen at both an arginyl-serine and methionyl-lysine residue to generate kallidin (Table IV). Kallidin may then react with receptors on the target tissue or be trimmed at the N-terminus to yield bradykinin. Bradykinin is associated with a host of biological activities including increases in vascular permeability and hypotension (19). Studies employing non-specific serine protease inhibitors indicate that the hypotension observed when converting enzyme is inhibited may be due to increases in circulating levels of kinins rather than the decreased rates of angiotensin I formation (20).

Research with synthetic kallikrein substrates indicates that peptides containing either the N-terminal or C-terminal sequences are recognized by the enzyme (21,22). Substrate mapping with analogs of the C-terminal portion of bradykinin has shown that the prolyl residue is important in cleavage of the arginyl-serine sequence. The pentapeptide Pro-Phe-Arg-Ser-Gln appears to be the minimal substrate for the enzyme and is thus analogous to the octapeptide found between positions 6 and 13 of angiotensinogen.

Current research from this laboratory (Figure 2) shows that the blocked hexapeptide Ac-Ser-Pro-Phe-Arg-Ser-Gln-NH_2 inhibits kallikrein in vitro (K_I = 61 μM) and demonstrates that the substrate analog approach is applicable to the design of inhibitors of kallikrein.

IgA_1 Protease

Various components of the secretory immune system prevent colonization and penetration of mucosal tissues by pathogenic bacteria. One of these, immunoglobulin IgA_1, is secreted onto mucosal surfaces where it is thought to prevent bacterial adherence. Pathogenic members of the the Neisseria, Streptococcus, and Haemophilus produce highly specific proteases that inactivate secretory IgA_1 by cleaving a peptide bond in the hinge region (4). Nonpathogenic commensal members of these bacteria do not make these enzymes. Several IgA_1 cleaving proteases which clip the peptide

Table IV. Sequences in the Kallikrein–Kininogen System

Kininogen -Ser-Leu-Met-Lys-Arg-Pro-Pro-Gly-Phe-Ser-Pro-Phe-Arg-Ser-Ser-Arg-

Kallikrein →

Kallidin Lys-Arg-Pro-Pro-Gly-Phe-Ser-Pro-Phe-Arg

→

Bradykinin Arg-Pro-Pro-Gly-Phe-Ser-Pro-Phe-Arg

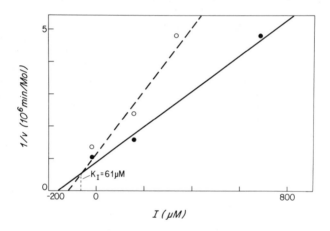

Figure 2. Dixon plot of the inhibition of human urinary kallikrein by the substrate analog KKI-6. Assay is done at pH 9.0,
37°C usingD-Val-Leu-Arg-pNA (S-2266, Kabi).

chain at slightly different locations have been isolated (Figure 3). Each IgA_1 protease is highly specific and splits a single peptide bond in the hinge region. No other protein tested is a substrate for the protease (23).

Initial research based on the substrate analog approach did not yield effective inhibitors (24). Sequences containing as many as 24 residues had IC_{50} values in the mM range, approximately three orders of magnitude higher than the K_M for the substrate. Modeling experiments indicate that the two immunoglobulin heavy chains in the hinge region of IgG_1 may be wrapped around each other in a poly-proline type of helix (25,26). Based on the limited homology found between the IgG_1 and IgA_1 hinge regions, we speculated that IgA_1 protease may need to bind both peptide chains before cleavage of either. This led to the synthesis of substrate analogs in which the two peptide chains are held in proximity by a disulfide link.

Synthesis of the IgA_1 protease inhibitors was completed by solid phase methods (27,28). After purification by chromatography on Sephadex G-25, the peptides were partly dimerized by air oxidation and subjected to a final purification by high performance liquid chromatography (HPLC) (Figure 4). In the system employed, the HPLC column is eluted through an HP-8450 spectrophotometer which measures and stores the u-v and visible region spectrum (200 - 800 nM) of the column effluent each second. For ease of interpretation, the absorbance at only one wave-length is plotted. The bottom half of Figure 4 however, compares the complete u-v spectra of one of the dimeric octapeptides taken during the begining and end of its elution from the column. The constant ratio of the two u-v spectra indicates that the dimer is homogeneous.

Results from the biological testing of the analogs obtained when each hydroxy amino acid in the octapeptide is replaced with cysteine are shown in Table V. IC_{50} values for inhibitors cross linked around the cleavage site are, like the long substrate analogs tested initially, in the mM range. When the disulfide link is displaced from the putative cleavage site, the peptides are considerably more effective inhibitors of IgA_1 protease. The best inhibitor is however, the blocked monomeric octapeptide which contains no cysteine and is not cross linked (29). These results prompted a closer look at the mechanism of cleavage of IgA_1. Studies in which the dimeric IgA_1 are treated with protease and then subjected to polyacrylamide gel electrophoresis show that the four F_{AB} units are removed independently from the immunoglobulin. Fragments containing three, two and one F_{AB} units linked to the dimeric $F_{C\alpha}$ have been identified (30). Computer modeling indicates that each F_{AB} unit is removed at the same rate. Cleavage of the hinge region peptide does not appear to require that both chains be present in the enzyme active site. Furthur evidence for the lack of tertiary structure is obtained from magnetic resonance studies of the free and blocked substrate analogs whose IC_{50} values differ by an order of magnitude. Ex-

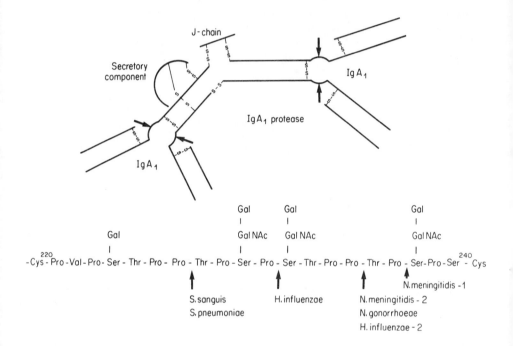

Figure 3.   Structure of IgA$_1$ and the amino acid sequence of the hinge region showing sites of cleavage by various IgA$_1$ proteases.

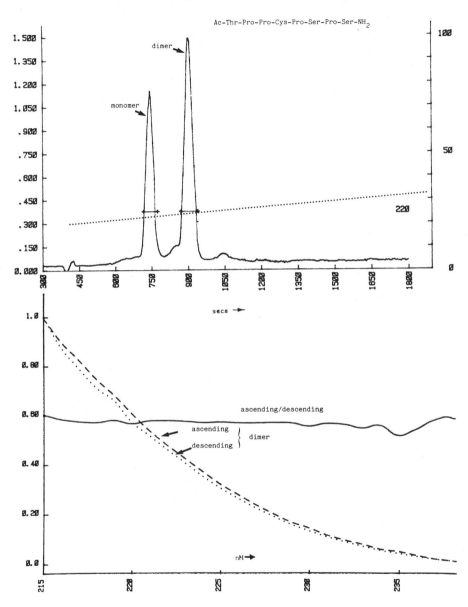

Figure 4. High performance liquid chromatography of the
octapeptide HRP-25 (Ac-Thr-Pro-Pro-Cys-Pro-Ser-Pro-Ser-
NH$_2$) on ODS (1.0 x 25 cm) using acetonitrile with a gradi-
ent of 0.1% TfaOH. Absorption at 220 nM (top) and u-v
spectra (bottom) taken during the beginning and end of
the elution of the dimer are shown. Constancy of the ratio
of the spectra indicates homogeneity of peptide in the peak.

Table V.   Substrate Analog Inhibitors of IgA$_1$ Protease

	N. Gonorrhoeae IC$_{50}$ (μM)
Thr-Pro-Pro-**Thr**-Pro-Ser-Pro-Ser	180
Ac————————————————NH$_2$	28
Ac—Cys————————————NH$_2$ S—S Ac—Cys————————————NH$_2$	800
Ac—————Cys————————NH$_2$ S—S Ac—————Cys————————NH$_2$	3000
Ac———————————Cys————NH$_2$ S—S Ac———————————Cys————NH$_2$	6000
Ac—————————————————Cys—NH$_2$ S—S Ac—————————————————Cys—NH$_2$	220

cept for the expected differences, the cmr spectra are virtually superimposable. In addition, temperature shift studies of amide protons in the blocked and unblocked octapeptides do not indicate that either contains hydrogen bonds. Neither peptide has a preferred conformation (31). Blockade of the N- and C-terminal functional groups may improve binding by removing unfavorable charge interactions between the peptide and the enzyme which prevent tight binding.

All Neisserial enzymes are inhibited by the substrate analogs even though the type I and type II IgA_1 proteases cleave at different positions. The IgA_1 proteases from both Haemophilus and Streptococci are not blocked by the peptides. The highly specific proteases from the latter organisms may have originated from different precursors than the Neisserial proteases and thus have very different active sites. DNA probes isolated from the Haemophilus protease do not bind to Neisserial DNA which also indicates that the enzymes are not homologous. The evolution of different highly specific proteases to perform the same function in pathogenic bacteria argues strongly for the importance of the enzyme in human disease.

Literature Cited

1. Holzer, H.; Heinrich, P.C. Ann. Rev. Biochem. 1980, 49, 63-91.

2. Peach, M.J. Physiol. Rev. 1977, 57, 313-70.

3. Prado, E.S.; Viel, M.S.; Sampaio, M.V.; Pavia, A.C.M.; Prado, J.L. Ciencia e Cultura 1974, 26, 384.

4. Plaut, A.G. Ann. Rev. Microbiol. 1983, 37, 603-22.

5. Muller-Eberhard, H.J. Ann. Rev. Biochem. 1975, 44, 697-724.

6. Davie, E.W.; Fujikawa, K.; Kurachi, K.; Kisiel, W. Adv. Enzymol. 1979, 48, 277-318.

7. Showe, M.K.; Isobe, E.; Onorato, L. J. Mol. Biol. 1976, 107, 55-69.

8. Burton, J.; Hyun, H.; TenBrink, R.E. in "Proc. 8th American Peptide Symp."; Hruby, V.J.; Rich, D.H. Eds.; Pierce Chem. Co.: Rockford, IL, 1983, In Press.

9. Skeggs, L.; Lentz, K.; Kahn, J.; Hochstrasser, H. J. Exp. Med. 1968, 128, 13-34.

10. Poulsen, K.; Burton, J.; Haber, E. Biochemistry 1973, 12, 3877-82.

11. Burton, J.; Cody, R.J.; Herd, J.A.; Haber, E. Proc. Nat. Acad. Sci, USA 1980, 77, 5476-79.

12. Zusman, R.; Christensen, D.; Burton, J.; Dodds, A.; Haber, E. Clin. Res. 1983, 31, In Press.

13. Szelke, M.; Leckie, B.J.; Hallett, A.; Jones, D.M.; Sueiras, J.; Atrash, B.; Lever, A.F. Nature, 1982, 299, 555-7.

14. Boger, J.; Lohr, N.S.; Ulm, E.H.; Poe, M.; Blaine, E.H.; Fanelli, G.M.; Lin, T.-Y.; Payne, L.S.; Schorn, T.W.; LaMont, B.I.; Bassil, T.C.; Stabilito, I.I.; Veber, D.F.; Rich, D.H.; Bopari, A.S. Nature 1983, 303, 81-4.

15. Aoyagi, T.; Morishima, H.; Nishizawa, R. J. Antibiot. 1972, 25, 689-94.

16. Drews, R.E.; Takaori, K.; Burton, J.; Donowitz, M. in "Proc. 8th American Peptide Symp."; Hruby, V.J.; Rich, D.H. Eds.; Pierce Chem. Co.: Rockford, IL, 1983, In Press.

17. Takaori, K.; Donowitz, M.; Burton, J. Fed. Proc. 1984, 42, In Press.

18. Matthews, D.M.; Payne, J.W. Current Topics in Membranes and Transport 1980, 14, 331-425.

19. Ryan, J.W.; Ryan, U.S. in "Chemistry and Biology of the Kallikrein-Kinin System in Health and Disease"; Pisano, J.J.; Austen, K.F. Eds.; DHEW Publication 76-791, 1974, pp. 315-334.

20. Muira, K.; Abe, Y.; Yamamoto, K. J. Pharm. Exp. Therap. 1982, 222, 246-250.

21. Feidler, F. in "Chemistry and Biology of the Kallikrein-Kinin System in Health and Disease"; Pisano, J.J.; Austen, K.F. Eds.; DHEW Publication 76-791, 1974, pp. 93-95.

22. Morris, D.H.; Stewart, J.M. Adv. Exp. Med. Biol. 1979, 120A, 213-8.

23. Kornfeld, S.J.; Plaut, A.G. Rev. Infect. Dis. 1981, 3, 521-34.

24. Plaut, A.G.; Gilbert, J.V.; Burton, J. in "Host-Parasite Interactions in Periodontal Diseases"; Genco, R.J.; Mergenhagen, S.E., Eds.; Am. Soc. Microbiol.: Washington, DC, 1982; pp. 193-201.

25. Marquart, M.; Deisenhofer, J.; Huber, R.; Palm, W. J. Mol. Biol. 1980, 141, 369-91.

26. Klein, M; Haeffner-Cavaillon, N.; Isenman, D.E.; Rivat, C.; Navia, M.A.; Davies, D.R.; Dorrington, K.J. Proc. Nat. Acad. Sci. USA 1981, 78, 524-8.

27. Merrifield, R.B. J. Am. Chem. Soc. 1964, 86, 304-5.

28. Burton, J.; Poulsen, K.; Haber, E. Biochemistry, 1975, 14, 3892-98.

29. Malison, R.T.; Burton, J.; Gilbert, J.; Plaut, A.G. in "Proc. 8th American Peptide Symp."; Hruby, V.J.; Rich, D.H. Eds.; Pierce Chem. Co.: Rockford, IL, 1983, In Press.

30. Plaut, A.G., personal communication.

31. Blumenstein, M., personal communication.

RECEIVED December 8, 1983

Structure–Behavioral Activity Relationships of Peptides Derived from ACTH
Some Stereochemical Considerations

J. W. VAN NISPEN and H. M. GREVEN

Organon Scientific Development Group, 5340 BH Oss, The Netherlands

The influence of chain length and side-chain modifications of ACTH-derived peptides on active avoidance behaviour in rats will be discussed. H-Met(O_2)-Glu-His-Phe-D-Lys-Phe-OH (Org 2766) emerged from these studies as an orally active peptide with an increased potency and selectivity of action. Physico-chemical data (from the literature) on the reference peptide ACTH-(4-10) did not point to a preferred conformation in solution, whereas in the crystalline state an antiparallel β-pleated sheet structure was found. At the receptor site we suggested an α-helical conformation in which the Phe and Met residues are close together. Additional support for this suggestion came from the behavioural activity of [des-Tyr[1], Met[5]]enkephalin and of cyclo-(-Phe-Met-εAhx-), εAhx merely serving as a spacer.

The relationship between the structure of a series of peptides derived from the adrenocorticotropic hormone ACTH, and the behavioural activity in an active avoidance behaviour test, has been studied over the past 10-20 years. The results obtained were quite different from those in which endocrine activity relationships were studied. From the outcome of a quantitative study on the structure-behavioural activity of the ACTH-related peptides, suggestions about the spatial interactions at the receptor site were made. This receptor-bound conformation differed from those suggested by solution experiments or found in crystal structures.

In this paper we will illustrate the line of research that was followed in the structure-behavioural activity work and that resulted

0097-6156/84/0251-0153$06.00/0

in a modified hexapeptide with an increased selectivity of action;
dissociation of active avoidance behavioural activity from other
activities will be mentioned briefly. We will also describe the
arguments that have led to the proposal of an α-helical conformation
for this hexapeptide at the receptor site.

Strategy and results of the structure-behavioural activity studies

ACTH, a straight-chain peptide of 39 amino acid residues (Figure 1),
has been the subject of extensive studies by many groups. In addition to stimulation of the adrenal cortex in vertebrate animals and
man, lipolytic and melanotropic effects are important, systemic,
extra-adrenal activities (1, 2). In the fifties it was found that ACTH
also affected behaviour in intact (3) and hypophysectomized animals
(4). The melanocyte-stimulating hormones α-MSH (comprising the
N-terminal 13 amino acid residues of ACTH but with blocked end
groups, see Figure 1) and β-MSH (containing, in general, the
sequence 4-10 of ACTH) were also able to correct behavioural
impairment in rats after removal of the pituitary or only its anterior
lobe (5). Since that time the influence of structural modifications
of these peptides on behaviour in rats has been investigated,
especially by de Wied and co-workers.

The first step in these studies has been the search for the shortest fragment of the ACTH chain that is essential for (maintenance
of) activity. Next, changes in the peptide backbone and modification of the side-chains of the amino acid residues have been studied.
As a test system the delay of extinction of an active avoidance
response in rats as measured in a pole-jumping test after subcutaneous administration has been used (7); this assay method
gives a graded dose-response relationship which allows the estima-
tion of an ED_{50} and thus potency ratio's. The heptapeptide ACTH-
-(4-10) has been used as the reference peptide (8). For a more
extensive review see ref. 9.

Influence of chain length. The fragments 1-24 and 1-10 were as
active as the whole molecule (weight basis) in delaying extinction
of the active avoidance response, whereas the C-terminal fragments
25-39, 18-39 (both porcine sequence) and 11-24 possessed 1/10th
of that potency. Stepwise shortening from the N- and, separately,
from the C-terminal end resulted in fragment 4-7 which contained
all the essential elements for a full response (10). ACTH-(7-10)
exerted a complete response only at a 10 times higher dose; this

residual potency could be increased to the same level as the reference peptide by extension to ACTH-(7-16)-NH_2 (11). It was concluded that regions other than the 4-7 also contain information for pole-jumping activity but that this is present in a latent form which needs chain elongation in order to become fully expressed (11).

H-Ser[1]-Tyr-Ser-Met-Glu-His-Phe-Arg-Trp-Gly-Lys-Pro-Val-Gly-

-Lys-Lys-Arg-Arg-Pro-Val-Lys-Val-Tyr-Pro[24]-Asn-Gly-Ala-Glu-

-Asp-Glu-Ser-Ala-Glu-Ala-Phe-Pro-Leu-Glu-Phe[39]-OH

Figure 1.   Amino acid sequence of human ACTH (6). α-MSH is [Ac-Ser[1], Val-NH_2[13]]ACTH-(1-13). The underlined sequence is ACTH-(4-10). Standard abbreviations are used for amino acids : IUPAC-IUB Commission on Biochemical Nomenclature, Eur. J. Biochem. 1975, 53, 1-14; 1972, 27, 201-7.

Influence of D-amino acids. As was found in an early stage of this work, the Arg[8] residue could be replaced by Lys[8] (which is simpler in a synthetical sense) without loss of activity. Therefore, the L/D replacements have been carried out on the Lys[8]-containing hexa-peptide 4-9, i.e. H-Met-Glu-His-Phe-Lys-Trp-OH (which is as potent as the sequence 4-10). The analogues with D-Met[4], D-Glu[5], D-His[6] or D-Trp[9] were as active as or more active than the all-L reference peptide. Incorporation of D-Arg[8] in ACTH-(4-10) resulted in a 3-fold increase in potency whereas incorporation of D-Lys[8] in the sequence 4-9 resulted in a 10-30 times more active compound. Replacement of Phe[7] by D-Phe[7] however, gave a compound which showed a reversal of the effect i.e. acceleration instead of delay of extinction (12). Other ACTH analogues containing a D-amino acid residue in position 7 also showed acceleration of extinction (9). Combinations of two D-amino acid residues had different effects. For instance, combining D-Glu[5] or D-His[6] with D-Lys[8] resulted in somewhat more active compounds. However, [D-Met[4], D-Lys[8]]-ACTH-(4-9) was less active than the reference peptide, meaning a loss of the potentiating contribution of D-Lys[8]. The combination of D-Met[4] and D-Phe[7] (in the L-Lys[8] containing 4-9 peptide) resulted in a loss of acceleration of extinction (typical for D-Phe[7] modifications), the new analogue being as active as ACTH-(4-10) in retarding extinction. Also when combining D-Phe[7] and D-Lys[8] as in [D-Phe[7], D-Lys[8], Phe[9]]ACTH-(4-9) a delay of extinction was observed with a relative potency of only 2.

Modifications of side-chains. Oxidation of the Met[4] residue to Met(O)[4] in ACTH-(4-10) resulted in a 3-10 times more potent peptide. Further oxidation to the corresponding sulfone increased the potency to 10 times that of the reference peptide. Finally, in [D-Lys[8], Phe[9]]ACTH-(4-9) oxidation of Met[4] to the sulfone gave a product that was 1000 times as active as ACTH-(4-10) while the corresponding sulfoxide analogue was slightly more active [3000 times ACTH-(4-10)]. Replacement of Met[4] by β-Ala, Aib, or Val did not yield peptides with potencies greater than that of the Met(O$_2$)[4] modification. Protection against an aminopeptidase-type of degradation by replacement of Met[4] by desaminomethionine (Dam) or of Met(O$_2$)[4] by Dam(O$_2$), resulted in an increase of potency by a factor of 3. Similarly, protection against a carboxy-peptidase-type of degradation by introducing tryptamine (descarboxy-tryptophan, Tra) or amphetamine (replacement of the COOH of Phe by a CH$_3$ group) at the C-terminal gave a 3-fold increase in potency. A combination of both types of modification, [Dam(O$_2$)[4], D-Lys[8], Tra[9]]ACTH-(4-9), resulted in a 10-fold potentiation; this new analogue is 10,000 times as potent as ACTH-(4-10).

Although removal of Trp[9] from unmodified ACTH-(4-9) or removal of Met[4] from ACTH-(4-10) resulted in no and some loss of activity, respectively, leaving out the N- or C-terminal amino acid residue in [Met(O$_2$)[4], D-Lys[8], Phe[9]]ACTH-(4-9) resulted in a considerable loss of activity (by a factor of 1000 and 30-100, respectively). So for potentiation the presence of the side-chains of Met(O$_2$)[4], D-Lys[8] and Phe[9] seems to be of prime importance.

As mentioned above, elongation of the sequence 7-10 to ACTH--(7-16)-NH$_2$ increased the potency to that of the reference peptide 4-10. Replacement of Arg[8]-Trp[9] by D-Lys[8]-Phe[9] resulted in a 100--fold increase in potency. C- or N-terminal shortening of this 7-16 analogue by only one amino acid residue resulted, again, in a large decrease of activity, as did omission of the Gly[10] residue (11). The potency of [D-Lys[8], Phe[9]]ACTH-(7-16)-NH$_2$ was increased a further 100-fold when Lys[11] was replaced by D-Lys[11]. An additional 10-fold increase in potency was observed after N-terminal elongation of the latter analogue with Met(O$_2$)-Glu-His; the new peptide was 100,000 times as active as reference ACTH-(4-10) on a weight basis. The most potent analogue reported to date is H-Met(O_2)-Ala--Ala-Ala-Ala-D-Lys-Phe-Gly-D-Lys-Pro-Val-Gly-Lys-Lys-NH_2 which is 3 million times as active as ACTH-(4-10), i.e. more than 4 million times on a molar base.

Discussion. The tetrapeptide H-Met-Glu-His-Phe-OH is the shortest sequence which was as active as ACTH-(1-39) on a weight basis. Additional information for extinction of pole-jumping avoidance behaviour seems to be stored, in a latent form, in the ACTH molecule in fragments 7-10, 11-13 and 25-39 (11). A similar finding was reported by Eberle and Schwyzer for melanocyte--stimulating activity of α-MSH fragments; they found two discrete message sequences for melanin dispersion, i.e. the fragments 4-10 and 11-13-NH_2 (13).

The effects of L/D substitutions in ACTH-(4-10) or (4-9) on pole-jumping behaviour were quite different from those on hormonal activities. While Arg^8 may be replaced by Lys^8 without loss of behavioural potency, a drastic decrease in steroidogenic and lipolytic effects was observed when the same modification was introduced in ACTH-(1-24) (14). $D-Arg^8$ and also $D-His^6$ substitutions showed an increase in behavioural potency but resulted in inactive compounds when tested for melanocyte-stimulating activity (in the 6-10 fragment) (15). [$D-Phe^7$]ACTH-(6-10) has been reported to be 30 times (15) and 5-10 times (16) more active than the all-L-peptide in the latter test. Ac-[Nle^4, $D-Phe^7$]ACTH-(4-10)--NH_2 was 10 times as active as the L-analogue when measured in the frog skin assay but about 160 times more potent in the lizard skin assay (17). An increase in potency was also observed in the mouse melanoma adenylate cyclase assay (17). In the pole--jumping test, only the L-/D-Phe^7 replacement resulted in a reversal of action i.e. acceleration instead of delay of extinction. [$D-Glu^5$, Lys^8]ACTH-(4-9) was slightly more active than the all--L-peptide in the pole-jumping test. When tested for lipolytic activity, [$D-Glu^5$]ACTH-(4-10) possessed only 2% of the activity of its L-Glu^5 analogue (18). These results clearly indicated a dissociation between requirements for behavioural activity on the one hand and melanocyte-stimulating or lipolytic activities on the other. Further evidence for this statement came from data of other substitutions : oxidation of the Met residue in ACTH or α-MSH resulted in a marked decrease of corticotropic (19) and melanocyte--stimulating (20) activity but to more active compounds in the behavioural assay. Trp^9, also important for the corticotropic

activity of ACTH (21, 22), cannot be replaced by Phe without a
marked loss of steroidogenic potency; this is in contrast to a 3-fold
potentiation in the pole-jumping test.

The introduction of a D-Lys in position 8 in ACTH-(4-9) resulted
in a 10-30 fold increase in pole-jumping activity, by far the largest
increase of the L/D substitutions; interestingly, D-Arg[8] gave only a
3-fold potentiation. Since the same metabolic stabilization may be
expected for those two compounds, the higher potency for the D-Lys
analogue might be attributed to an increase in receptor affinity. It
was suggested by Greven and de Wied that the flexible side-chain of
the D-Lys residue can function more efficiently as an electrostatic
anchor at the receptor site than the more bulky and rigid D-Arg[8]
side-chain (23).

Biological and physico-chemical properties of ACTH-(4-10) and
Org 2766

Biological activities in animals. In order to see how the 1000-fold
increase in potency of the modified hexapeptide H-Met(O_2)-Glu-
-His-Phe-D-Lys-Phe-OH, coded Org 2766, to delay extinction of
pole-jumping behaviour was related to its endocrine activities, the
effects on corticotropic, lipotropic and melanocyte-stimulating
activity were compared with those of ACTH-(4-10). Only 1% or less
of these mentioned activities was present (Table I). Studies
comparing ACTH-(4-10) and Org 2766 in other (behavioural) test
situations clearly showed different structure-activity relationships
(Table I). In most cases a clear difference in potency (Org 2766
being more potent) and in some cases even a reversed action was
found (social interaction); when tested for grooming behaviour, both
peptides showed no effect. Recent studies of Fekete and de Wied
showed that Org 2766 had a longer time course of action in the active
and passive avoidance tests than ACTH-(4-10) after subcutaneous
administration (24). In these latter two tests, Org 2766 was also
found to be active after oral administration (a dose of approx.
10 μg/kg showed oral activity in the active avoidance test; ACTH-
-(4-10) was not active when given orally). When dose-response
relationships were studied after intracerebroventricular, subcutaneous and oral administration of these two peptides and the super-
active H-Met(O_2)-Ala-Ala-Phe-D-Lys-Phe-Gly-D-Lys-Pro-Val-
-Gly-Lys-Lys-NH$_2$ [1,000,000 times as active as ACTH-(4-10) on
a weight basis], the relative potency ratio's remained fairly constant irrespective of the route of application (23). This indicates

Table I.   Comparison of activities of Org 2766 and the reference peptide ACTH-(4-10) in rats.

Activity[a]	ACTH-(4-10)	Org 2766	Ref.
Corticotropic (cell suspension)	1	0.01	25
Lipolytic (in vitro, rabbits)	1	0.01	i
Melanocyte-stimulating (lizard)	1	0.001	i
Pole-jumping	1	1000[b]	10
Passive avoidance (pre-retention[c])	1	1000[b]	24
Attenuation of CO_2-induced amnesia	1	1000[d]	26
Acquisition shuttle-box (hypox. rats)	1	100	27
Affinity for opiate receptor	yes, weak	no	28
Grooming[e]	inactive	inactive	29
Social interaction[f]	decrease; 1	increase; 1000	30
Self-stimulation[f]	1	1000	31
Stress-induced motor activity	inactive	prevents decline in activity	32
Analeptic[g]	inactive	active	33
Synaptic membrane phosphorylation[h]	stimulation	stimulation	34
Axonal nerve regeneration	1	1	35
ibid. in adrenalectomized rats	active 4-10 ng	inactive in these doses	36

a. Subcutaneous administration unless stated otherwise.
b. Effect was of longer duration. Also active after oral administration.
c. Post-trial : ACTH-(4-10) no effect, Org 2766 effective.
d. Also active after oral administration.
e. Intraventricular administration.
f. Administration in septum.
g. Reversing pentobarbital-induced sedation; intraperitoneal and intracisternal administration.
h. Stimulation of diphosphoinositide (DPI) formation, in vitro.
i. Unpublished data.

that the combination of metabolic stability and transport characteristics is about the same for the three peptides, and suggests that the increase in potency for the two analogues of ACTH-(4-10) is mainly due to an increased affinity for the relevant receptor site.

Studies in man. The animal studies with ACTH-(4-10) and Org 2766 have suggested that these peptides enhance attention or motivation and that they also may improve memory consolidation (for a review see 37). Studies using acute systemic administration of ACTH-(4-10) (subcutaneously, intramuscularly or intravenously) indicated increased selective attention and or motivation both in volunteers and in patients (38, 39). Inconsistent effects of ACTH--(4-10) on tests of memory and other tests of cognitive performance have been found (38). Subcutaneous or oral administration of Org 2766 (acute studies) have led to essentially the same results (38, 39). These peptides differ from (other) psychostimulant drugs in that they do not show any unwanted side-effects.

Recent findings after subchronic, oral administration of Org 2766 in daily doses of 10-40 mg, showed a decrease in anxiety and depression (self-rated) and an improvement of feelings of competence, sociability and ward behaviour (observer-rated) (39). No side-effects like influence on autonomic activity and appetite, and no sedative effects were reported. It seems that Org 2766 may be a drug to be used in treating disturbances of mood in the elderly as well as symptoms of dementia. Many studies in these areas are underway.

Physico-chemical properties. In the fifties and sixties, several studies on the conformation of ACTH in solution were carried out. Among the used techniques were ORD, CD, fluorescence depolarization studies and kinetics of deuterium hydrogen exchange (for a review see ref. 2). The results pointed to a highly flexible random coil in solution; however, Eisinger (40) found that the distance between Tyr^2 and Trp^9 [in ACTH-(1-24)] as measured by excitation spectroscopy, was in better agreement with some form of loop or helical structure. In addition, Squire and Bewley noted 11-15% helical content, located in the N-terminal 1-11 part of the molecule, when measuring the ORD of ACTH at pH 8.1 (41) (a random coil was found at neutral and acidic pH values, 2).

Prediction of the secondary structure of ACTH using the rules of Chou and Fasman (42) by Löw et al. (43), Jibson and Li (44) and Mutter et al. (45), revealed a preference for an α-helical structure for the fragments 3-9 ($\underline{43}$) or 2-9 ($\underline{44}$, $\underline{45}$) and 27-35 ($\underline{43}$, $\underline{44}$) or 29-34 ($\underline{45}$) and indications for a β-turn at 23-26 ($\underline{43}$, $\underline{44}$, $\underline{45}$) and 12-15 ($\underline{44}$) or 14-17 ($\underline{45}$). Applying Tanaka and Scheraga's method ($\underline{46}$), Mutter et al. calculated the α-helical region to be fragment 2-9 ($\underline{45}$).

In the mid-seventies, Löw et al. studying ACTH-(1-39) and fragments, found a transition from random coil to a helix structure when the solvent water was gradually replaced by trifluoroethanol (TFE) ($\underline{43}$). This latter solvent had been shown to favour the establishment of ordered structures (β-sheet or α-helix) like a membrane-receptor environment ("membrane-receptor mimetic" properties) ($\underline{47}$). Subsequent work of the groups of Löw and Fermandjian on ACTH-(1-39) and several large fragments and analogues making use of ^{1}H- and ^{13}C-NMR spectroscopy, IR hydrogen-deuterium exchange kinetics and CD all pointed to helical structures of sequences in ACTH ($\underline{48}$, $\underline{49}$ and references therein).

Small ACTH fragments related to ACTH-(4-10) have also been investigated for the presence of ordered structure. CD of ACTH-(5-10) in TFE showed a random structure ($\underline{50}$) as was found with ^{1}H-NMR for fragment 4-10 ($\underline{51}$). The addition of anionic or cationic surfactants to an aqueous solution of ACTH-(4-11) dit not promote any α-helix or β-form in this peptide (CD experiments; $\underline{52}$). When ACTH-(1-14) and 1-10 were measured by CD and NMR respectively, indications for a helical or ordered structure were found ($\underline{50}$, $\underline{51}$). Thus it seems that the addition of the non-helix "prone" fragment 1-3 or 1-4 can promote the formation of a helical structure in the adjacent sequence. Arguments in favour of this come from the theoretical work of Argos and Palau ($\underline{53}$) on amino acid distribution in protein secondary structures. They found that Ser and Thr frequently occur at the N-terminal helical position (cf. Ser^{3} in ACTH) to provide stability; the position adjacent to the helical C-terminus is often occupied by Gly or Pro (adjacent to Trp^{9} in ACTH we have Gly^{10}); acidic amino acid residues are frequently found at the helix N-terminus (cf. Glu^{5} in ACTH) and/or basic residues at the C-terminus (cf. Arg^{8}).

Crystal structure(s) of ACTH-(1-39) or 1-24 are not known. Suitable crystals for X-ray diffraction experiments could be obtained however, for the heptapeptide 4-10 ($\underline{54}$, $\underline{55}$) and the smaller tetrapeptide 4-7 ($\underline{54}$, $\underline{56}$). In the former case, an anti-parallel β-pleated sheet structure of the backbone was found with clustering of hydrophobic (Met, Phe and Trp) and hydrophilic (Glu, His, Arg) side-chains as remarkable features. ACTH-(4-7) crystallizes as a monohydrate horseshoe-like structure which is again characterized by the proximity of the hydrophobic Phe and Met and the hydrophilic Glu and His residues, but now via intra- and inter-chain interactions. So in two quite different conformational structures of ACTH-(4-10) and 4-7 a striking common feature is that the Phe and Met side-chains are close together. Org 2766 has not yet yielded crystals suitable enough for structure determination.

In summary, theoretical approaches point to the potential for an α-helical structure for the fragment 4-10 and the conformation found in solutions of this and several other fragments of ACTH seem to be confirmatory; the crystal structure reveals an antiparallel β-pleated sheet.

Suggestion for conformation at the receptor site for pole-jumping activity

In 1977 a quantitative study on the relationship between the structure and pole-jumping behaviour of ACTH-derived peptides (only those that delayed extinction), was performed (11, 57) according to method of Free and Wilson as modified by Fujita and Ban (58). Apparently the data on 55 peptides satisfied the conditions for such a mathematical approach which means that the potencies of the analogues could be considered to be composed of the product of independent group contributions from individual substitutions in the peptide chain. For instance, the combination of D-Lys^8 with either D-Glu^5 or D-His^6 gave the same actual and calculated activities. However, when D-Lys^8 was combined with D-Met^4 as in H-D-Met--Glu-His-Phe-D-Lys-Trp-OH, the observed potency was much lower than the calculated one. Since this is one of the very few exceptions where the calculation failed, i.e. the condition of independent group contributions was no longer fulfilled (outlier), it was suggested by Greven and de Wied (11) that this could be due to steric interference of the D-Met^4 and D-Lys^8 residues, which in turn implies that positions 4 and 8 are close together at the receptor site. The amino acids in between seem to serve merely as a spacer as was shown by replacement of these amino acids by simple, neutral alanine residues (11). This close proximity of the side--chains of residues 4 and 8 is possible when the backbone assumes an α-helical conformation (11). In this helical structure the Met^4 and Phe^7 residues are extra-chain neighbours.

The β-lipotropin fragments H-Tyr-Gly-Gly-Phe-Met-OH (Met--enkephalin) and H-Gly-Gly-Phe-Met-OH show the presence of Phe and Met as intra-chain neighbours. When these two molecules were tested for delay of extinction in the pole-jumping test, they were found to be approx. as active as ACTH-(4-10) (23, 9). In addition, oxidation of Met to Met(O) resulted in a similar potentiation as that found in the ACTH series. The hypothesis that the close proximity of a Phe and Met residue in ACTH- and enkephalin-like peptides is essential for a delay in extinction was further checked by testing a cyclic peptide containing Phe, Met and a spacer ε-aminohexanoic acid (εAhx) to close the ring [εAhx was chosen since it contains no functional groups and does not distort the peptide groups significantly from planarity or force them into the cis conformation (59)]. Cyclo-(-Phe-Met-εAhx-) (60) was found to be as active as ACTH--(4-10) in delaying extinction (9), thus supporting the hypothesis of Greven and de Wied (11).

As mentioned before (section 1), introduction of the D-Lys residue in the ACTH fragment 4-10 or 4-9 resulted in a higher increase in active avoidance behaviour than the 3-fold increase in activity when L-Arg was replaced by D-Arg, suggesting an additional function of the D-Lys residue at the receptor site. The mere presence of D-Lys, Met(O) or Met(O_2) and Phe in one molecule as in Org 2766 is not sufficient, however, for high activity in the pole-jumping test. When H-Gly-Gly-Phe-Met(O)-D-Lys-Phe-OH was tested, acceleration instead of delay of extinction was found. The corresponding all-L hexapeptide delayed extinction and was as active as ACTH-(4-10) (Greven and de Wied, unpublished results). A special spatial arrangement of these three residues at the receptor for pole-jumping activity therefore appears to be a requirement for high activity in delaying extinction of a conditioned avoidance response.

Suggested preferred conformations can be fixed by cyclization. Cystine has been used to obtain cyclic analogues of Org 2766 viz. H-Cys-Glu-His-Cys-D-Lys-Phe-OH, H-Cys-Ala-Ala-Cys-D-Lys--Phe-OH and H-Cys-Ala-Ala-Phe-D-Lys-Cys-OH (patent application 0052028 of Roussel-Uclaf), and the peptides were tested for activity in the pole-jumping test. Unfortunately, one cannot conclude from their data if cyclization has resulted in an increase or decrease in activity since no reference peptide has been included to compare potencies. In the literature cyclization of [Lys[5]]ACTH--(5-10) (the COOH group of Gly[10] with the ε-NH_2 function of Lys[5]) has been reported; the resulting peptide was inactive in steroidogenesis (61). Increase of the ring size with three atoms (a Gly residue), however, resulted in a peptide that was more active than the linear unmodified 5-10 sequence (61), indicating the importance of the ring size. Cyclization of the message sequence for steroidogenic activity by replacement of Glu^5 and Gly^{10} by a cystine residue in $[2$-δ-aminovaleric acid$]$ACTH-(2-19) resulted in a 50-fold decrease in steroidogenic activity and 10-fold decrease in lipolytic activity (62). When a cystine molecule was incorporated into α-MSH in place of Met^4 and Gly^{10}, a very potent analogue was obtained with a potency $> 10,000$ times that of α-MSH in stimulating frog skin darkening and about 30 times more potent when measured in vitro in lizard skin (63).

Thus strong potentiation of biological activity can be obtained either by substitutions which allow or enhance a preferred conformation at the receptor site or by fixation of such a preferred conformation via cyclization of the backbone.

Concluding remarks

For activity of ACTH-derived peptides at the receptor for pole-jumping activity, the basic requirement seems to be the presence of a Phe and Met residue in close proximity. It is interesting to see that Phe and Met are close together in an α-helical structure in ACTH peptides (and as intra-chain neighbours in Met-enkephalin) and in the crystalline state in ACTH-(4-10) as a β-pleated sheet and in ACTH-(4-7) in the form of a horseshoe; this close proximity is in line with the results of a Free-Wilson type of analysis.

In H-Met(O_2)-Glu-His-Phe-D-Lys-Phe-OH (Org 2766), the large increase in activity in the pole-jumping test and the longer duration of action can only partly be explained by an increase in stability. It is suggested that in the form of an α-helix or loop-like structure at the receptor site, the presence of D-Lys^8 as well as $Met(O_2)^4$ and Phe^9 contributes to an increase of receptor affinity.

Literature Cited

1. Hofmann, K. in "Handbook of Physiology, Section 7 : Endocrinology, vol. IV, The pituitary gland and its neuroendocrine control, Part 2; Greep, R.O.; Astwood, E.B., Eds.; Waverly Press : Baltimore, 1974; pp. 29-58.

2. Schwyzer, R. Ann. N.Y. Acad. Sci. 1977, 297, 3-26.

3. Mirsky, I.A.; Miller, R.; Stein, M. Psychosom. Med. 1953, 15, 574-88.

4. Applezweig, M.H.; Baudry, F.D. Psychol. Rep. 1955, 1, 417-20.
5. De Wied, D. in "Frontiers in Neuroendocrinology"; Ganong, W.F.; Martini, L., Eds.; Oxford Univ. Press : London; 1969, pp. 97-140.
6. Riniker, B.; Sieber, P.; Rittel, W.; Zuber, H. Nature (New Biol.) 1972, 235, 114-5.
7. De Wied, D. Proc. Soc. Exp. Biol. Med. 1966, 122, 28-32.
8. Greven, H.M.; de Wied, D. Eur. J. Pharmacol. 1967, 2, 14-6.
9. Nispen, J.W. van; Greven, H.M. Pharmac. & Ther. 1982, 16, 67-102.
10. Greven, H.M.; de Wied, D. in "Progress in Brain Research"; Zimmermann, E.; Gispen, W.H.; Marks, B.H.; de Wied, D., Eds.; Elsevier : Amsterdam, 1973; Vol. 39, pp. 429-41.
11. Greven, H.M.; de Wied, D. in "Frontiers of Hormone Research"; van Wimersma Greidanus, Tj. B., Ed.; Karger : Basel, 1977; Vol. 4, pp. 140-152.
12. Bohus, B.; de Wied, D. Science 1966, 153, 318-20.
13. Eberle, A.; Schwyzer, R. Helv. Chim. Acta 1975, 58, 1528-35.
14. Tesser, G.I.; Maier, R.; Schenkel-Hulliger, L.; Barthe, P.L.; Kamber, B.; Rittel, W. Acta Endocrinol. 1973, 74, 56-66.
15. Yajima, H.; Kubo, K.; Kinomura, Y.; Lande, S. Biochim. Biophys. Acta 1966, 127, 545-9.
16. Schnabel, E.; Li, C.H. J. Am. Chem. Soc. 1960, 82, 4576-9.
17. Sawyer, T.K.; Hruby, V.J.; Wilkes, B.C.; Draelos, M.T.; Hadley, M.E.; Bergsneider, M. J. Med. Chem. 1982, 25, 1022-7.
18. Draper, M.W.; Rizack, M.A.; Merrifield, R.B. Biochemistry 1975, 14, 2933-8.
19. Dedman, M.L.; Farmer, T.H.; Morris, G.J.O.R. Biochem. J. 1955, 59, xii.
20. Lo, T.-B.; Dixon, J.S.; Li, C.H. Biochim. Biophys. Acta 1961, 53, 584-6.
21. Hofmann, K.; Andreatta, R.; Bohn, H.; Moroder, L. J. Med. Chem. 1970, 13, 339-45.
22. Nispen, J.W. van; Tesser, G.I. Int. J. Peptide Prot. Res. 1975, 7, 57-67.

23. Greven, H.M.; de Wied, D. in "Hormones and the Brain"; de Wied, D.; van Keep, P.A., Eds.; MTP : Falcon House, 1980; pp.115-127.
24. Fekete, M.; de Wied, D. Pharmacol. Biochem. Behav. 1982, 16, 387-92.
25. Krieger, D.T., communication to Organon.
26. Rigter, H.; Janssens-Elbertse, R.; van Riezen, H. Pharmacol. Biochem. Behav. 1976, 5 (suppl. 1), 53-8.
27. Fekete, M.; Bohus, B.; de Wied, D. Neuroendocrinol. 1983, 36, 112-8.
28. Gispen, W.H.; Terenius, L., communication to Organon.
29. Gispen, W.H.; Wiegant, V.M.; Greven, H.M.; de Wied, D. Life Sci. 1975, 17, 645-52.
30. Clarke, A.; File, S.E. Br. J. Pharmacol. 1981, 74, 277P.
31. Fekete, M.; Bohus, B.; van Wolfswinkel, L.; van Ree, J.M.; de Wied, D. Neuropharmacol. 1982, 21, 909-16.
32. Saint-Côme, C.; Acker, G.R.; Strand, F.L. Peptides 1982, 3, 439-49.
33. Bissette, G.; Nemeroff, C.B.; Loosen, P.T.; Prange A.J., Jr.; Lipton, M.S. Pharmacol. Biochem. Behav. 1976, 5 (suppl. 1), 135-8.
34. Jolles, J.; Bär, P.R.; Gispen, W.H. Brain Res. 1981, 224, 315-26.
35. Bijlsma, W.A.; Jennekens, F.G.I.; Schotman, P.; Gispen, W.H. Eur. J. Pharmacol. 1981, 76, 73-9.
36. Smith, C.M.; Strand, F.L. Peptides 1981, 2, 197-206.
37. Bohus, B. Pharmacol. 1979, 18, 113-22.
38. Gaillard, A.W.K., in "Endogenous Peptides and Learning and Memory Processes"; Martinez, J.L.; Jensen, R.A.; Messing, R.B.; Rigter, H.; McGaugh, J.L., Eds.; Academic : New York, 1981; pp.181-196.
39. Pigache, R.M.; Rigter, H. in "Frontiers of Hormone Research"; van Wimersma Greidanus, Tj.B.; Rees, L.H., Eds.; Karger : Basel, 1981; Vol. 8, pp.193-207.
40. Eisinger, J. Biochemistry 1969, 8, 3902-7.
41. Squire, P.G.; Bewley, T. Biochim. Biophys. Acta 1965, 109, 234-40.
42. Chou, P.Y.; Fasman, G.D. Biochemistry 1974, 13, 222-45.
43. Löw, M.; Kisfaludy, L.; Fermandjian, S. Acta Biochim. et Biophys. Acad. Sci. Hung. 1975, 10, 229-31.
44. Jibson, M.D.; Li, C.H. Int. J. Peptide Prot. Res. 1979, 14, 113-22.

45. Mutter, H.; Mutter, M.; Bayer, E. <u>Z. Naturforsch.</u> 1979, <u>34b</u>, 874-85.
46. Tanaka, S.; Scheraga, H.A. <u>Macromolecules</u> 1977, <u>10</u>, 305-16, and references therein.
47. Urry, D.W.; Masotti, L.; Krivacic, J.R. <u>Biochim. Biophys.</u> <u>Acta</u> 1971, <u>241</u>, 600-12.
48. Toma, F.; Dive, V.; Lam-Thanh, H.; Piriou, F.; Lintner, K.; Fermandjian, S.; Löw, M.; Kisfaludy, L. <u>Biochimie</u> 1981, <u>63</u>, 907-10.
49. Toma, F.; Fermandjian, S.; Löw, M.; Kisfaludy, L. <u>Bio-polymers</u> 1981, <u>20</u>, 901-13.
50. Greff, D.; Toma, F.; Fermandjian, S.; Löw, M.; Kisfaludy, L. <u>Biochim. Biophys. Acta</u> 1976, <u>439</u>, 219-31.
51. Rawson, B.J.; Feeney, J.; Kimber, B.J.; Greven, H.M. <u>J. Chem. Soc. Perkin Trans. II</u> 1982, 1471-7.
52. Wu, C.-S.; Yang, J.T. <u>Biochem. Biophys. Res. Commun.</u> 1978, <u>82</u>, 85-91.
53. Argos, P.; Palau, J. <u>Int. J. Peptide Prot. Res.</u> 1982, <u>19</u>, 380-93.
54. Admiraal, G. Ph. D. Thesis, Groningen State University, Groningen, 1981.
55. Admiraal, G.; Vos, A. <u>Int. J. Peptide Prot. Res.</u>, in press.
56. Admiraal, G.; Vos, A. <u>Acta Crystallogr.</u>, Sect. C 1983, <u>C39</u>, 82-7.
57. Kelder, J.; Greven, H.M. <u>Recl. Trav. Chim. Pays-Bas</u> 1979, <u>98</u>, 168-72.
58. Fujita, T.; Ban, T. <u>J. Med. Chem.</u> 1971, <u>14</u>, 148-52.
59. Némethy, G.; McQuie, J.R.; Pottle, M.S.; Scheraga, H.A. <u>Macromolecules</u> 1981, <u>14</u>, 975-84.
60. Nispen, J.W. van; Greven, H.M. <u>Recl. Trav. Chim.</u> <u>Pays-Bas</u> 1982, <u>101</u>, 451-5.
61. Romanovskis, P.J.; Siskov, I.V.; Liepkaula, I.K.; Porunkevich, E.A.; Ratkevich, M.P.; Skujins, A.A.; Chipens, G.I. <u>Proc. 7th American Peptide Symp.</u> 1981, pp. 229-32.
62. Blake, J.; Rao, A.J.; Li, C.H. <u>Int. J. Peptide Prot. Res.</u> 1979, <u>13</u>, 346-52.
63. Sawyer, T.K.; Hruby, V.J.; Darman, P.S.; Hadley, M.E. <u>Proc. Natl. Acad. Sci. USA</u> 1982, <u>79</u>, 1751-5.

RECEIVED November 15, 1983

Design of Novel Cyclic Hexapeptide Somatostatin Analogs from a Model of the Bioactive Conformation

ROGER M. FREIDINGER and DANIEL F. VEBER

Merck Sharp & Dohme Research Laboratories, West Point, PA 19486

Novel cyclo retro isomers and N^α-methyl lysine analogs of somatostatin cyclic hexapeptides were designed from a model of the bioactive conformation. Compounds of greater potency and stability than somatostatin were prepared. The analogs furnished additional information about the receptor bound conformation which was consistent with the working conformational model. Conformational information from solution studies using NMR and CD was generally consistent with inferences from the biological data. These studies illustrate the utility of a conformation-activity approach to peptide analog design.

The naturally-occurring biologically active peptides represent an almost untapped potential source of new therapeutic agents. The spectrum of activities already known is large and new structures with novel biology are continually being elucidated. The increasing understanding of biochemical processes in which these peptides are involved suggests numerous areas for new drug development. The challenge to the medicinal chemist is to learn how to develop useful agents based on these peptide leads.

There are a number of problems associated with the use of peptides as drug molecules. Peptides are rapidly degraded by proteases and, therefore, their biological half lives are normally too short to be useful in a therapeutic sense. Most peptides exhibit more than one type of biological effect making lack of specificity a problem to be overcome. The size of even "small" peptides is larger than most common drug molecules, and it is usually desirable, if for no other reason than ease of synthesis, to simplify the structures as much as possible. Finally, for the small number of peptides which have been studied by the oral route, poor bioavailability has been a problem.

0097–6156/84/0251–0169$06.00/0
© 1984 American Chemical Society

Conformational Approach to Peptide Analog Design

The traditional approach to peptide modification has entailed systematic substitution for the various amino acids in the molecule and determining the resultant effect on biological activity. After a large number of these changes have been completed, the most successful ones can be combined to produce a peptide with improved properties. This approach still has its place; however, in our laboratories, we have also been emphasizing the importance of information pertaining to the peptide bioactive conformation in the design process (1). The bioactive conformation is defined as the conformation of the peptide bound to a given receptor at the instant that a specific response is elicited. If important features of the bioactive conformation can be ascertained, it should be possible to modify peptide structures in a more rational manner.

Conformational Constraints. How is information about the bioactive conformation obtained? An approach which we have emphasized involves constraining the peptide backbone in various ways and gauging the effect on biological activity (2). The conformational constraints may be noncovalent in nature such as D-amino acids or N^{α}-methyl amino acids. Alternatively, covalent constraints such as cyclic amino acids, bridged dipeptides, or cyclic peptides may be utilized. Normally a combination of several different modifications is necessary to develop a hypothesis for the peptide bioactive conformation. Computer modeling of peptide structures has been an integral part of this approach in our laboratories (3).

Besides obtaining information pertaining to the bioactive conformation, there are other advantages to be gained from successful application of conformational constraints. Potency may be increased through stabilization of a biologically active conformer (1). Degradation by peptidases may be decreased by destabilizing metabolized conformers. Biological selectivity may also be improved by increasing the preference for a conformer which interacts with a specific receptor but not with others which lead to different responses (4, 5).

Conformationally Restricted Somatostatin Analogs. For several years, we have been applying this conformation-activity approach to the design of analogs of the tetradecapeptide somatostatin (1). Somatostatin is a hypothalamic peptide which inhibits the release of insulin, glucagon, and growth hormone and also inhibits gastric acid secretions (6). These properties suggest potential utility in the therapy of diabetes and ulcers (7). Somatostatin has several shortcomings, however, deriving from peptide limitations already discussed. It is inactive after oral

administration and has a short duration of action after intra-
venous dosing. Multiple biological effects are produced with the
inhibition of insulin release being possibly the most serious
limitation. Finally, the size of the molecule makes its availability through chemical synthesis difficult and expensive. A
goal of the work in our laboratories was to obtain simplified
analogs with improved stability to proteases and oral activity.
A further objective was to develop compounds with selectivity for
inhibition of release of glucagon and/or growth hormone.

Studies leading to the development of highly active bicyclic
analogs of somatostatin such as 2 have been reported (8, 9).
Based on the potency of these conformationally constrained
structures, a working model for the bioactive conformation of
somatostatin emerged (10). Using this model as a basis with
input from computer modeling, further simplified cyclic hexapeptide analogs such as 3 with potency greater than somatostatin
were designed (11). These analogs have increased resistance to
protease degradation and show activity after oral administration.
Only five of the original fourteen amino acids of somatostatin
remain in 3 and synthesis of these cyclic hexapeptides is much
simplified compared to that of somatostatin. The present discussion will focus on recent results involving two types of conformational modifications of 3 designed from the hypothesized
bioactive conformation. These cyclo retro isomers and N^{α}-methyl
lysine analogs would be expected to possess additional protease
stability which could prolong duration of action. These studies
also provide a further test for the utility of the working
bioactive conformational model in analog design.

```
H-Ala-Gly-Cys-Lys-Asn-Phe-Phe-Trp
              |                   |
          HO-Cys-Ser-Thr-Phe-Thr-Lys
```

1

```
        ┌Cys-Phe-D-Trp
    Aha │    |         |
        └Cys- Thr- Lys
```

2

```
    X-Phe-D-Trp
    |        |
    Phe-Thr-Lys
```

3a, X=Pro
3b, X=N^{α}-Me-Ala

Retro Peptides

One approach to extending the duration of action of peptides
through stabilization of the structure to the action of proteases
has involved retro enantiomeric peptides (12) (see Figure 1). In
these compounds, the direction of the peptide backbone is
reversed and the chirality of each α-amino acid is inverted.
Linear peptides modified in this manner are termed "retro
inverso" analogs (13). The assumption underlying this approach,
which may not be generally true, is that only the side chains and
not the peptide backbone are important for eliciting the biological response at a given receptor. If good topographic correspondence between side chains of the parent peptide and its retro
enantiomer is possible, similar biological activities would be
expected for the two compounds. The latter structure containing
a number of D-amino acids should be more stable, if not totally
stable, to proteolytic degradation. In addition, a successful
application of this approach will yield considerable information
about the bioactive conformation.

Limitations. There are several limitations to the retro enantiomer approach (12, 13). If the amide linkages are involved in
important interactions with the receptor, reversal of the peptide
links would be expected to decrease receptor binding affinity and
therefore potency. For linear peptides, reversal of end groups
will be a problem; this is not the case for cyclic peptides such
as will be described in the present study. Secondary amino acids
such as proline or N^{α}-methyl alanine cannot be accommodated
directly by the approach since the substituent attached to the
α-amino group will always be misplaced. There is no guarantee
that the peptide backbone conformation of the retro enantiomer
will be similar to that of the parent peptide. A different set
of low energy conformations may be preferred in the modified
analog (14). Finally, even if conformation does not change,
nonequivalence of side chain topography may be a problem due to
small differences in corresponding peptide backbone bond lengths
and bond angles. We have demonstrated this nonequivalence with
the least squares fitting of the cyclic hexapeptide cyclo-(Ala-
Ala-Gly-Gly-Ala-Gly) and its retro enantiomer (15). Similar
comparisons using crystal structure data gave deviations from
topographic equivalence of similar magnitude (16). In spite of
the limitations of the retro enantiomer approach, we theorized
that its successful application should be possible through design
based on the overall shape of the molecules. The confirmation of
this idea through the design of modified somatostatin analogs
termed cyclo retro isomers (not enantiomers) (13) has now been
achieved (17).

Design of Cyclo Retro Isomeric Somatostatin Analogs. We have
described our working computer-generated model for the bioactive

conformation of cyclo-(Pro-Phe-D-Trp-Lys-Thr-Phe), **3a** (Figure 2)
(**18**). Key conformational features of this model believed important for biological potency include Phe-D-Trp-Lys-Thr and Thr-
Phe-Pro-Phe β-turns of Types II' and VI, respectively, the latter
containing a cis peptide bond between Phe[11] and Pro[6]. The model
of **3b** is very similar with N^α-methyl alanine replacing proline
(**19**) (see Reference **20** for definition of β-turns). In designing
cyclo retro isomeric analogs of **3**, we wished to retain the
overall shape of the molecule resulting from these turns and
their attendant side chain relationships. The analog of **3b**
obtained by reversing the peptide backbone and inverting all
amino acids is cyclo-(D-Phe-D-Thr-D-Lys-L-Trp-D-Phe-N^α-Me-D-Ala)
4 which would be expected to adopt a different shape due to
misplacement of the alanine N^α-methyl group (Figure 3) as has
been already discussed. Indeed, compound **4** was synthesized and
found to be about 0.1% as potent as **3b** (Table I) for inhibition
of growth hormone release in vitro. The misplaced N-methyl
probably results in a change in preferred conformation away from
the bioactive conformation. In particular, the crucial cis
peptide bond is likely to be trans in **4**.

  Examination of molecular models revealed that the desired
two β-turn conformation might be restored by moving the N-methyl
group from D-Ala[6] to D-Phe[11] in **4**. This change would permit the
key cis peptide bond to form in the proper location in the
backbone and should as a result achieve better overall side chain
correspondence with **3b**. The resultant structure, cyclo-(N^α-Me-D-
Phe-D-Thr-D-Lys-L-Trp-D-Phe-D-Ala) **5**, was prepared and in fact,
displayed a full biological response and had about 10% of the
potency of **3b** and 25% of somatostatin itself.

  At this point, we considered that good topographical correspondence to the Type VI β-turn of **3b** had been achieved in **5**, but
that adjustments to the β-turn containing the key tryptophan and
lysine residues at the other end of the molecule were still

Table I. Potencies Cyclo Retro Isomeric Somatostatin Analogs[a]

Cpd	Hormone Release Inhibition[b]				
	Growth Hormone in vitro		Insulin		Glucagon
3b	3.5	(2.6,4.5)	6.0 (3.8,10.9)		16.7 (4.3,200)
4	0.003	(0.001,0.005)	0.08 (0.03,0.17)		0.09 (0.0,0.50)
5	0.27	(0.2,0.36)	0.67 (0.31,1.3)		0.17 (0.04,0.4)
6	0.88	(0.7,1.10)	1.02 (0.41, 2.3)		0.3 (0.15,0.51)
7	2.4	(1.4,4.0)	0.8 (0.5,1.5)		1.3 (0.5,3.1)
8	1.59	(1.33, 1.92)	4.5 (2.3, 25.0)		6
9	Inactive		Inactive		Inactive

[a]Relative to somatostatin=1.
[b]For a description of assay methods, see Reference **11**.

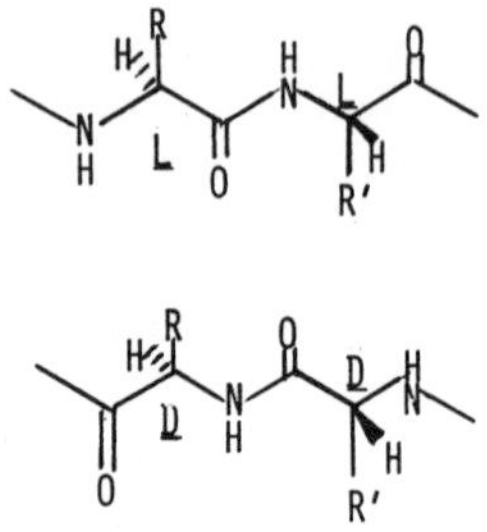

Figure 1. Retro enantiomeric peptides.

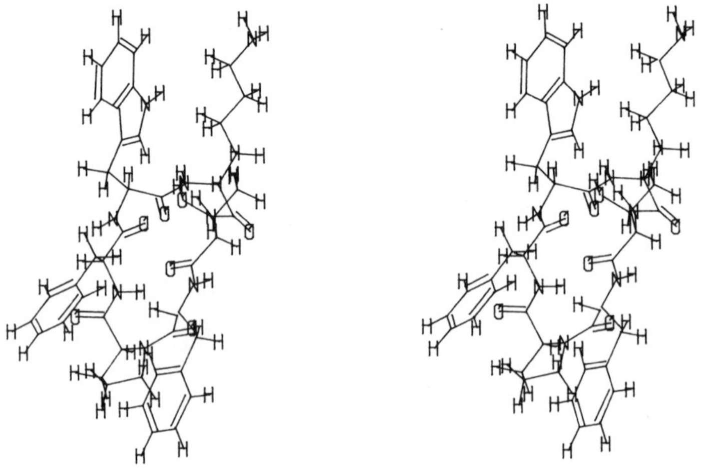

Figure 2. Bioactive conformational model of **3a**. (From Reference
19 with permission. Copyright 1983 by Munksgaard
International Publishers Ltd., Copenhagen, Denmark.

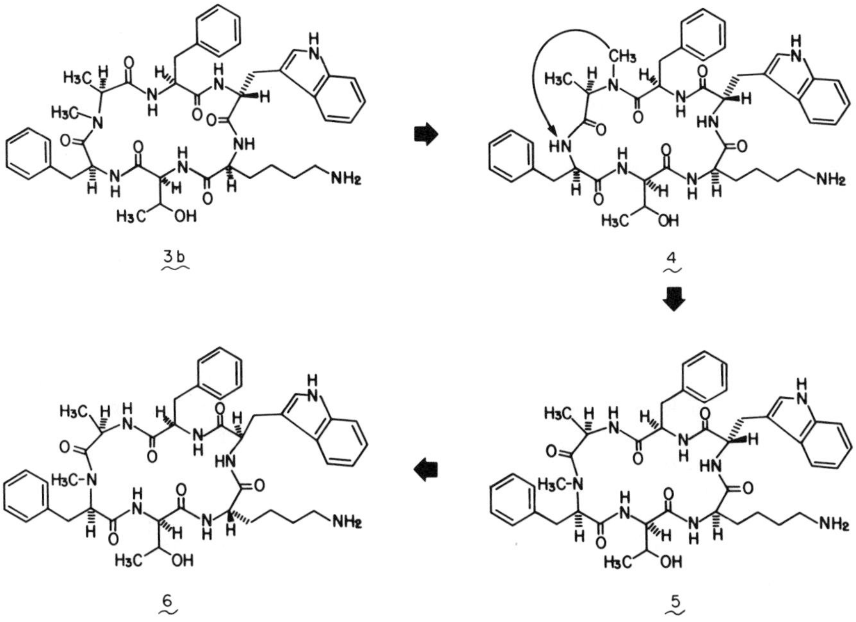

Figure 3.   Cyclo retro isomers of **3b**.

required. The D-Lys-Trp-containing turn in 5 would be predicted
to be Type II' (20). By inverting the chirality of these two
residues, a Type II β-turn should be favored. This turn is the
mirror image of the Type II' turn in 3b and might be expected to
provide a closer side chain correspondence to 3b. Such is
apparently the case since the analog cyclo-(N$^\alpha$-Me-D-Phe-D-Thr-L-
Lys-D-Trp-D-Phe-D-Ala) 6 displays 25% of the potency of 3b and
is of comparable potency to somatostatin. The correspondence in
side chain topography for the bioactive conformations of 3b and 6
must be quite good because these relative potencies reflect a
difference of less than 1 Kcal/mole of receptor binding energy.

The potencies of 4-6 for inhibition of release of insulin
and glucagon in vivo follow trends similar to the growth hormone
data although the absolute magnitudes are somewhat different.
The in vitro potencies are most likely to reflect relative
receptor affinities since protease degradation in this system is
minimized. Improved metabolic stability should, therefore, not
appear as enhanced potency.

The potency of 6 is still not equal to that of 3b and this
remaining difference could be due to the effect on conformation
of small differences in backbone bond lengths and angles for each
pair of corresponding amino acids (15). Alternatively, a hydrogen bonding contribution from the backbone may have been lost in
6. The results do indicate that the peptide backbone contributes
at most a small amount to receptor binding by somatostatin and
its analogs. Incorporation of known potency-enhancing modifications into 6 gave 7, cyclo-(N$^\alpha$-Me-D-Phe-D-Val-Lys-D-Trp-D-Tyr-D-
Abu), the most potent cyclo retro isomer of 3b prepared to date.
This analog is more potent than somatostatin and nearly as potent
as the parent structure 3b in the growth hormone assay.

It has been reported that the L-Trp analog of 3a cyclo-(Pro-
Phe-Trp-Lys-Thr-Phe) (8) and 3a itself are equipotent (21). In
light of the results with 5 and 6, it was of interest to prepare
the cyclo retro isomer cyclo-(N$^\alpha$-Me-D-Phe-D-Thr-D-Lys-D-Trp-D-
Phe-D-Ala) (9). This compound, however, was not active. This
difference in potency may be a consequence of 8 and 9 adopting
noncomplementary conformations (especially in the Trp-Lys
regions) in which correspondence of side chain topography is
poor. Even if 8 and 9 adopt the predicted Type I and I' turns
for Phe-Trp-Lys-Thr and D-Thr-D-Lys-D-Trp-D-Phe, respectively,
our analysis shows that the inherent shape differences are
greater than for the flatter Type II' and II turns of 3b and 6.
Such differences have also been observed in a comparison of
different types of β-turns in cyclic hexapeptide crystal structures (16). Additional studies will be required to elucidate the
degree of generality of the approaches described here for various
β-turn types.

Solution Conformation. Knowledge of solution conformation of
constrained peptide analogs has proven very useful for corre-

lating inferences about the bioactive conformation (18). In the present example, evidence has been obtained from proton NMR studies for the side chain topographic correspondence of 3 and 5 and 3 and 6 in solution. The NMR spectrum of 6 is shown in Figure 4. The upfield shift of the γ-methylene protons of lysine due to shielding by the indole of tryptophan has been postulated as important for good biological potency. As illustrated in Table II, this shift is observed for each of compounds 3-6 and provides evidence for similar side chain relationships for the Trp and Lys residues. Another diagnostic shift is that of the Ala β-methyl which for 3b is observed shifted upfield by 1.3 ppm due to proximity of the 11-position aromatic side chain. Both 5 and 6 also exhibit the high field methyl, but the major conformer of 4 does not. We conclude that for the two key β-turn regions of 5 and 6, the side chain relationships in water are very similar to those found in 3. The two β-turn structure for 6 is also supported by the observation of two solvent shielded N-H's (slow exchange in D_2O) assigned to D-Thr and D-Phe. A similar pattern was observed for 3 and is evidence for internally oriented possibly intramolecularly hydrogen bonded protons which are expected for the postulated β-turns (20). The NMR spectra of 8 and 9 also show shielded lysine γ-protons and 6-position β-protons, although the magnitude of the upfield shift for the former protons of 8 is less than for the other analogs. In this case, it appears that the solution data, which favor appropriate side chain relationships for bioactivity, do not correlate with the observed biological results (9 is inactive). Less information regarding the conformation of 8 than for 3 is currently available, however, and it would be premature to draw direct conclusions from these results.

Table II. Chemical Shifts of Upfield Shifted Protons in D_2O[a]

Cpd	Lys[9] γ-CH_2	Ala[6]-β-CH_3	Pro[6]-β-CH_2
3b	0.33, 0.52	0.20	–
4b	0.48, 0.98	1.28	–
5c	0.62, 1.05	0.20	–
6	0.53, 0.99	0.18	–
8	1.08	–	0.77 (1 H)
9	0.64, 0.79	0.35	–
Usual Position (22)	1.25	1.5	2.0

[a]Parts per million (ppm) relative to sodium trimethylsilylpropanesulfonate as internal standard. [b]Major conformer (∼75%); the minor conformer has a high field methyl resonance at 0.59 ppm. [c]One of 2 conformers observed (∼1:1 ratio); the second conformer does not exhibit shifts of this magnitude.

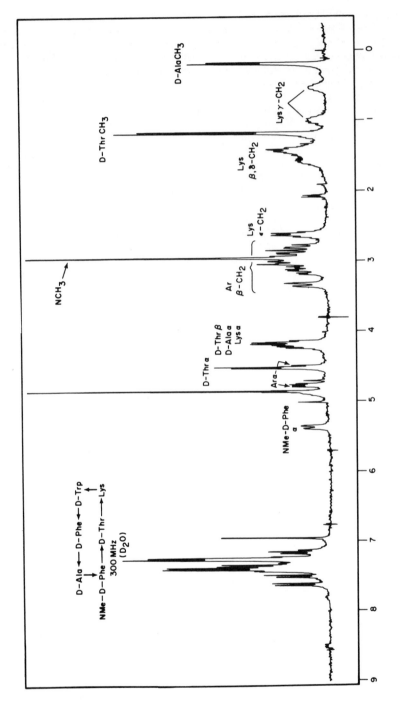

Figure 4.   Proton NMR spectrum of 6.

Both biological and solution data indicate that **3** and its cyclo retro isomers **5** and especially **6** have similar shapes, thus providing further support for the proposed bioactive conformation of D-tryptophan-containing cyclic hexapeptide analogs. These results show that the retro enantiomer concept can be applied successfully through design based on the overall topography of the molecules when sufficient conformational information about the parent peptide is available. The key modification in these examples was transferring the N^α-methyl from the 6- to the 11-position residue to circumvent the secondary amino acid problem discussed under <u>Limitations</u> and properly position the necessary Type VI β-turn. Chirality changes in the other β-turn further improved the overall topographical correspondence. Thus, through conformational modification, it has been possible to apply the concepts of Shemyakin (<u>12</u>) in spite of the inherent topographical differences between retro enantiomers.

Analogs **5-7** were stable to trypsin degradation under conditions where **3b** was cleaved with a half life of 80 hrs. This increased stability was not reflected in an increase in duration. Other processes, therefore, must be controlling the duration of action of these peptides <u>in vivo</u>.

<u>Synthesis</u>. The synthesis of cyclo retro enantiomer **6** is outlined in Scheme 1. Compounds **4, 5, 7,** and **9** were prepared by an analogous route. Initially, a protected linear hexapeptide was prepared by solid phase synthesis on 2% crosslinked polystyrene resin beginning with a protected lysine resin. The peptide was then removed from the polymer by hydrazinolysis. Cyclization was

Scheme 1. Synthesis of **6**

$$\text{H-D-Trp-D-Phe-D-Ala-}N^\alpha\text{-Me-D-Phe-D-Thr-L-Lys-O}\textcircled{R}$$

with Bzl and 2-Cl-Cbz protecting groups above Thr and Lys respectively.

↓ NH_2NH_2

$$\text{H-D-Trp-D-Phe-D-Ala-}N^\alpha\text{-Me-D-Phe-D-Thr-L-Lys-NH-NH}_2$$

with Bzl and 2-Cl-Cbz protecting groups above Thr and Lys respectively.

↓ 1) Isoamyl Nitrite
  2) Dilute
  3) Base
  4) HF, anisole

$$\text{Cyclo-(D-Trp-D-Phe-D-Ala-}N^\alpha\text{-Me-D-Phe-D-Thr-L-Lys)}$$

6

achieved using the azide method followed by anhydrous HF/anisole deblocking. The crude product was purified by silica gel chromatography and/or gel filtration on Sephadex G-25. Products were characterized by amino acid analysis and ^{1}H NMR and gave the expected M + H molecular ions by fast atom bombardment mass spectrometry. HPLC purity was >92% for all compounds except 9 which was 86% pure. For a detailed experimental procedure describing synthesis of cyclic hexapeptide somatostatin analogs, see Reference 19.

N^{α}-Methyl Lysine Somatostatin Analogs

The working model for the bioactive conformation of 3 accommodates a methyl group on the α-amino of lysine without obvious steric interactions. This noncovalent constraint should further restrict the conformation perhaps leading to greater protease stability and/or increased biological selectivity. It would also be another test for the necessity for the lysine N-H in receptor binding. In addition, a biologically active N^{α}-methyl lysine analog would provide further support for the proposed model of 3.

One precaution should be kept in mind for N^{α}-methyl amino acids. N-methylation of the peptide linkage results in the energy of the usual trans amide becoming comparable to that of the cis (23). The trans to cis transformation at a point in the peptide backbone results in a significant conformational change. This possibility must be considered in interpreting results based on incorporation of N^{α}-methyl amino acids.

To fully explore the potential of the novel N^{α}-methyl lysine in somatostatin cyclic hexapeptides, the four possible analogs containing D- and L-tryptophan and D- and L-N^{α}-methyl lysine combinations were prepared (See Table III). As predicted from the working model, the D-Trp-N^{α}-Me-L-Lys analog 10 was comparable in potency for inhibition of growth hormone release in vitro to the parent compound 3a. Surprisingly, the D-Trp-N^{α}-Me-D-Lys analog 11 was just as active. This result is in contrast to the D-Lys analog of 3a (12) which has about 3% the potency of the parent compound. Both L and D-N^{α}-methyl lysine analogs of 8 (13 and 14, respectively) are considerably less potent than 8 itself. The D-lysine analog of 8 (15) also shows low potency. As observed for the cyclo retro isomers, the insulin and glucagon results in vivo follow the same trends as the in vitro data with some differences in absolute potencies.

Solution Studies. The solution data for the N^{α}-methyl lysine analogs show conformational trends similar to those deduced from the biological data. Evidence pertaining to side chain and backbone conformation favors similar shapes for 10 and 3a in water. Proton NMR spectra for both compounds show high field lysine γ-methylenes (0.02, 0.33 for 10; 0.40, 0.55 for 3a) and single proline β- and γ-methylene protons (0.91, ∿1.1 for 10;

Table III. Relative Potencies of N^{α}-Methyl Lysine Analogs and Reference Peptides cyclo-(Pro-Phe-X-Y-Thr-Phe)[a]

Analog	X-Y	Growth Hormone in vitro	Hormone Release Inhibition Insulin	Hormone Release Inhibition Glucagon
10	D-Trp-N-Me-L-Lys	1.6 (0.7, 3.4)	0.5 (0.1, 1.8)	Active
3a	D-Trp-L-Lys	1.71 (1.31, 2.32)	5.2 (2.4, 11)	8.0 (1.4, 60.2)
11	D-Trp-N-Me-D-Lys	1.5 (1.2, 1.9)	0.4 (0.01, 1.9)	0.4 (0.1, 0.7)
12	D-Trp-D-Lys	0.05 (0.03, 0.08)	<0.07	<0.07
13	L-Trp-N-Me-L-Lys	0.1 (0.09, 0.2)	0.3 (0.1, 0.7)	0.2 (0.1, 0.7)
8	L-Trp-L-Lys	1.59 (1.33, 1.92)	4.5 (2.3-25.0)	6
14	L-Trp-N-Me-D-Lys	0.05 (0.04, 0.07)	<0.07	Low Activity
15	L-Trp-D-Lys	0.02 (0.01, 0.03)	<0.07	Low Activity

[a]See footnotes, Table I.

0.83, 1.0 for 3a) as well as proline α-methines (3.64 for 10; 3.54 for 3a). The circular dichroism (CD) curves have very similar shapes and intensities with the minimum for 10 at 6-7 nm higher wavelength than that for 3a (see Figure 5). The NMR spectrum of the N^α-methyl-D-lysine analog 11 shows high field absorption in 0.4-0.5 ppm range indicative of lysine γ-methylene shielding by tryptophan. In contrast, CD comparisons show the backbone conformation of 11 to be different from that of 3a, and also different from the D-lysine compound 12. Compound 13 exhibits multiple conformations in water based on the NMR spectrum and comparisons with the more potent 8 are not possible. Compound 14 shows largely a single conformer by NMR, and it does show high field Lys γ and Pro β and γ protons. There are a number of atypical chemical shifts in both the aliphatic and aromatic regions of the spectrum, however, indicative of changes from the usual conformational preferences in these cyclic hexapeptides.

Conformational Inferences. The biological activity and solution conformation results with analog 10 provide further support for the bioactive conformational model of 3 and for its utility in novel analog design. This same type of conformational modification (N^α-methylation of leucine) was successful in LHRH (24) which also contains a proposed Type II' β-turn in the receptor bound conformation (1). The high potency of the N^α-methyl D-lysine analog 11 was unexpected. Based on literature precedents (20), this compound would be predicted to assume a different β-turn from either the Type II' turn in the conformational model of 3 or the Type I β-turn which is likely in the active L-tryptophan analog 8. It also must be assuming a conformation different from that of the D-lysine compound 12, since this analog is much less potent and displays different chemical shifts in solution. The most likely explanation of these results is that the peptide bond between D-Trp and N^α-Me-D-Lys has become cis. Models indicate that this backbone conformation has side chain topography similar to that found in the model of 3. This type of cyclic hexapeptide conformation with two cis amides has been observed previously (25), although the L-X-L-Pro and D-Y-N^α-Me-D-Z combination is apparently unique.

As with the cyclo retro isomers, these studies have shown that there may be more than one peptide backbone conformation which can produce similar side chain topography. The N^α-methyl lysine analogs have also further confirmed that the N^α-H of lysine has no important role in receptor binding or conformational stabilization. These compounds did not, however, provide any advantage over 3 in biological selectivity or duration of action.

Synthesis. The novel synthesis of N^α-Fmoc N^ϵ-2-Cl-Cbz-protected N^α-methyl-DL-lysine was recently described (26). The synthesis

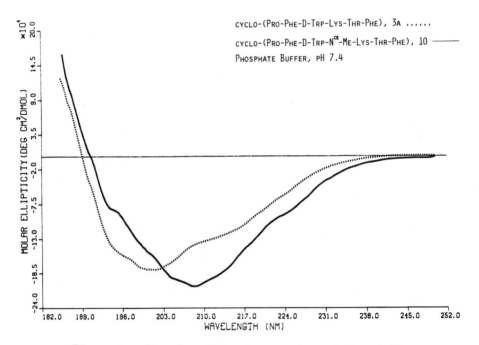

Figure 5.   Circular dichroism spectra of **3a** and **10**.

of the cyclic hexapeptides containing N^{α}-methyl lysine is shown
in Scheme 2. A standard solid phase synthesis through incorporation of the N^{α}-methyl lysine residue was followed. The Fmoc
protection was removed by treating twice, for 2 hr, with a 1:1
mixture of diisopropyl amine-DMF. The degree of completion of
this reaction was monitored by measuring the liberated dibenzo-
fulvene by UV determination at 255 nm. The hindered secondary
amine base was used rather than the more common piperidine to
avoid the possibility of any cleavage of the benzyl ester linkage
to the resin. Recent results indicate that this precaution may
have been unnecessary (27). After Fmoc removal, the resin was
divided into two batches for incorporation of D- and L-tryptophan, respectively. The remaining solid phase synthesis,

Scheme 2.   Synthesis of N^{α}-Methyl Lysine Cyclic Hexapeptides

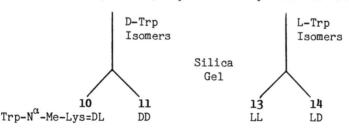

                    2-Cl-Cbz Bzl
                       | |
        Fmoc-N^{α}-Me-DL-Lys-Thr-Phe-Pro-O(R)

                    ↓   1:1 Diisopropylamine/DMF
                    ↓   2 x 2 hrs.

                    2-Cl-Cbz Bzl
                       | |
        H-N^{α}-Me-DL-Lys-Thr-Phe-Pro-O(R)

                    ↓ Solid Phase Synthesis

                            2-Cl-Cbz Bzl
                               | |
TFA•H-Phe-[D- or L]-Trp-N^{α}-Me-DL-Lys-Thr-Phe-Pro-O(R)

                    1) NH_2NH_2/MeOH
                    2) Isoamyl nitrite, DMF
                    3) Dilute
                    4) Base
                    5) HF

    c-(Phe-[D- or L]-Trp-N^{α}-Me-DL-Lys-Thr-Phe-Pro)

              D-Trp   L-Trp
              Isomers   Isomers

                        Silica
                         Gel

        10   11   13   14
Trp-N^{α}-Me-Lys=DL   DD   LL   LD

hydrazinolysis, azide cyclization, and HF deblocking followed standard procedures (19). The two pairs of diastereomers were purified and the isomers were separated by silica gel chromatography. Products were characterized by amino acid analysis and ^{1}H NMR. HPLC purity was >92% for 10, 11, and 14; 13 was 85% one component.

Conclusions

The utility of a bioactive conformational model has been illustrated for the design of novel cyclic hexapeptide analogs of somatostatin. Emphasis is on manipulation of the peptide backbone to eliminate undesired properties while maintaining necessary side chain topography. The working conformational model is re-evaluated on a continuing basis. This approach has the potential for more rational design of peptide analogs with improved properties as possible drug molecules. Carried to the ultimate, it would lead to the design of completely nonpeptide agonists or anagonists of the original biologically active peptide. Experience will tell whether this degree of modification will be required in order to obtain molecules with therapeutically useful properties.

Acknowledgments

We wish to acknowledge our colleagues who contributed to the ideas expressed here and to the synthesis, characterization, and biological testing of the compounds: C. D. Colton, D. S. Perlow, W. L. Whitter, W. J. Paleveda, B. H. Arison, R. Saperstein, C. D. Bennett, W. C. Randall, C. Homnick, S. L. Fitzpatrick, D. W. Cochran, J. L. Smith. We also thank M. Z. Banker for typing the manuscript and P. S. Anderson for his support.

Legend of Symbols

Abbreviations generally follow the IUPAC-IUB Commission recommendations. Abu, α-amino butyric acid; LHRH, luteinizing hormone releasing hormone; Fmoc, 9-fluorenylmethyloxycarbonyl; DMF, dimethylformamide. Numbering of amino acids in cyclic hexapeptides follows somatostatin numbering.

Literature Cited

1. Freidinger, R. M.; Veber, D. F.; Perlow, D. S.; Brooks, J. R.; Saperstein, R. Science 1980, 210, 656.
2. Marshall, G. R.; Gorin, F. A.; Moore, M. L. Annu. Rep. Med. Chem. 1978, 13, 227.
3. Freidinger, R. M. in "Peptides: Synthesis-Structure-Function"; Rich, D. H.; Gross, E., Eds.; Pierce Chemical Company: Rockford, IL, 1981; p 673.

4. Schiller, P. W.; DiMaio, J. Nature 1982, 297, 74.
5. DiMaio, J.; Nguyen, T. M.-D.; Lemieux, C.; Schiller, P. W.
    J. Med. Chem. 1982, 25, 1432.
6. Koerker, D. J.; Ruch, W.; Chideckel, E.; Palmer, J.;
    Goodner, C. J.; Ensinck, J.; Gale, C. C. Science 1974, 184,
    482.
7. Unger, R. H. Diabetes 1976, 25, 36.
8. Veber, D. F.; Holly, F. W.; Paleveda, W. J.; Nutt, R. F.;
    Bergstrand, S. J.; Torchiana, M.; Glitzer, M. W.;
    Saperstein, R.; Hirschmann, R. Proc. Nat. Acad. Sci. U.S.A.
    1978, 75, 2636.
9. Veber, D. F.; Holly, F. W., Nutt, R. F., Bergstrand, S. J.;
    Brady, S. F.; Hirschmann, R.; Glitzer, M. S.; Saperstein, R.
    Nature 1979, 280, 512.
10. Veber, D. F. in "Peptides: Proceedings of the 6th American
    Peptide Symposium"; Gross, E.; Meienhofer, J., Eds; Pierce
    Chemical Company: Rockford, IL, 1979; p 409.
11. Veber, D. F.; Freidinger, R. M.; Perlow, D. S.; Paleveda, W.
    J.; Holly, F. W.; Strachan, R. G.; Nutt, R. F.; Arison, B.
    H.; Homnick, C.; Randall, W. C.; Glitzer, M. S.; Saperstein,
    R.; Hirschmann, R. Nature 1981, 292, 55.
12. Shemyakin, M. M.; Ovchinnikov, Y. A.; Ivanov, V. J. Angew.
    Chem. Int. Ed. Engl. 1969, 8, 492.
13. Goodman, M.; Chorev, M. Acc. Chem. Res. 1979, 12, 1.
14. Momany, F. A.; Au Buchon, J. R. Biopolymers 1978, 17, 2609.
15. Freidinger, R. M.; Veber, D. F. J. Am. Chem. Soc. 1979, 101
    6129.
16. Van der Helm, D.; Hossain, M. B. in "Peptides 1982:
    Proceedings of the 17th European Peptide Symposium"; Blaha,
    K.; Malon, P., Eds.; Walter de Gruyter & Co.: Berlin, 1983;
    p 91.
17. Freidinger, R. M.; Colton, C. D.; Perlow, D. S.; Whitter, W.
    L.; Paleveda, W. J.; Veber, D. F.; Arison, B. H.;
    Saperstein, R. in "Proceedings of the Eighth American
    Peptide Symposium"; Hruby, V. J.; Rich, D. H., Eds; Pierce
    Chemical Company: Rockford, IL, in press.
18. Veber, D. F., in "Peptides: Synthesis-Structure-Function";
    Rich, D. H.; Grosse, E., Eds.; Pierce Chemical Company:
    Rockford, IL, 1981; p 685.
19. Freidinger, R. M.; Perlow, D. S., Randall, W. C.;
    Saperstein, R.; Arison, B. H.; Veber, D. F. Int. J. Pept.
    Prot. Res., in press.
20. Smith, J. A.; Pease, L. G. CRC Crit. Rev. Biochem. 1980, 8
    315.
21. Veber, D. F.; Randall, W. C.; Nutt, R. F.; Freidinger, R.
    M.; Brady, S. F; Perlow, D. S.; Curley, P.; Paleveda, W. J.;
    Strachan, R. G.; Holly, F. W.; Saperstein, R., in "Peptides
    1982: Proceedings of the 17th European Peptide Symposium";
    Blaha, K.; Malon, P., Eds.; Walter de Gruyter & Co.:
    Berlin, 1983; p 789.

22. Roberts, G. C. K.; Jardetzky, O. Advances in Protein Chemistry 1970, 24, 452.
23. Tonelli, A. E. Biopolymers, 1976, 15, 1615.
24. Ling, N.; Vale, W. Biochem. Biophys. Res. Commun. 1975, 63, 801.
25. Gierasch, L. M.; Deber, C. M.; Madison, V.; Niu, Chien-Hua; Blout, E. R. Biochemistry 1981, 20 4730.
26. Freidinger, R. M.; Hinkle, J. S.; Perlow, D. S.; Arison, B. H. J. Org. Chem. 1983, 48, 77.
27. Heimer, E. P.; Chang, Chi-Deu; Lambros, T.; Meienhofer, J. Int. J. Pept. Prot. Res. 1981, 18, 237.

RECEIVED December 5, 1983

Design of Kinase Inhibitors
Conformational and Mechanistic Considerations

GEORGE L. KENYON and REBECCA E. REDDICK

Department of Pharmaceutical Chemistry, University of California, San Francisco, CA 94143

General aspects of enzymatic reactions catalyzed by kinases are briefly mentioned. Many alternate substrates, competitive inhibitors and affinity labels based either on the structure of ATP or on the structure of the non-ATP kinase substrates are described. Several examples are presented that should be of particular interest to the medicinal chemist. Finally, the design of an affinity label for creatine kinase is reviewed as an example of how such information can be used in the search for agents directed at an enzyme's active site.

The design of a drug that acts by altering the activity of a kinase must begin with the study of the interactions of this class of enzymes with their nucleotide substrates, their co-substrates and regulatory molecules such as cyclic nucleotides. Once such interactions are adequately understood, enzymes can potentially be exploited in rational drug design in at least three ways. The most often used is that of enzyme inhibition, the main subject of this chapter. The second possibility is for the enzyme to be involved in the conversion of a biologically inactive molecule to one which is biologically active, i.e., the conversion of prodrug to drug. The third possibility, which has not yet been exploited, at least in a direct way, is that of activation of enzymes.

This chapter will briefly cover some important requirements and properties of the general enzymatic reaction catalyzed by kinases. There are many examples of the use of analogs of the common substrate, ATP, as probes of the conformational and steric requirements of kinase active sites. ATP analogs that function as affinity labels have been used as tools for pinpointing amino acid residues present at or near the active site. The kinases can be divided into three groups based on the type of non-ATP substrate phosphorylated enzymatically. Selected kinases from these three groups will be discussed with respect to studies using substrate analogs and inhibitors. These studies can be used in the design

0097-6156/84/0251-0189$06.25/0

of specific substrates or inhibitors of potential use as drugs. Lastly, the rationale for the design of a specific irreversible inhibitor of creatine kinase, namely epoxycreatine, will be reviewed.

Kinases are proteins whose catalytic function is the transfer of the γ-phosphoryl moiety of ATP to a particular acceptor:

$$R-X-H + ATP^{4-} \rightleftharpoons ADP^{3-} + R-X-PO_3^{2-} + H^+$$

Both ATP and the phosphoryl acceptor become reversibly and selectively bound to the enzyme during catalysis. So far, kinases that have been shown to react by direct phosphoryl transfer between ATP and the co-substrates show strict inversion of configuration at phosphorus, while those with a phosphorylated enzyme intermediate show retention of configuration at phosphorus ($\underline{1},\underline{2}$).

All known ATP-utilizing enzymes have a requirement of divalent metal cations for activity ($\underline{3}$), although the roles that these metal ions play have not been fully elucidated. Typically Mg^{2+} and Mn^{2+} are activating whereas other metal ions such as Ca^{2+} and Ba^{2+} are either less activating or inhibitory ($\underline{4-6}$). For all kinases one divalent cation is nucleotide bound. In addition, a few kinases have been shown to bind a second divalent cation that may be either activating as with pyruvate kinase ($\underline{7},\underline{8}$) or inhibiting as with cAMP dependent protein kinase ($\underline{9}$). It is the presence of this pair of cations at the active sites of these latter two enzymes that has allowed detailed NMR studies to be carried out and has aided in the formulation of detailed working models of their active-site geometries ($\underline{10-13}$). These studies will be discussed elsewhere in the chapter.

ATP: The Common Substrate

ATP and numerous ATP analogs have been extensively studied as substrates, inhibitors and as various other probes of the active sites of kinases. Efforts have been made to pinpoint the conformational and steric requirements of ATP at the active site of kinases in order to distinguish between general and specific characteristics of ATP binding.

ATP Triphosphate Chain Conformation. Much of the work in the area of ATP triphosphate chain conformation has been performed by Cleland and co-workers ($\underline{14-16}$). Their studies on metal(III)ATP interactions with kinases have led to the classification of kinases according to the stereochemistry of the polyphosphate chain as it binds to the active site. For the kinases they studied (hexokinase, glycerokinase, creatine kinase, phosphofructokinase, 3-phosphoglycerate kinase, acetate kinase, arginine kinase, adenylate kinase and pyruvate kinase) it was found that β, γ-bidentate chromium(III)-ATP (CrATP) and not α,β,γ-tridentate CrATP is a substrate. However, the tridentate isomer is a strong competitive inhibitor of some kinases (e.g., creatine kinase, phosphofructokinase, 3-phosphoglycerate kinase, and acetate kinase)(14). In addition, the two screw sense isomers of β,γ-bidentate CrATP (Figure 1a) were distinguished by the enzymes (14). Thus, hexokinase, glycerokinase, creatine kinase and arginine kinase are specific for the Λ isomer (Figure 1a-1) whereas pyruvate kinase, adenylate kinase and phosphofructokinase are specific for the Δ isomer (Figure 1a-2). Recently, cAMP dependent protein kinase has also been found to be specific for the Δ isomer (17).

Inhibition studies with CrADP complexes allowed these workers to conclude that hexokinase and glycerokinase both release MgADP as the β-monodentate form, whereas creatine kinase, pyruvate kinase, adenylate kinase, acetate kinase, 3-phosphoglycerate kinase, and phosphofructokinase all release MgATP as the bidentate form (14). Creatine kinase was specifically inhibited by isomer I (Figure 1a-3)(16) of bidentate CrADP, which is believed to be the Δ isomer. Thus, the mechanism for phosphoryl transfer with respect to the nucleotide bound metal appears to proceed according to two pathways. The first is the reaction of β,γ-bidentate MgATP to form β-monodentate MgADP and the second is the reaction of the bidentate MgATP to form α,β-MgADP (Figure 1b)(16).

Nucleotide Base Conformation. Using NMR data, a relationship between the degree of specificity and the conformation of bound ATP at the active site has been shown for a number of ATP utilizing enzymes. Two examples of these are cAMP-dependent protein kinase and pyruvate kinase (18,19). It appears that enzymes that exhibit higher nucleotide triphosphate specificity bind ATP so that the glycosidic bond angle(χ)(Figure 2a) is greatly distorted from its free solution value of 40-44°. Based on x-ray data cited in reference (18) hexokinase also appears to conform to this trend.

8-BrATP (Figure 2b) is an ATP analog in which the glycosidic bond angle (χ) is restricted such that the syn conformation of the base is greatly preferred (19,20). This compound has been found to be an alternate substrate, albeit a rather poor one, for several kinases (pyruvate kinase, hexokinase, phosphofructokinase, and adenylate kinase)(22,23). Isoenzymes sometimes display differential specificities for this analog (22). 8,5'-Cyclo-AMP and 8,5'-cyclo-ADP are analogs locked in the anti conformation (Figure 2c)(24). They are substrates for adenylate kinase and pyruvate kinase, respectively (25). In the case of adenylate kinase, 8,5'-cyclo-AMP is actually a better substrate than AMP itself, supporting the idea that the enzyme preferentially binds AMP in the anti conformation.

Non-hydrolyzable ATP analogs such as adenylyl imidodiphosphate (AMP-PNP, Figure 2d) and β,γ-adenylyl methylene bisphosphonate (CH$_2$-ATP,Figure 2e) have been used as inhibitors of kinases because they can bind in a similar manner to the natural substrate

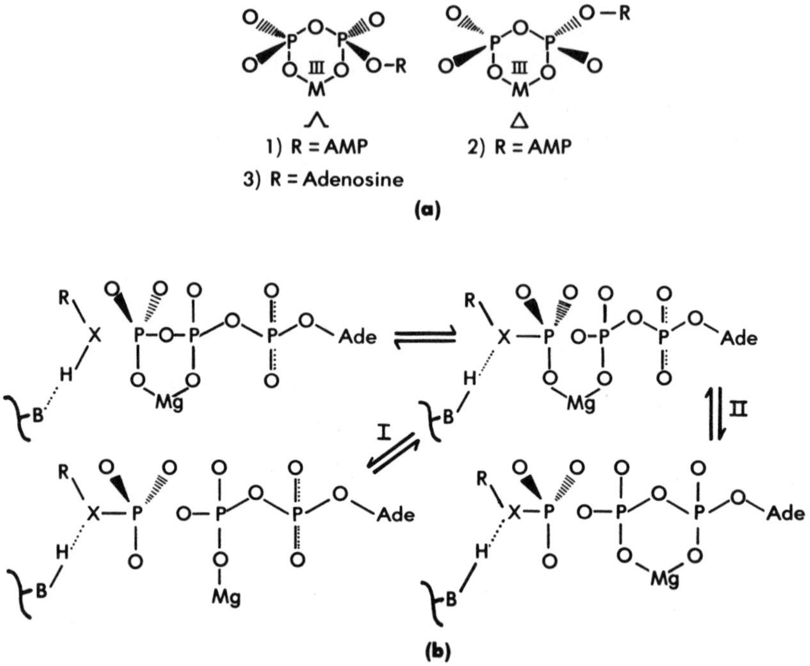

Figure 1. a) Structural isomers of β,γ-bidentate M(III)ATP and
     α,β-bidentate M(III)ADP complexes; b) Proposed mechanisms of
     kinases.

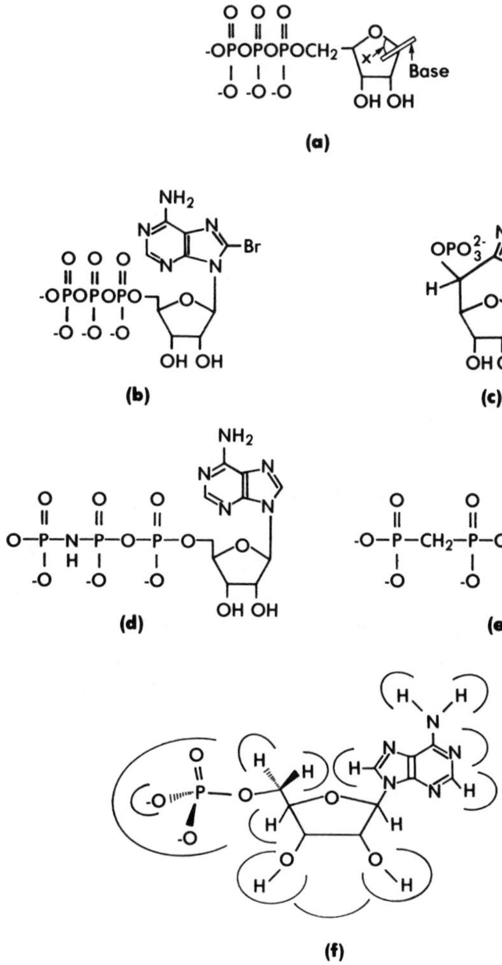

Figure 2.   a) Glycosidic bond angle(χ) in nucleotide triphos-
phates; b) 8-BrATP; c) 8,5'-Cyclo-AMP; d) Adenylyl imidodiphosphate; e) β,γ-Adenylyl methylene bisphosphonate; f) Regions of bulk tolerance explored by Hampton et
al(28-31).

yet do not undergo the phosphoryl transfer reaction (24). These analogs allow close-to-normal binding of the co-substrate and regulatory molecules so that the mode of binding of other substrates or co-factors can be investigated in the absence of phosphoryl transfer.

Exploration of Bulk Tolerance at ATP Sites. Non-covalent type inhibitors have also been used to study bulk tolerance around the ATP binding sites. In this vein Hampton and co-workers have both synthesized and tested as inhibitors a large number of adenine nucleotide analogs (Figure 2f) to probe the bulk tolerance at a number of positions on the parent compound (28-31). These compounds have been used to study systematically the isoenzyme selectivity of adenylate kinases, hexokinases, thymidine kinases and pyruvate kinases with respect to bulk tolerance at many sites on the ATP molecule. Some of the most isoenzyme specific results were obtained with pyruvate kinase isoenzymes K,L and M using ADP derivatives. Here 3'-OMe-ADP was found to inhibit pyruvate kinase preferentially with a ratio of inhibitory potency of 7.6:6.0:1.0 for the K,M and L isoenzymes ,respectively. Another compound, 8-NHEt-ADP, was selective for the M isoenzyme, giving a ratio of 7.1:1.2:1.0 for the M, K and L forms, respectively.

Affinity Labeling of Catalytic ATP Sites. Residues involved in ATP binding are potentially revealed by the use of affinity labels that are based on ATP's structure. Perhaps the most systematically studied of these compounds is 5'-fluorosulfonylbenzoyladenosine (5'-FSBA) (Figure 3a), which has been reported to label at least six kinases (32-41). In the case of rabbit muscle pyruvate kinase such work has indicated the presence of a tyrosine residue within the metal nucleotide binding site and an essential cysteine residue located at or near the free metal binding site (32). A similar reagent, 5'-FSBGuanosine, revealed the presence of two cysteine residues at the catalytic site of this same enzyme, both distinct residues from those modified by 5'-FSBA (33,34). With yeast pyruvate kinase both tyrosine and cysteine residues were modified by 5'-FSBA at the catalytic site (35), and with porcine cAMP-dependent protein kinase a lysine residue was labeled at the active site (36).

Unfortunately, as yet there emerges no clear pattern of a general role for these residues either in binding ATP or in catalyzing phosphoryl transfer. Indeed 5'-FSBA is not necessarily specific for the catalytic ATP site but rather has been shown in some cases to bind preferentially to regulatory ATP sites of kinases (37,38). Nevertheless, such labeling experiments do offer the possibility of characterization and comparison of peptide fragments from the site modified, whether it be catalytic or regulatory. A review of the use of 5'-FSBA with kinases and other ATP-utilizing enzymes has very recently appeared (42).

The affinity labeling reagent ATP-dialdehyde (Figure 3b) has

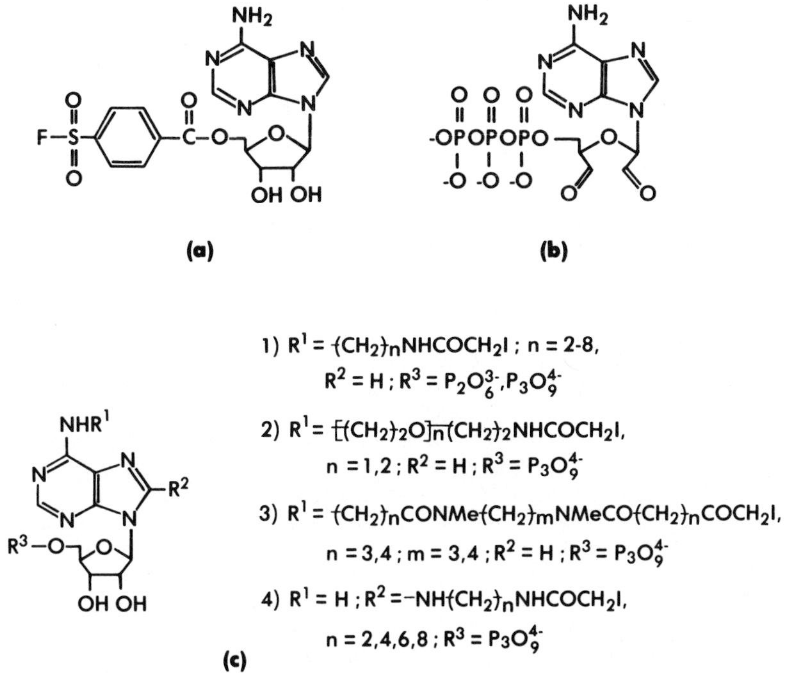

(a)

(b)

1) $R^1 = \{CH_2\}_n NHCOCH_2I$; $n = 2\text{-}8$,
$R^2 = H$; $R^3 = P_2O_6^{3-}, P_3O_9^{4-}$

2) $R^1 = \{(CH_2)_2O]_n(CH_2)_2NHCOCH_2I$,
$n = 1,2$; $R^2 = H$; $R^3 = P_3O_9^{4-}$

3) $R^1 = \{CH_2\}_nCONMe\{CH_2\}_mNMeCO\{CH_2\}_nCOCH_2I$,
$n = 3,4$; $m = 3,4$; $R^2 = H$; $R^3 = P_3O_9^{4-}$

4) $R^1 = H$; $R^2 = -NH\{CH_2\}_nNHCOCH_2I$,
$n = 2,4,6,8$; $R^3 = P_3O_9^{4-}$

(c)

Figure 3.   a) 5'-Fluorosulfonylbenzoyladenosine; b) Dialdehyde ATP; c1-c4) Potential exo-active-site-directed agents investigated by Hampton et al(47-50).

also been used for the purpose of identifying basic amino acid
residues at or near the ribose binding site(s) of creatine kinase,
pyruvate kinase and phosphofructokinase (43-45). It appears to
label a lysine residue in each case. With the latter two enzymes
it does not act as a straightforward affinity label since more
than one residue per active site is modified. Inactivation with
these two enzymes has been found to occur in the absence of either
$NaBH_4$ or $NaBH_3CN$; thus the product of the reaction of this reagent[4] with lysine is proposed to be a dihydroxy morpholine-like
adduct rather than a Schiff's base as has been found with other
enzymes (46).

Isoenzyme specificity for other parts of the ATP binding site
has also been examined . Thus ATP derivatives (Figures 3c1-3c4)
bearing an iodoacetamide on C-8 or N^6 with a spacer arm of varying
length (2-19 atoms) consisting of methylene, amide or ether
linkages were designed to inactivate specific isoenzymes (47-50).
These exo-active-site-directed reagents were tested for tissue
specificity on isoenzymes including the L, K and M rat pyruvate
kinases, four rat hexokinases and three rat adenylate kinases.
They were also tested for species specificity by comparing adenylate kinases from rabbit, pig and carp and adenylate kinases,
thymidine kinases, and hexokinases from yeast and bacteria. The
most isoenzyme-specific results were obtained for pyruvate kinase
isoenzymes M,K and L with compound 3c1(n=8), where the L isozyme
was inactivated to the extent of 80% while the M and K isoenzymes
were not affected (48). Similarly, with adenylate kinase from
rabbit, carp, and pig only the rabbit muscle enzyme (76% inactivation) was affected by interaction with compound 3c1(n=6), whereas
the other two isoenzymes remained unaffected (47).

Nucleic Acids As Cosubstrates

Of the kinases whose non-ATP substrates are nucleic acid derivatives thymidine kinase and adenylate kinase are perhaps the most
studied. Thymidine kinase is of interest because of the existence
of a specific cellular isoenzyme induced by herpes simplex virus-
I(HSV-I)(51). The strategy in drug design here is to search for
compounds that would both act as substrates for this enzyme and
exert their pharmacologic activities as their phosphorylated products (52,53). Analogs of thymidine, cytosine, uridine, guanidine
and adenine have all been investigated. Bulk tolerance and phys-
icochemical requirements of nearly all possible sites of these
analogs have been studied, and, as a result, a figure similar to
Figure 2f could be drawn.(54-58). For many of these a correlation
between the ability to function as substrates and as anti-HSV-1
agents has been examined (55,57,58).

Acyclovir is a particularly important alternate substrate for thymidine kinase:

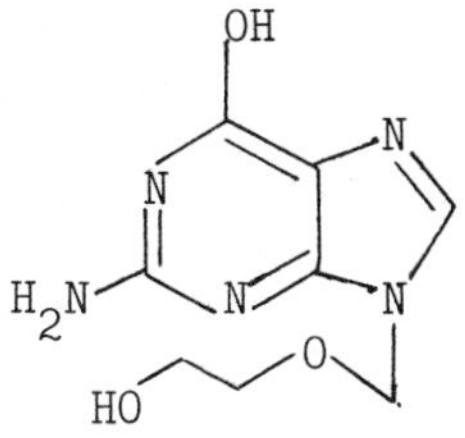

Because it exhibits such good antiviral activity along with low host toxicity, the binding, substrate and antiviral activities of many guanosine analogs differing in their 9-ring substituent have been investigated (57). Some compounds that are closely related to acyclovir, namely those differing by either addition of one or two methylene linkages on either side of the ether linkage, by a branched methyl on the distal side of the ether oxygen, or by substitution of -S or -CH$_2$ for the ether oxygen, were substrates. In contrast, those either with added branched hydrocarbon groups on the proximal side or with an amino functionality replacing the acyclic hydroxyl were not substrates. Analogs bearing cyclic 9-ring substituents on guanosine were also tested. Those with ribose and deoxyribose moieties were found to have low substrate activity, whereas those with arabinose (differing by having opposite stereochemistry at the 2'-OH) were found to have none. Adenosine and xanthine derivatives of acyclovir were inactive, with the exception of 9-(2-hydroxyethoxymethyl)-2-methylthioadenine. Mono- or dimethylation of N-2 of the guanosine moiety or substitution of N-2 by thiomethyl left reasonable activity (38-55%). It is interesting to note that for the pyrimidine bases the enzyme is quite specific for the natural deoxyribose moiety, whereas for analogs of the purine base guanosine, which is quite different from the natural substrate, the selectivity is altered greatly. Thus, it seems that the acyclovir analogs must be binding in a fundamentally different way from the natural substrate when they exhibit substrate activity.

Proteins and Other Polypeptides as Cosubstrate

The next class of cosubstrates for kinases consists of proteins. Protein kinases are very important in the regulation of cellular processes. Investigations of both these mechanisms and the roles that the protein kinases play might be aided by the use of selective inhibitors of these kinases. One indication of just how little is known about the characteristics of protein kinase-substrate interactions is the fact that many of these enzymes are named by their activators rather than by their substrates.

One protein kinase, namely cAMP-dependent protein kinase, has been extensively studied to relate primary polypeptide structure to substrate activity. The peptide sequences surrounding the phosphorylation sites (serine residues) in several protein substrates for cAMP-dependent protein kinases have been determined (59-61). Small peptide analogs of these have been synthesized and found to be substrates (60,62-64). Systematic substitutions, modifications and deletions of individual residues in these small peptides have revealed that multiple basic residues on the amino-terminal side of the phosphorylated serine residue are important in determining the substrate specificity of the enzyme (65).

NMR and kinetic studies have been conducted with the hope of providing more details about the position and conformation of the polypeptide substrate in cAMP-dependent protein kinase. These have served to narrow down the possible spatial relationships between enzyme bound ATP and the phosphorylated serine. Thus, a picture of the active site that is consistent with the available data can be drawn (12,13,66,67). Although these studies have been largely successful at eliminating some classes of secondary polypeptide structure such as α-helices, β-sheets or an obligatory β-turn conformation (66), the precise conformation of the substrate is still not known. The data are consistent with a preference for certain β-turn structures directly involving the phosphorylated serine residue. However, they are also consistent with a preference or requirement for either a coil structure or some nonspecific type of secondary structure. Models of the ternary active-site complexes based on both the coil and the β_{3-6} turn conformations of one alternate peptide substrate have been constructed (12). These two models are consistent with the available kinetic and NMR data.

The number of degrees of rotational freedom present in polypeptide substrates produces a staggering number of possibilities for substrate conformation, even when the peptide is small and many regular structures are eliminated. One way further to pinpoint the substrate conformation needed for optimal substrate or binding activity is to use conformationally restricted analogs (20). This idea has already been exploited in the use of proline and hydroxyproline in some of the synthetic peptide analogs mentioned earlier. However, no work has yet been done on nonpolypeptide analogs, and in particular, conformationally restricted analogs, but this may be a fruitful area for future research.

Studies similar to the substrate specificity studies outlined for cAMP-dependent protein kinase have already begun for other protein kinases such as cGMP-dependent protein kinase (68), phosphorylase kinase (69-71) and two tyrosine-specific protein kinases (72-75).

Small Molecules as Cosubstrates

The third class of cosubstrates for kinases encompasses substrates that are neither nucleic acid derivatives nor proteins, but are small molecules which serve many functions, often in energy metabolism. Rather than review substrate specificity for one representative enzyme of this class it may be more useful to give examples of some the most recent work on a few kinases with small, non-nucleotide substrates. Three enzymes mentioned in this section are involved in glycolysis (hexokinase, 3-phosphoglycerate kinase and pyruvate kinase) and one (creatine kinase) is involved in maintaining the energy reservoir in muscle cells which use large bursts of energy. Creatine kinase has been the most systematically studied of these enzymes with respect to its bulk tolerance and conformation of the non-ATP co-substrates. This will be discussed in detail later in this chapter as an example of how these types of studies can be used to map out the active site.

Hexokinase and pyruvate kinase constitute potential targets for chemotherapy since the predominant isoenzymes in highly neoplastic rat tissue in both cases are the fetal rather than the adult isoenzymes ($\underline{48}$). Isoenzymes of these targeted kinases have been compared and contrasted in their specificity for ATP analogs. But the search for agents selective for one kinase isoenzyme could also be conducted with analogs of the non-nucleotide cosubstrates. These substrates are more likely to be selective for single enzymes than are ATP analogs, which may affect many kinases and other ATP-utilizing enzymes. For example, there are significantly fewer enzymes which utilize PEP as substrate than ATP.

The substrate specificities of both mammalian and yeast hexokinases have been extensively studied ($\underline{76,77}$). Nevertheless, work in this area continues both in the search for isoenzyme specific inhibitors and in increasingly detailed investigations of the catalytic mechanism. Recently potential transition state analogs P1-(adenosine-5')-P3-glucose-6 triphosphate (Ap_3-glucose) and P1-(adenosine-5')-P4-glucose-6 triphosphate (Ap_4-glucose) were tested as inhibitors of four hexokinase isoenzymes. However, they were found to exhibit less affinity for the enzyme than either of the natural substrates alone ($\underline{78}$).

Nine other glucose analogs were systematically studied with yeast and mammalian brain hexokinases ($\underline{79}$). Five of these analogs exhibited substrate activity with the yeast isoenzyme, and two were found to be competitive inhibitors. Two of the alternate substrates were studied with the mammalian enzyme, but no significant differences were found.

In another recent study it was concluded that both the pyranose and the furanose forms of the alternate substrate 5-keto-D-fructose act as substrates. The pyranose form can be compared to glucose lacking hydroxyl at C-1 and having a second hydroxyl at C-2 (ketohydrate form). The furanose form is comparable to fructose but bears an extra hydroxyl moiety at C-5. Correcting for the amount of 5-keto-D-fructose in the pyranose form (98%), a K_m value for the furanose form could be calculated that is more than an order of magnitude smaller than that for fructose. This suggests that there is a favorable interaction between the enzyme and the additional C-5 hydroxyl. However, since no conclusive data for C-

5 specificity have been reported, more work is needed to assess accurately the effect of the extra C-5 hydroxyl (80).

The x-ray structure for yeast hexokinase is also available. Thus, glucose analogs are now being used to elucidate minute details of the catalytic mechanism. Recently D-xylose was used in crystallographic work to show that the 6-hydroxymethyl group of the natural substrate is necessary for substrate-induced closure of the active-site cleft (81). This induced closure, which is observed with glucose binding (82), is believed to be a part of the induced fit mechanism postulated for hexokinase (83).

Since the discovery that glycolate was an alternate substrate for pyruvate kinase (84), several other α-hydroxy acids have also been found to be substrates for this enzyme (85). This class of alternate substrates provides a new approach the problem of substrate specificity for pyruvate kinase. 3-Nitrolactate is one such alternate substrate. Interestingly, the phosphorylated product of this reaction inactivates the enzyme (86). However, 3-nitrolactate does not behave as a straightforward affinity label since covalent modification occurs nonspecifically. It is hoped that this new information may lead to the design of an affinity label of this enzyme, further serving to pinpoint amino acid groups at the active site.

Recently, it was reported that the fasciolicide MK-401 (4-amino-6-trichloroethenyl-1,3-benzenedisulfonamide) acts by inhibiting both phosphoglycerate kinase and phosphoglycerate mutase, thus effectively blocking glycolysis (87,88). This agent is a potent competitive inhibitor of phosphoglycerate kinase. In fact, the K_i value of 0.29 mM is three-fold lower than the K_m value for 1,3-diphosphoglycerate. Using computer-generated models (89), the structures of the natural substrate, 1,3-diphosphoglycerate, and the inhibitor, MK-401, were compared. The structures matched well when tne carbon skeleton of the substrate was conformed to fit the arrangement of the benzyl carbons of the inhibitor. Thus, this inhibitor may be considered a conformationally restricted analog of the natural substrate. Limited modifications of the MK-401 structure at the 6-position revealed a positive correlation between the size of ring substituent and potency as an inhibitor.

Affinity Labeling of Creatine Kinase: Rationale for the Design of Epoxycreatine

In the course of studying the mechanism of action of creatine kinase from rabbit skeletal muscle (M.M isoenzyme), Kenyon and co-workers (4,90) have been involved in the design of specific irreversible inhibitors that are active-site-directed (affinity labels). Creatine kinase catalyzes the reversible transfer of a phosphoryl group (the elements of "PO$_3$") from ATP to creatine, as shown in the following reaction:

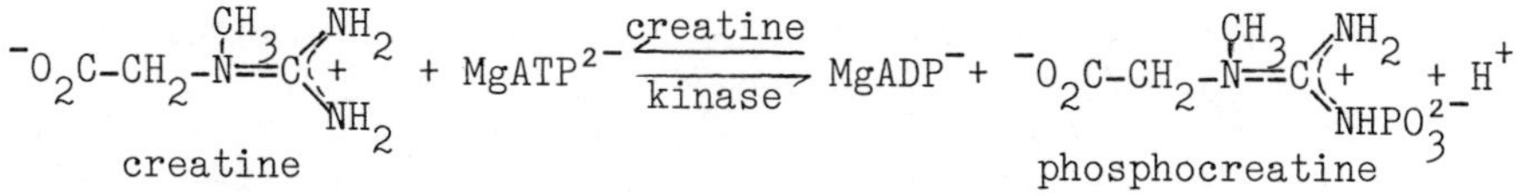

$$^-O_2C-CH_2-N=\!\!=\!\!C\Big\langle^{\substack{CH_3 \\ NH_2}}_{\substack{+ \\ NH_2}} + MgATP^{2-} \xrightarrow[\text{kinase}]{\text{creatine}} MgADP^- + {}^-O_2C-CH_2-N=\!\!=\!\!C\Big\langle^{\substack{CH_3 \\ NH_2}}_{\substack{+ \\ NHPO_3^{2-}}} + H^+$$

creatine   phosphocreatine

Efforts to synthesize an affinity label structurally related to creatine were stimulated by the lack of detailed information about the active site of creatine kinase. At the time of this writing, the complete primary amino acid sequence of rabbit muscle creatine kinase has not yet been published, although it may soon be forthcoming owing to developments in recombinant DNA methodology that should permit isolation and sequencing of the complementary DNA to its messenger RNA. But even when the primary sequence is known, the type of information provided by affinity labeling is important in pinpointing the substrate binding site(s) on the enzyme's surface.

The ability to inactivate creatine kinase with high selectivity in vivo should also permit detailed investigations concerning the bioenergetics of ATP-utilization in muscle action without the complicating features of the ATP-phosphocreatine interconversion. This has provided a second motivating force for finding an affinity label for the enzyme.

Designing specific enzyme inhibitors on a rational basis when one does not have a detailed three-dimensional crystal structure to which to relate is a rather sophisticated challenge. Some viable approaches to such a challenge are discussed in a review chapter by Santi and Kenyon (91). This discussion will focus on our rationale for the design of an affinity label for creatine kinase, namely N-(2,3-epoxypropyl)-N-amidinoglycine (epoxycreatine):

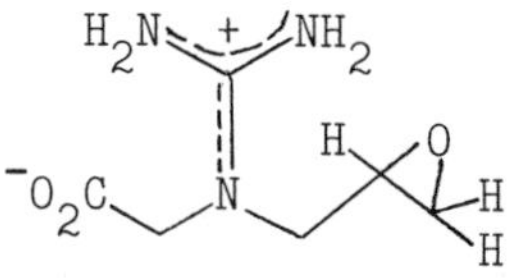

Exploration of Bulk Tolerance. Most affinity labels contain functional groups added to the substrate's basic structure. Discerning just where added bulk can be tolerated by the enzyme is therefore crucial information. In the case of creatine, it has been determined (92,93) that the structures below, for example, are good substitutes for creatine in the creatine-kinase reaction ($V_{max} \geqq 25\%$ that of creatine itself):

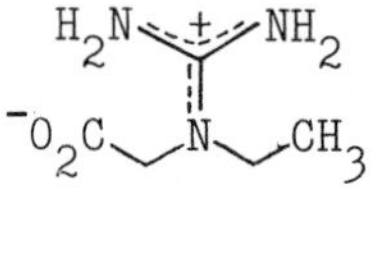

N-ethyl-   D-N-methyl-   cyclo-   D-N-
N-amidinoglycine   N-amidinoalanine   creatine   amidinoazetidine-
                                                      2-carboxylic acid

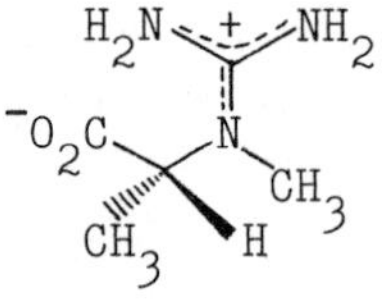

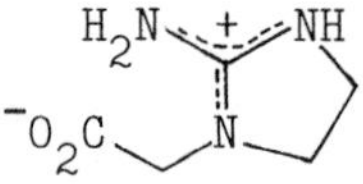

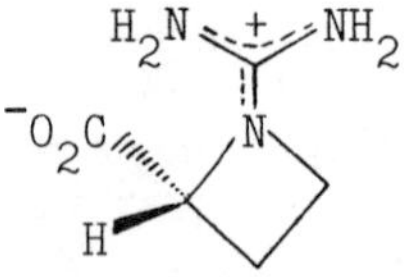

On the other hand, the following structures are some examples
that are very poor substrates at best:

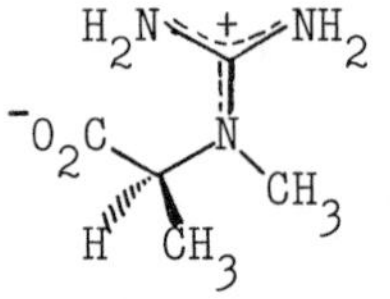

L-N-methyl-   N-methylamidino-   L-N-
N-amidinoalanine   N-methylglycine   amidinoazetidine-
                                               2-carboxylic acid

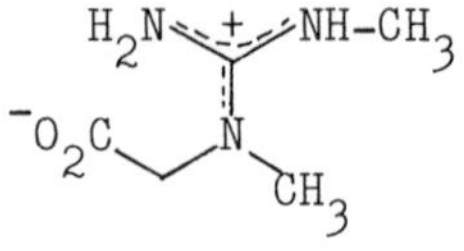

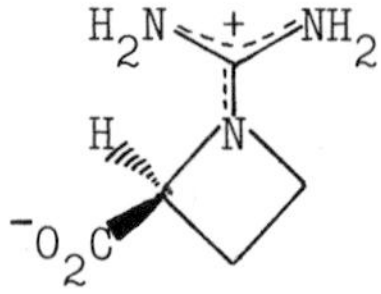

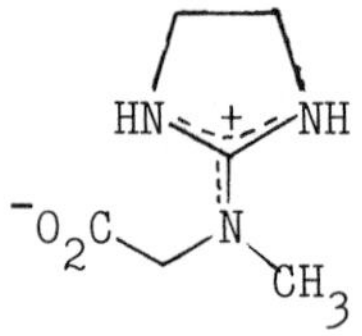

N-[2-(4,5-dihydroimidazolyl)]   D,L-2-imino-3-methyl-
       sarcosine   imidazolidine-4-carboxylic acid

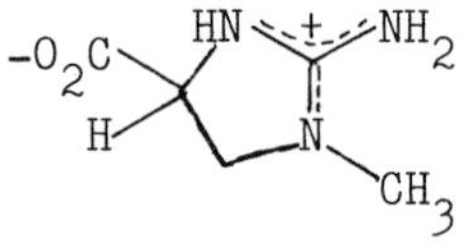

From these and other data, it is possible to propose a putative three-dimensional picture (see below)

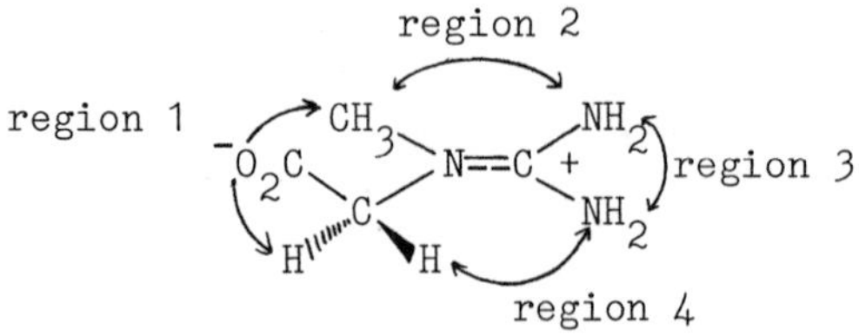

of creatine as it is bound to creatine kinase, and, moreover,
pinpoint regions where steric bulk, in the form of methylene
groups, can and cannot be tolerated (94). It should be emphasized
that this picture represents an absolute stereochemical projec-
tion.
       When single methylene groups are added to regions 1 and 2,
and four- and five-membered rings are formed, good substrate ac-

tivity is retained.   The   addition of methylene groups to regions
3 and 4 destroys all detectable substrate binding.   Even   an   N-
propyl can be added to the central, tertiary nitrogen atom, without obliterating activity.   With this steric information in hand
the stage was set for the placement of a reactive, alkylating
moiety (an epoxypropyl group) on this same tertiary nitrogen to
generate the affinity label, epoxycreatine.

Target Funtional Groups at the Enzyme's Active Site.   Shown in
Figure 4 is a possible structure of the   transition   state   for
phosphoryl transfer in the creatine kinase reaction.   The picture
in Figure 4 is a summary of most of the facts about the   enzyme's
active site (4) that are known at present.   Of particular interest
here is the tentative placement of a carboxylate group of the
enzyme juxtaposed against the guanidinium moiety of the   creatine
structure.   This carboxylate group is presumably that of either. an
aspartate or glutamate residue, although the carboxyl terminus of
the polypeptide chain cannot be ruled out.   This carboxylate
group has been implicated in the binding of creatine to the enzyme
by pH studies on the kinetic mechanism (95).   It may be involved
in polarizing the positive charge density on the guanidinium group
toward the tertiary nitrogen and, thus, away from the primary
nitrogen, the nucleophilic species that attacks the γ-phosphoryl
group of ATP in the transition state (4,95). Epoxycreatine, shown
below, has the indicated degrees of rotational freedom about its

$$H_2N \diagdown \overset{+}{\diagup} NH_2$$

$$^-O_2C \diagdown N \diagdown \diagdown \overset{H \diagdown O}{\diagdown} \overset{H}{\underset{H}{\diagup}}$$

epoxypropyl moiety.   It was felt that it could, by such rotations,
seek out an appropriate nucleophile at the active site.

Evidence that Epoxycreatine is an Affinity Label.   All the available evidence is consistent with the hypothesis that epoxycreatine
behaves like an affinity label for the enzyme and that it is
attacked by a carboxylate group of the enzyme.   That is, it inactivated the enzyme rapidly at 0°C.   Inactivation was complete and
activity did not return upon exhaustive dialysis.   Creatine was
shown to give protection against the inactivation in the expected
manner. Most importantly, though, the irreversible binding of the
inhibitor was shown to be stoichiometric using [^{14}C]-epoxycrea-
tine; that is, one and only one inhibitor molecule becomes bound
per active site, even in the presence of excess inhibitor.
       Additional evidence that epoxycreatine is capable of interac-
tion with the active site of creatine kinase is provided by the
observation that epoxycreatine can serve as a substrate in the

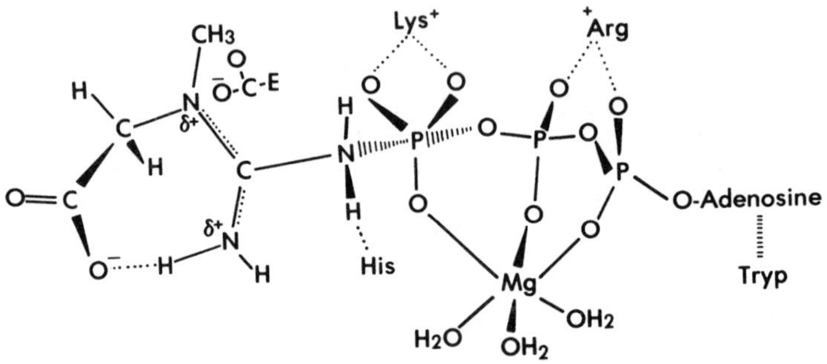

Figure 4. Possible structure of the transition state for phosphoryl transfer in the creatine kinase reaction. Adapted from Cook et al(95).

enzymic reaction. By coupling of the ADP production with the pyruvate kinase and lactate dehydrogenase reactions, Marletta and Kenyon (90) were able to compare the rate of the reaction of epoxycreatine as a substrate (turnover to generate phosphoepoxy-creatine) and the rate of inactivation by epoxycreatine. At 25°C a ratio of fifteen turnovers per inactivating event was found.

The enzyme could hydrogen bond to the oxygen of the epoxide ring and therefore mimic, to some extent, an acid-catalyzed reaction. This is illustrated below:

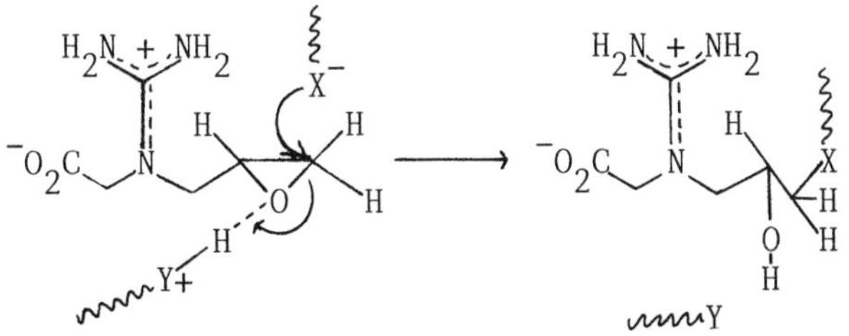

Here the group Y hydrogen bonds to the oxygen and the group X reacts with the epoxide ring carbon. The attack of X is shown at the least sterically hindered position on the ring; however, considering the potential constraints at the active site, reaction at the other position is certainly possible.

The evidence so far for epoxycreatine, although not definitive, suggests that a carboxylate group of the enzyme is the X⁻ group in the above scheme, generating an ester linkage (90). This is consistent with the finding that soluble carbodiimides rapidly inactivate the enzyme (96). Efforts are currently underway to isolate radioactive peptides from [^{14}C]-epoxycreatine-blocked creatine kinase and determine the amino acid sequence surrounding this putative ester linkage.

Literature Cited

1. Knowles, J., Ann. Rev. Bioch. 1980,49, 877.
2. Sheu, K.-F.R.; Richard, J.P.; Frey, P.A., Biochemistry 1979, 18, 5548-5556.
3. Mildvan, A.S., NMR Bioch. Symp. Opella, S.J.; Lu, Ponzy, Eds.; Dekker: New York, N.Y., 1979, Chapter 20, pp.345-56.
4. Kenyon, G.L.; Reed, G., Adv. Enz. Relat. Areas Mol. Biol. 1983, 54, 367-426.
5. Bloxham, D.P.; Lardy, H.A., in "The Enzymes"; Boyer, P.D., Ed.; Academic:New York, 1973; 8, p.247.
6. Scopes, R.K., in "The Enzymes"; Boyer, P.D., Ed.; Academic :New York, 1973; 8, p.349.
7. Gupta, R.K.; Fung, C.H.; Mildvan, A.S., J. Biol. Chem. 1976, 251, 2421-2430.
8. Gupta, R.K.; Oesterling, R.M.; Mildvan, A.S., Biochemistry 1976, 15,2881-2887.

9. Armstrong, R.N., Biochemistry 1979, 18, 1230-1238.
10. Gupta, R.K.; Benovic, J.L., J. Biol. Chem. 1978, 253, 8878-8886.
11. Gupta, R.K.; Mildvan, A.S., J. Biol. Chem. 1977, 252, 5967.
12. Granot, J.;Mildvan, A.S.; Bramson, N.H.; Thomas, N.; Kaiser, E.T., Biochemistry 1981, 20, 602-610.
13. Granot, J.; Mildvan, A.S.; Bramson, H.N.; Kaiser, E.T. Biochemistry 1980, 19, 3537-3543.
14. Dunaway-Mariano, D.; Cleland, W.W., Biochemistry 1980, 19, 1506-1515.
15. Cornelius, R.D.; Cleland, W.W., Biochemistry 1978, 17, 3279-3286.
16. Dunaway-Mariano, D.; Cleland, W.W. Biochemistry 1980, 19, 1496-1505.
17. Granot, J.; Mildvan, A.S., FEBS Letters 1979, 103, 265-269.
18. Mildvan, A.S., Phil. Trans. R. Soc. Lond.B 1981, 293, 65-74.
19. Granot, J.; Kondo, H; Armstrong, R.N.; Mildvan, A.S.; Kaiser, E.T., Biochemistry 1979, 18, 2339.
20. Kenyon, G.L.; Fee, J.A., in "Physical Organic Chemistry"; Streitweiser, Jr., A.; Taft, R.W., Eds.; John Wiley & Sons, Inc., 1973; 10, pp.381-410.
21. Tavale, S.S.; Sobell, H.M., J. Mol. Biol. 1970, 48, 109-123.
22. Lascu, I.; Kezdi, M.; Goia, I.; Jebeleanu, G.; Barzu, O.; Pansini, A.; Papa, S.; Mantsch, H.H., Biochemistry 1979, 18, 4818-4826.
23. Danenberg, K.; Cleland, W.W., Biochemistry 1975, 14, 28-39.
24. Yount, R.G.,Adv.Enz. Relat. Areas Mol. Biol. 1975, 43, 1-56.
25. Hampton, A.; Harper, P.J.; Sasaki, R., Biochemistry 1972, 11, 4965-4969.
26. Yount, R.G.; Babcock, D.; Ballantyne, W.; Ojala, D., Biochemistry 1971,10, 2484-2489.
27. Glöggler, K.G.; Fritzsche, T.M.; Huth, H.; Trommer, W.E., H-S Z. Physiol. Chem. 1981, 362, 1561-1565.
28. Hampton, A.; Slotin, L.A.; Kappler, F.; Sasaki, T.; Perini, F., J. Med. Chem. 1976,19, 1371-1377.
29. Hampton, A.; Picker, D., J. Med. Chem. 1979, 22, 1529-1532.
30. Hai, T.T.; Picker, D.; Abo, M.; Hampton, A., J. Med. Chem. 1982, 25, 806-812.
31. Hai, T.T.; Abo, M.; Hampton, A.S., J. Med.Chem. 1982, 25, 1184-1188.
32. Annamalai, A.E.; Colman, R.F., J. Biol. Chem. 1981, 256, 10276-10283.
33. Tomich, J.M.; Marti, C.; Colman, R.F., Biochemistry 1981, 20, 6711-6720.
34. Annamalai, E.A.; Tomich, J.M.; Mas, M.T.; Colman, R.F., Arch. Biochem. Biophys. 1982, 219, 47-57.
35. Likos, J.J.; Hess, B.; Colman, R.F., J. Biol. Chem. 1980, 255, 9388-9398.
36. Zoller, M.J.; Taylor, S.S., J. Biol. Chem. 1979, 254, 8363-8368.

37. Pettigrew, D.W.; Frieden, C., J. Biol. Chem. 1978, 253, 3623-3627.

38. Mansour, T.E.; Martensen, T.M., J. Biol. Chem. 1978, 253, 3628-3634.

39. King, M.M.; Carlson, G.M., FEBS Letters 1982, 140, 131-134.

40. Hixson, C.G.; Krebs, E.G., J. Biol. Chem. 1979, 254,7509-7514.

41. Buhrow, S.A.; Cohen, S.; Staros, J.V., J. Biol. Chem. 1982, 257, 4019-4022.

42. Colman, R.F., Ann. Rev. Biochem. 1983, 52,67-91.

43. Hinrichs, M.V.; Eyzaguirre, J., Bioch. Bioph. Acta 1982, 704, 177:185.

44. Gregory, M.R.; Kaiser, E.T., Arch. Bioch. Bioph. 1979, 196, 199-208.

45. Nevinsky, G.A.; Gazaryants, M.G.; Mkrtchyan, Z.S., Bioorg. Khim. 1983, 9, 487-495.

46. Evans, C.T.; Goss, N.H.; Wood, H.G., Biochemistry 1980, 19, 5809-5814.

47. Hampton, A.; Slotin, L.A.; Chawla, R.R., J. Med. Chem. 1976, 19, 1279-1283.

48. Hampton, A.; Kappler, F.; Maeda, M.; Patel, A.D., J. Med. Chem. 1978, 21,1137-1140.

49. Hampton, A.; Picker, D.; Nealy, K.A.; Maeda, M., J. Med. Chem. 1982, 25, 382-386.

50. Hampton, A.; Patel, A.D.; Chawla, R.R.; Kappler, F.; Hai, T.T., J. Med. Chem. 1982, 25, 386-392.

51. Cheng, Y.-C., in "Antimetabolites in Biochem., Biol., and Medicine"; Skoda, J.; Langen, P.; Pergamon Press, Ltd.: Oxford, 1979; pp.263-274.

52. Cheng, Y.-C.; Ostrander, M.; Derse, D.; Chen, J.-Y., in "Nucleoside Analogs: Chemistry, Biology and Medical Applications", Walker, R.T.; Clercq, Eric de; Eckstein, F., Eds.; NATO Adv. Study Inst. Ser., Ser. A A26, NATO Adv. Study Inst., 1979, pp.319-336.

53. Cheng, Y.-C., Grill, S.; Ruth, J.; Bergstrom, D.E., Antimicrob. Agents and Chemother. 1980, 18, 957-961.

54. Hampton, A.; Kappler, F.; Chawla, R.R., J. Med. Chem. 1982, 25, 621-631.

55. Cheng, Y.-C.; Dutschman, G.; Fox, J.J.; Watanabe, K.A.; Machida, H., Antimicrob. Agents Chemother. 1981, 20, 420-423.

56. Hampton, A.; Kappler, F.; Chawla, R.R., J. Med. Chem., 1979,22, 1524-1528.

57. Keller, P.M.; Fyfe, J.A.; Beauchamp, L.; Lubbers, C.M.; Furman, P.A.; Schaeffer, H.J.; Elion, G.B., Biochem. Pharmac. 1981, 30, 3071-3077.

58. Ashton, W.T.; Karkas, J.D.; Field, A.K.; Tolman, R.L.,Bioch. Biophys. Res. Comm. 1982, 108, 1716-1721.

59. Hjelmquist, G.; Andersson, J.; Edlund, B.; Engström, L., Biochem. Biophys. Res. Commun. 1974, 61, 559-563.

60. Kemp, B., J. Biol. Chem. 1979, 254, 2638-2642.

61. Cohen, P.; Rylatt, D.B.; Nimmo, G.A., FEBS Letters 1977, 76, 182-186.
62. Zetterquist, Ö.; Ragnarsson, U.; Humble, E.; Berglund, L.; Engström, L., Bioch. Bioph. Res. Comm. 1976, 70, 696-703.
63. Matsuo, M.; Huang, C.-H.; Huang, L.C., Bioch. J. 1978,173, 441-447.
64. Kemp, B.E.; Rae, I.C.; Minasian, E.; Leach, S.J., in "Pept. Struct. Biol. Funct.", Gross, E.; Meienhofer, J., Eds.; Proc. Am. Pept. Symp., 6th, 1979, Pierce Chem. Co.: Rockford, Ill., pp.169-172.
65. Kemp, B.E.; Graves, D.J.; Benjamini, E.; Krebs, E.G., J. Biol. Chem. 1977, 252, 4888-4844.
66. Granot, J.; Mildvan, A.S.; Kaiser, E.T., Arch. Bioch. Bioph. 1980, 205, 1-17.
67. Kaiser, E.T.; Armstrong, R.N.; Bolen, D. W.; Bramson, H.N.; Kondo, H.; Stingelin, J.; Thomas,N.; Granot, J.; Mildvan, A.S., in "Protein Phosphorylation"; Rosen, O.M.; Krebs, E.G., Eds.; Cold Spring Harbor Conf. on Cell Prolif. 19, Cold Spring Harbor Laboratory 1981; pp.67-81.
68. Glass, D.B.; Krebs, E.G., J. Biol. Chem. 1982, 257, 1196-1200.
69. Viriya, J.; Graves, D.J., Bioch. Biophys. Res. Comm. 1979, 87, 17-24.
70. Tessmer, G.W.; Shuster, J.R.; Tabatabai, L.B.; Graves, D.J., J. Biol. Chem. 1977, 252, 5666-5671.
71. Chan, J.K.-F.; Hurst, M.O.; Graves, D.J., J. Biol. Chem. 1982, 257, 3655-3659.
72. Hunter, T., J.Biol. Chem. 1982,257, 4843-4848.
73. Casnellie, J.E.; Harrison, M.L.; Pike, L.J.; Hellström, K.E.; Krebs, E.G., Proc. Natl. Acad. Sci., USA 1982, 79, 282-286.
74. Kilimann, M.W.; Heilmeyer, Jr., M.G., Biochemistry 1982, 21, 1735-1739.
75. Wong, T.W.; Goldberg, A.R., J. Biol. Chem. 1983, 258, 1022-105.
76. Purich, D.L.; Fromm, H.J.; Rudolph, F.B., Adv. Enz. Relat. Areas Mol. Biol. 1973, 39, 250-319.
77. Colowick, S.P. in "The Enzymes", Boyer, P.D., Ed.; 3rd Ed.; Acad. Press, N.Y. 1973, 9, 1-46.
78. Hampton, A.; Hai, T.T.; Kappler, F.; Chawla, R.R.,J. Med. Chem. 1982, 25, 801-805.
79. Machado, E.E.; Sols, A., FEBS Letters 1980, 119, 174-176.
80. Blanchard, J.S.; Brewer, C.F.; Englund, S.; Avigad, G., Biochemistry 1982, 21, 75-81.
81. Shoham, M.; Steitz, T.A., Bioch. Biophys. Acta 1982, 705, 380-384.
82. Bennett, Jr., W.S.; Steitz, T.A., Proc. Natl. Acad. Sci. 1978, 75, 4848-4852.
83. Koshland, D.E., in "The Enzymes", Boyer, P.D.; Lardy, H.; Myrbäck, K., 2nd Ed., Acad. Press, 1959, 1, 305-346.
84. Kayne, F.J., Bioch. Biophys. Res. Comm. 1974, 59, 8-13.

85. Ash, D.E.; Goodhart, P.J.; Řeed, G.H., <u>Arch. Bioch.Biophys.</u>, in press.
86. Porter, D.J.T.; Ash, D.E.; Bright, H.J., <u>Arch. Bioch. Biophys.</u> 1983, <u>222</u>, 200-206.
87. Schulman, M.D,; Valentino,D., <u>Exp. Parasitol.</u> 1980, <u>49</u>, 206-215.
88. Schulman, M.D.; Ostlind, D.A.; Valentino, D., <u>Mol. Bioch. Parasit.</u> 1982, <u>5</u>, 133-145.
89. Gund, P.; Andose, J.D.; Rhodes, J.B.; Smith, G.M., <u>Science</u> 1980, <u>280</u>, 1425-1431.
90. Marletta, M.A.; Kenyon, G.L., <u>J. Biol. Chem.</u> 1979, <u>254</u>, 1879-1886.
91. Santi, D.V.; Kenyon, G.L., in "Burger's Medicinal Chemistry"; Wolff, M.E., Ed.; Wiley-Interscience; New York, 1980; 4th Edition, Vol.I, pp.349-391.
92. Rowley, G.L.; Greenleaf, A.L.; Kenyon, G.L., <u>J. Am. Chem. Soc.</u> 1971, <u>93</u>, 5542-52.
93. McLaughlin,A.D.; Cohn, M.; Kenyon, G.L., <u>J. Biol. Chem.</u> 1972, <u>247</u>, 4382.
94. Dietrich, R.F.; Miller, R.B.; Kenyon, G.L.; Leyh, T.S.; Reed, G.H., <u>Biochemistry</u> 1980, <u>19</u>, 3180.
95. Cook, P.F.; Kenyon, G.L.; Cleland, W.W., <u>Biochemistry</u> 1981, <u>20</u>, 1204-1210.
96. Nguyen, A.C.; Kenyon, G.L., unpublished data.

RECEIVED November 15, 1983

Design and Discovery of Aspartyl Protease Inhibitors
Mechanistic and Clinical Implications

DANIEL H. RICH, FRANCESCO G. SALITURO, and MARK W. HOLLADAY

School of Pharmacy, University of Wisconsin–Madison, Madison, WI 53706

PAUL G. SCHMIDT

Oklahoma Medical Research Foundation, Oklahoma City, OK 73104

The synthesis and mechanism of action of four new aspartyl protease inhibitors related to pepstatin are described. A lysine side-chain analog of statine (DAHOA) in a pepstatin derivative increases binding to penicillopepsin 100-fold but decreases binding to pepsin 100-fold. Statine is an analog of a dipeptide reaction pathway intermediate because a hydroxyethylene isostere of a dipeptide can replace statine in inhibitors without diminishing binding to pepsin or renin. Pepstatin analogs containing the new statine derivative, 3-methylstatine, inhibit aspartyl proteases most effectively when C-3 has the R configuration, suggesting a new mechanism for inhibition of this enzyme class. NMR studies of ^{13}C labeled ketone analogs of statine bound to porcine pepsin provide evidence for a general acid-general base catalyzed mechanism for hydrolysis of peptide substrates by aspartyl proteases.

0097–6156/84/0251–0211$07.75/0

Novel protease inhibitors are needed in increasing numbers for
medical and biochemical applications. The successful treatment
of hypertension with angiotensin converting enzyme inhibitors
(e.g., Captopril) (1) and the use of protease inhibitors to
elucidate mechanisms of enzyme action (2) and peptide biosynthesis provide three examples where these compounds have proven
most valuable. New strategies for designing protease inhibitors are needed in addition to a greater understanding of how
known inhibitors bind to enzymes. Together these efforts can
lead to signficant advances in enzymology and medicinal
chemistry.

At the present time, most efforts at designing protease
inhibitors start by synthesizing analogs of enzymatic reaction
intermediates, e.g., tetrahedral intermediates, collected substrates or collected products. Several potent inhibitors of
proteases have been prepared in this way, including Captopril
and Enalapril (3), two clinically useful inhibitors of angiotensin converting enzyme, and KetoACE, a ketomethylene analog
of an inhibitor of ACE.(4) The former two compounds are related to a stable combination of the two products derived from
hydrolysis of angiotensin I by ACE more than to the transition
state or tetrahedral intermediate for amide bond hydrolysis and
thus can be classified as collected-product (bi-product) enzyme
inhibitors.(2) Other protease inhibitors have been designed to
more closely mimic a presumed tetrahedral intermediate for
amide hydrolysis. Examples of these include the peptide phos-
phoramide derivatives described by Galardy (5) and Bartlett.(6)
Inhibitors of other enzymes, e.g., enkephalinases (7) also have
been developed by these approaches.

An alternative approach for designing inhibitors begins
with naturally occurring inhibitors. The objective is to modify the parent structure to achieve selectivity for a particular enzyme without sacrificing the potency of the parent structure. This approach has been applied less often because only a
few naturally occurring inhibitors of proteases have been discovered (e.g., pepstatin, bestatin and amastatin, phosphoramidon, and the peptide aldehydes related to leupeptin) (8) and
because the relationships between most naturally-occurring inhibitor structures and the structure of either substrates or
reaction pathway intermediates are not always apparent. For
example, pepstatin [Iva-Val-Val-Sta-Ala-Sta, 1; Sta=statine:
(3S,4S)-4-amino-3-hydroxy-6-methylheptanoic acid, 2] inhibits
most aspartyl proteases with dissociation constants generally
in the range of 0.1 to 1 nM, renin being a notable exception
($K_i \sim 10^{-6}$M). The central Sta residue contains structural
features, particularly a tetrahedral carbon at C-3 bearing a
hydroxyl group in the pro-S position, which are essential for
tight-binding inhibition.(9) On the basis of structural similarities between the central Sta and the tetrahedral intermediate for amide bond hydrolysis, it has been postulated that

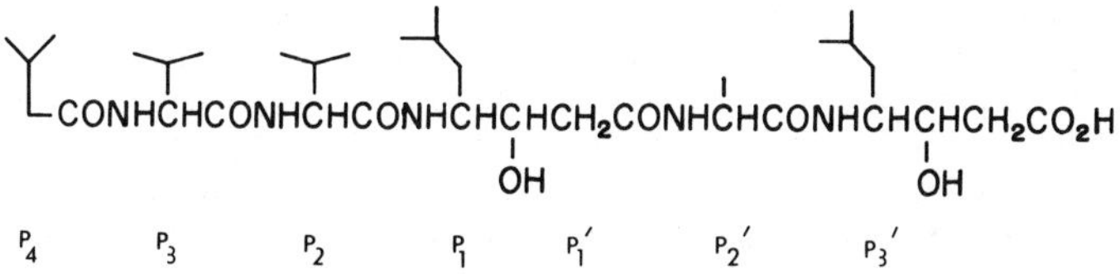
CONHCHCONHCHCONHCHCHCH2CONHCHCONHCHCHCH2CO2H
OH
OH
P4
P3
P2
P1
P1′
P2′
P3′

1

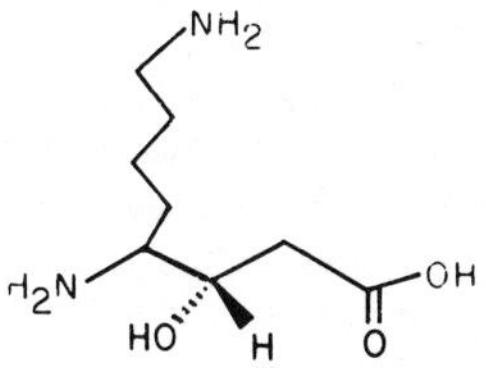
NH2
H2N
HO
H
OH
O

20

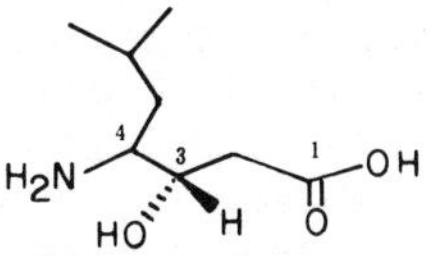
H2N
HO
H
OH
O
4
3
1

2

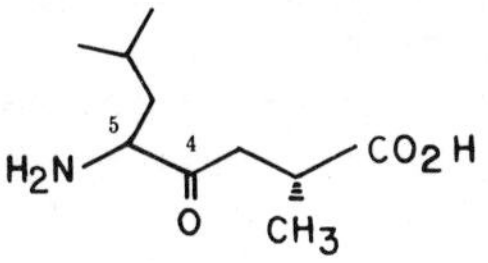
H2N
5
4
O
CH3
CO2H

7

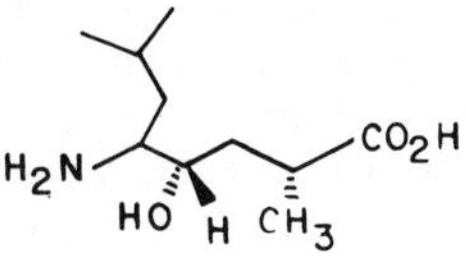
H2N
HO
H
CH3
CO2H

8

pepstatin acts as a transition-state analogy inhibitor.(10,11)
Here we reevaluate and clarify the evidence that statine-
containing peptides bind to aspartyl proteases in complexes
structurally related to the tetrahedral intermediate for substrate hydrolysis, and, in so doing, raise the likelihood that
much of the inhibitory potency of pepstatin is attributable to
a collected-substrate type of mechanism. We also demonstrate
how these peptides can be used to elucidate the mechanism of
aspartyl proteases and provide important lead structures for
the development of selective and potent inhibitors of aspartyl
proteases with potential for clinical application.

Is Pepstatin a Transition-State Analog Inhibitor?

Pepstatin analogs lacking a pro-S C-3 hydroxyl group, e.g.,
dideoxypepstatin 3 and the (3R,4S) diastereomer 4 (Table I) are
much weaker inhibitors of aspartyl proteases than inhibitors
containing the pro-S hydroxyl group found in natural statine.(12,13) The importance of this hydroxyl group is rein-
forced by the x-ray crystal structure of the complex between
pepstatin and R. chinensis aspartyl protease which shows that
this C-3 hydroxyl group is within hydrogen bonding distance of
the carboxyl groups of the catalytically essential Asp-32 and
Asp-220 residues of the enzyme (Figure 2).(14) A remarkably
similar structure is observed for the complex between Iva-Val-
Val-Sta-OET (5) and penicillopepsin, which includes hydrogen
bonds from the inhibitor hydroxyl group to the carboxyl groups
of Asp-33 and Asp-213.(15) Moreover, recent high resolution
refinements of these data (16) have revealed that the final
resting point of the hydroxyl group in tripeptide 5 is nearly
identical to the site occupied by a water molecule oxygen that
is hydrogen bonded to Asp-33 and Asp-213 in native penicillopepsin;(17) thus inhibitor binding must be accompanied by
displacement of an enzyme-bound water molecule, a process
illustrated schematically in Figure 1.
     The significance of this result becomes apparent when one
considers the extent to which the positive entropy change associated with water displacement will contribute to the strength
of inhibitor binding. Jencks (18) has estimated that the return of a "bound" water molecule to bulk solvent increases entropy from 10-16 eu to produce 3-5 kcal of energy favorable to
inhibitor binding. It should be emphasized that the hydrogen
bonds formed between the statine hydroxyl group and the enzyme
must be considered only as replacements for the hydrogen bonds
between the bound water molecule and the native enzyme, so that
the net enthalpic change for the water displacement process
would be comparatively small.
     Thus, although pepstatin still may be considered a
transition-state analog inhibitor owing to the tetrahedral
geometry at C-3 of statine, pepstatin is also a collected-

Table I. Inhibition of Aspartyl Proteases by Pepstatin Analogs

#	Compound[a]	Ki, nM	
		Porcine Pepsin	Penicillopepsin
1	Iva-Val-Val——Sta——Ala-Sta-OH	.056	.15
3	Iva-Val-Val-dSta——Ala-dSta-OH[b]	210	-
4	Iva-Val-Val-(3R,4S)——Sta——Ala-Iaa	2000	-
5	Iva-Val-Val——Sta——OEt	10	47
6	Iva-Val——Sto——Ala-Iaa[c]	56	-
9	Iva-Val —Leu^{K}—Ala-Iaa[d]	970	-
10	Iva-Val —Leu^{K}—Ala-Ala-Iba[d]	110	-
11	Iva-Val-Val——Sto——Ala-Iaa[c]	10	85
12 a	Iva-Val-Leu^{OH}—Ala—Iaa (4S)[e]	27	-
b	(4R)	750	-
13 a	Iva-Val-Val-Leu^{OH}—Ala—Iaa (4S)[e]	9.2	-
b	(4R)	500	-
14	Iva-Val-Leu^{OH}—Ala-Ala-Iba[e,f]	3	-
15	Iva-Val-Leu^{OH}—Ala—Gly-Iba[e,f]	53	0.4
18	Iva-Val——Sta——Gly-Iaa	56	1.0
22	Iva-Val-Val-DAHCA——OEt	>1000	0.08
23	Iva-Val-Val——Sta——Phe-OMe	-	500
24	Iva-Val-Val-DAHOA——Phe-OMe	-	7600
25	Iva-Val-Val-DAHOA(Z)——Phe-OMe	500	6.5
16	Iva-Val——Sta——Ala-Iaa	3	
17	Iva-Val-Val——Sta——Ala-Iaa	0.1	

[a] All statine analogs have the (3S,4S) configuration.
[b] dSta, 4-amino-6-methylheptanoic acid.
[c] Sto, 4-Amino-3 oxo-6-methylheptanoic acid.
[d] K = -CO-CH$_2$-
[e] OH = -CHOH-CH$_2$-
[f] Iba, isobutylamide.

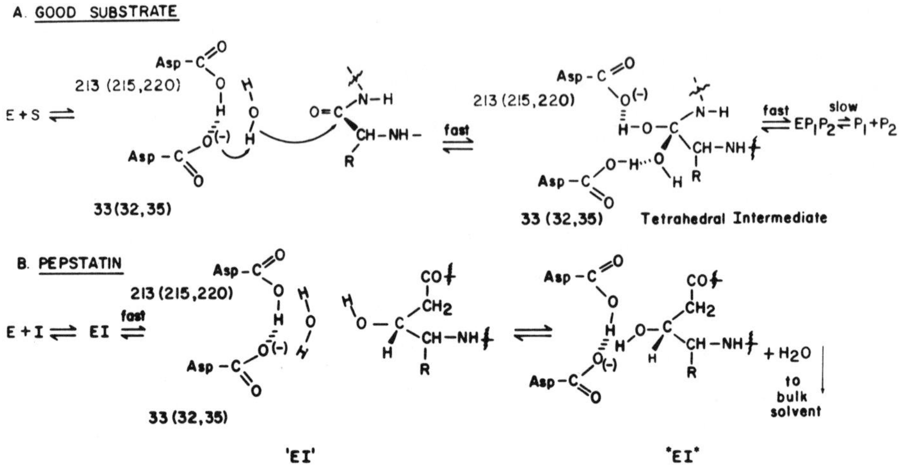

Figure 1. Schematic representation of the relationships be-
    tween proposed catalytic and inhibitory mechanisms. A.
    Postulated general acid-general base catalyzed mechanism
    for substrate hydrolysis by an aspartyl protease. The
    water molecule indicated is extensively hydrogen bonded to
    both aspartic acid residues plus other sites in the active
    site (see Reference 16 for details). Hydrogen bonds to
    water are omitted here. B. Kinetic events associated
    with the inhibition of pepsin by pepstatin. The pro-S
    hydroxyl group of statine displaces the enzyme immobilized
    water molecule shown in Figure 1A. Variable aspartyl se-
    quence numbers refer to penicillopepsin (pepsin, Rhizopus
    pepsin), respectively.

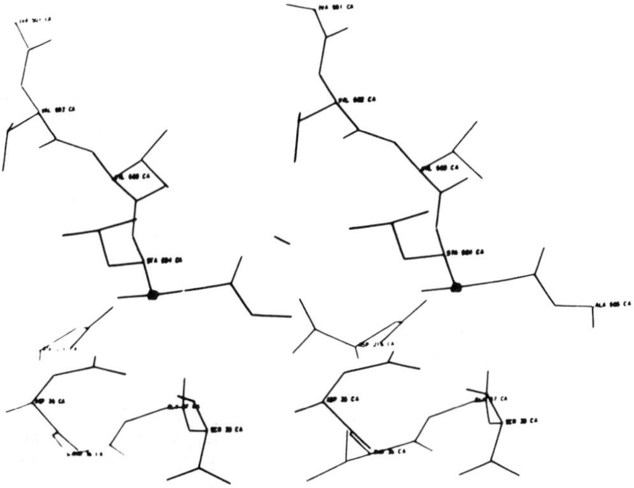

Figure 2. Stereo view of pepstatin bound in the R. chinensis pepsin active site. C-3 of statine carrying an OH group is indicated by the ■ . Availability for hydrogen bonding is indicated by closeness of carboxyl groups of Asp-220 and Asp-32 to the statine hydroxyl and to each other.

substrate inhibitor because the statine pro-S hydroxyl group
mimics the enzyme-bound water molecule. The dissociation constant for dideoxy pepstatin, 3, ($K_i = 10^{-7}M$) is about 10-100
fold smaller than K_s for comparable substrates, and addition of
a pro-S hydroxyl group to C-3 contributes an additional 1000-
4000 fold to inhibition binding (Table I, cf. 1 vs 3). It is
reasonable to attribute much of the tighter binding of 3, compared with substrates, to the tetrahedral geometry of C-3, in
accord with transition state analog theory. To the extent that
steric interactions between a proton on C-3 of the central deoxy Sta residue and the bound water might interfere with optimal binding of 3, the contribution of tetrahedral geometry to
the binding of inhibitors (e.g., pepstatin) which displace
bound water (and thus do not encounter steric interference)
could be greater. Consequently, it is difficult to assign precisely the degree to which entropic considerations are responsible for the considerably tighter binding of 1 compared with
3; but as discussed above, this contribution is likely to be
substantial. It is worthwhile to point out here that similar
entropic considerations may be important to the binding of
other postulated transition state analog inhibitors. In particular, hydrolase or deaminase inhibitors often resemble
substrate plus water as well as a tetrahedral intermediate.

Statine is an Analog of a Dipeptide

The structures of statine and the tetrahedral intermediate for
amide hydrolysis are compared in Figure 1. It is readily apparent that statine is isosteric with the tetrahedral intermediate only from C-3 through C-7. Because of atoms C-1 and C-2,
statine is either two atoms too long to be isosteric with a
normal α-amino acid or one atom too short to be isosteric with
a dipeptide. Powers suggested on the basis of an extensive
comparison of pepsin substrate sequences that statine might be
closer to a dipeptide.([19]) Using the x-ray data for pepstatin
bound to R. chinensis aspartyl protease, Boger proposed a more
specific model in which statine is an analog of an enzyme-bound
dipeptide in its tetrahedral intermediate form.([20]) A comparison between pepstatin and the tetrahedral form of -Leu-Leu-Val-
Phe- generated by molecular modeling is shown in Figure 3.
Pepstatin residues are indicated by dashed lines and the tetrahedral intermediate of -Leu-Leu-Val-Phe- is indicated by solid
lines. It is clear that in this conformation, the isobutyl and
hydroxyl groups of statine and the first Leu residue in substrate can bind to the same enzyme site (S1) while, at the same
time, the isobutyl group of the second statine and the benzyl
group of the substrate Phe can bind to the S3' enzyme site, a
steric "match" possible only if statine serves as a dipeptide
replacement. The concept that statine is a dipeptide replacement was utilized to generate the series of potent renin inhib-

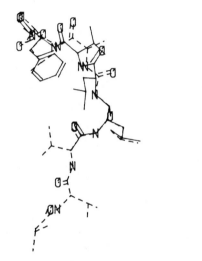
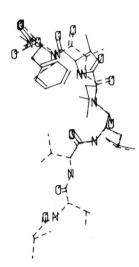

Figure 3. Ac-Leu*Leu-Val-Phe-NH$_2$ (solid), where * denotes a tetrahedral carbonyl (-CHOH-NH-), matched onto isovaleryl-Val-Val-Sta-Ala-Sta,1, (dashed, pepstatin) as in the complex with <u>R. chinensis</u> aspartyl protease.

Reprinted with permission from Ref. 20.

itors shown in Table 3 in which statine replaces the Leu-Val
unit in peptides derived from various renin angiotensinogen
sequences.(21) Szelke et al. recently described the synthesis
of a new series of renin inhibitors derived from the hydroxyethylene isostere for a dipeptide.(22) As shown in Table III,
replacement of the Leu-Leu or Leu-Val sequences in peptides
derived from renin angiotensinogen sequences by the hydroxyethylene isostere also produces very potent renin inhibitors,
and the close agreement between the hydroxyethylene- and
statine-based inhibitors is consistent with statine serving as
a dipeptide analog.

We synthesized the ketomethylene,7, and hydroxyethylene,8,
isosteres of a Leu-Ala dipeptide sequence in order to explore
the importance of the two extra atoms in statine relative
either to substrate or to the tetrahedral intermediate (Figure
1) in another aspartyl protease system. The compounds were
synthesized by the routes outlined in Scheme I. This route was
chosen so as to provide steric control at C-2 and C-5 of both 7
and 8 as well as to provide ready access to C-4 labeled analogs. Details of the synthesis have been described elsewhere.(23,24) Inhibitors were synthesized in which Leu-Ala
dipeptide isosteres replaced either Sta or Sta-Ala in known
pepstatin analogs. Inhibition of porcine pepsin was determined
using the reported spectrophotometric assay (Table I).(25)

Comparison of hydroxyethylene analogs 12 and 14 with the
Sta-containing inhibitor 16 reveals that the K_i for 14, in
which the hydroxyethylene isostere of Leu-Ala replaces Sta, is
remarkably similar to that of 16, whereas 12, in which the hydroxyethylene isostere of Leu-Ala replaces Sta-Ala, is a ca.
10-fold weaker inhibitor than 16. A similar pattern is found
for the ketone analogs (6 vs 9 and 10). Other parallels in
enzyme inhibitory properties support the conclusion that
isostere-containing and Sta-containing peptides are acting by
similar mechanisms. Hydroxyethylene analog 14 exhibits slow
binding properties similar to those observed for the more potent Sta-containing analogs, including 16. Moreover, replacement of Ala with Gly in 14 (to give 15) and in 16 (to give 18)
results in similar losses of binding potency and in loss of the
slow binding properties of both inhibitors. Finally, a change
in stereochemistry at the hydroxyl-bearing carbon results in
dramatic losses of binding potency for both Sta- and
hydroxyethylene analogs (cf. 1 vs 4 and 12a vs 12b).

In summary, the results with pepsin extend the renin data
reported by Szelke and Boger and strongly support the postulate
of Boger that statine is an analog of a dipeptide tetrahedral
intermediate.(20) The C-3 hydroxyl group hydrogen bonds to
Asp-213 (220) and Asp-33(35) and displaces a "bound" water molecule from the active site. The isobutyl side chain of statine
corresponds to the P1 substituent that binds to the S1 subsite
on the enzyme. The C-1 and C-2 atoms of statine serve to span

Table II. Effect of Inhibitor Chain Length on Inhibition Constant for Three Aspartyl Proteases.

#	P_4 P_3 P_2 P_1 P_1' P_2' P_3'	$K_i \times 10^9$ M		
		Pepsin $P_3 \rightarrow P_3'$	Cathepsin D $P_4 \rightarrow P_3'$	Penicillopepsin $P_4 \rightarrow P_2'$
26	Iva-Val-Val—Sta—Ala-Iaa	0.1	3.7	6.5
27	Boc-Val-Val—Sta-Ala-Iaa	1.5	1.1	4
38	Boc-Val—Sta-Ala-Iaa	170	270	6100
29	Ipoc-Val—Sta-Ala-Iaa	86	620	5700
16	Iva-Val—Sta-Ala-Iaa	3	220	7600
30	Et$_2$Ac-Val—Sta-Ala-Iaa	0.2	120	
31	Iva-Val—Sta—NHC$_3$H$_7$	300		3600
5	Iva-Val-Val—Sta—OEt	10	180	47
32	Iva-Val-Val—Sta—Ala—OMe	3.5	90	4.5

Table III. Substrate Derived Renin Inhibitors.

Compound No.	Structure	IC_{50} (M), Human Plasma Renin

	6 7 8 9 10 11 12 13	
33	H His Pro Phe His Leu Leu Val Tyr OH	(5.5×10^{-5})[a]
34	H Leu-Val-Ile-His-OH	
35	Pro- Phe-Phe	7×10^{-6}
36	D-His Leu$\overset{R}{-}$Leu	$1 \times 10\text{-}6$
37	Pro- Leu$\overset{R}{-}$Leu	1×10^{-8}
38	Iva-His —Sta---Ile-Phe-NH_2	1.9×10^{-9}
39	Iva-His —Sta---Ile-Phe-OMe	0.6×10^{-9}
40	Boc-His Leu$\overset{OH}{—}$Val-Ile-His	0.7×10^{-9}
41	Boc-Phe-His——----Sta—Ala-Sta-OMe	2.7×10^{-8}
1	Iva-Val-Val——----Sta—Ala-Sta	22×10^{-6}

[a] Km value for substrate $\underline{R}$ = -CH_2-NH- $\underline{OH}$ = -CH(OH)-CH_2-

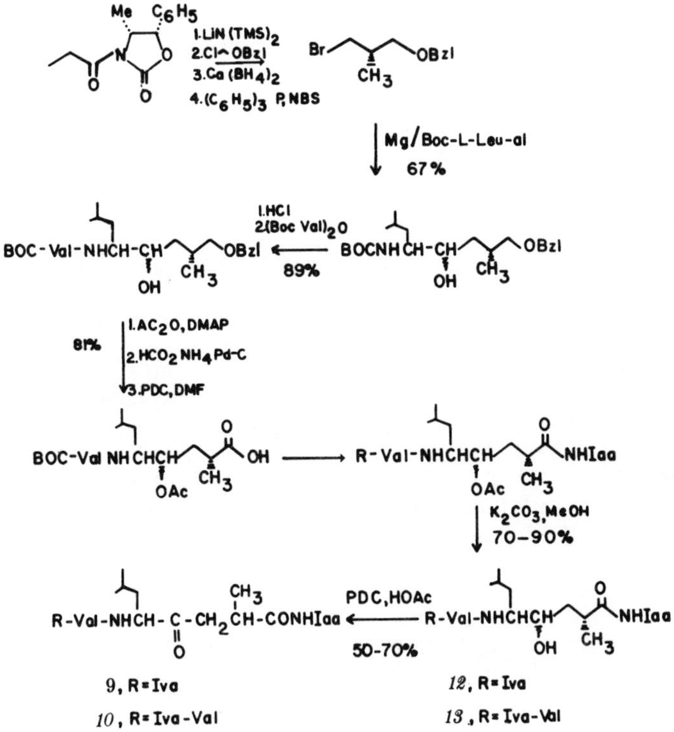
Me
C_6H_5
1. LiN(TMS)$_2$
2. Cl⌒OBzl
3. Ca(BH$_4$)$_2$
4. $(C_6H_5)_3$ P, NBS
Br
OBzl
CH_3
Mg/Boc-L-Leu-al
67%
1. HCl
2. (Boc Val)$_2$O
89%
BOC-Val-NHCH-CH
OBzl
OH
BOCNHCH-CH
1. AC$_2$O, DMAP
2. HCO$_2$NH$_4$Pd-C
3. PDC, DMF
81%
BOC-Val NHCHCH
OAc
OH
R-Val-NHCHCH
NHIaa
K_2CO_3, MeOH
70-90%
R-Val-NHCH-C-CH$_2$CH-CONHIaa
PDC, HOAc
50-70%
9, R = Iva
10, R = Iva-Val
12, R = Iva
13, R = Iva-Val

Scheme I.

the distance between the P1 and P2' sites. Thus, the alanine
methyl group in pepstatin binds approximately to the S2'site on
the enzyme and not to the S1' site. This pattern is repeated
in the renin inhibitors with the Sta-Ile-Phe sequence serving
approximately the same binding role as the -Leu($CHOHCH_2$) Leu-
Ile-His- sequence. Surprisingly, the Sta analogs 16 and 17
which lack an isobutyl group near the P1' site are as potent as
the hydroxyethylene isosteres which contain this group. It
must be noted that none of the side-chain substituents in analogs 10-18 correspond to substituents known to favor rapid
hydrolysis of substrate by pepsin, and better inhibitors of
aspartyl proteases derived from the ketomethylene and hydroxyethylene isosteres are likely to be found when the isobutyl and
methyl side chains in 10-18 are replaced by the hydrophobic
substituents known to favor binding to pepsin or other aspartyl
proteases.(26)

Specificity

Statine Side Chain. To explore the effect of structure in the
P1 position of pepstatin analogs on inhibition of aspartyl proteases, we carried out the synthesis of two new statine analogs, 4-amino-3-hydroxy-5-phenyl pentanoic acid (AHPPA) and
4,8-diamino-3-hydroxy-octanoic acid (DAHOA). These compounds
are variations of statine modified so that the side chain more
closely approximates the side chain of a good substrate for the
target enzyme. Replacement of statine with AHPPA produces the
inhibitor, Iva-Val-AHPPA-Ala-Iaa,19, which is a slightly
stronger inhibitor of pepsin than the parent compound 16.(12)
The difference between the two inhibitors is not as great as
would be expected from the 10-fold differences in k_{cat} or $k_{cat}/$
K_m for substrates in which Phe replaces a Leu residue in the P1
position.(26)
     A much more remarkable example of side-chain specificity
is found with inhibitors derived from the lysine side chain
analog of statine, DAHOA, 20. The rationale underlying the
synthesis of the lysine side-chain analog 20 comes from the
substrate specificity of fungal proteases. One major difference between mammalian aspartyl proteases (e.g., pepsin) and
those isolated from fungi (e.g., penicillopepsin) is that the
fungal proteases have the ability to activate trypsinogen, an
activation process which requires specificity for lysine.
Mammalian aspartyl proteases prefer to hydrolyze amide bonds
between hydrophobic residues. The best penicillopepsin substrate, N-Ac-Ala-Ala-Lys-Phe(NO_2)-Ala-Ala-NH_2, 21, is cleaved
by penicillopepsin at the Lys-Phe(NO_2) bond.(27) A specific
interaction between the positively charged ε-amino group of
lysine and some negatively charged group on the enzyme is indicated because penicillopepsin cleaves Lys-Phe bonds faster
than amide bonds between hydrophobic residues, and because the

kinetic parameters for cleavage of this substrate, K_m and k_{cat}, depend on pH. Using the refined crystal structure of the complex between penicillopepsin and Iva-Val-Val-Sta-OEt, 5, (15) and molecular graphics simulations, James and Hofmann examined a possible tetrahedral intermediate that would be formed during penicillopepsin catalyzed hydrolysis of a substrate that contains a Lys-Phe segment. These studies suggested it is possible to form a solvated ion pair from the bis-carboxylate pair, Glu16 and Asp115, and the ε-amino group of substrate lysine.(28)

If the model proposed by James and Hofmann is correct, then the pepstatin analog Iva-Val-Val-DAHOA-OEt, 22, formed from replacing the isobutyl side chain of the statine residue in 5 with a 4-aminobutyl side chain, should be a stronger inhibitor of penicillopepsin than the statine-containing inhibitor 5 owing to the additional ionic attraction. A schematic representation of the penicillopepsin-tripeptide inhibitor 22 complex is shown in Figure 4. The coordinates are based on the x-ray structure of tripeptide 5 but use the lysine side-chain in the DAHOA analog 22. The enzyme has been omitted here to permit visualization of the appropriate interactions between the side chain of inhibitor and the enzyme carboxyl groups.

(3S,4S)-4,8-Diamino-3-hydroxyoctanoic acid (DAHOA) derivatives were synthesized by the route shown in Scheme II using the known aldehyde Boc-Lys(Z)-CHO (29) and were converted to the DAHOA peptide analogs shown. Inhibition of penicillopepsin by all statine and DAHOA pepstatin analogs was measured using substrate 21. The results of these determinations are shown in Table I.

Replacement of (3S,4S)-statine in 5 with (3S,4S)-DAHOA leads to tripeptide 22 in which Ki has been decreased by a factor of about 100. Tetrapeptide 24 is 12 times more potent than the corresponding statine analog 23. The decrease in Ki for 22 relative to 5 corresponds to an increased binding interaction of 2-3 Kcal, a value close to the interaction expected for a solvated ion pair.(30) An ionic interaction also is suggested by the fact that Cbz protected DAHOA tripeptide 25, which cannot form an ion pair at the terminal nitrogen, is a much poorer inhibitor of penicillopepsin. There is evidence that the ionic interaction is with the acidic amino acid in position 115 because tighter binding is seen with penicillopepsin, a fungal protease, but not with pepsin, a mammalian aspartyl protease, in which amino acid 115 is tyrosine rather than aspartic acid.(28,31) The Ki of DAHOA tripeptide 22 is greater than 1000 nM on porcine pepsin even though the corresponding statine analog 5 has a Ki of 10 nM on porcine pepsin. This very weak binding of 22 to porcine pepsin relative to 5 suggests the positively charged ion may actually be repelled from the active site of pepsin.

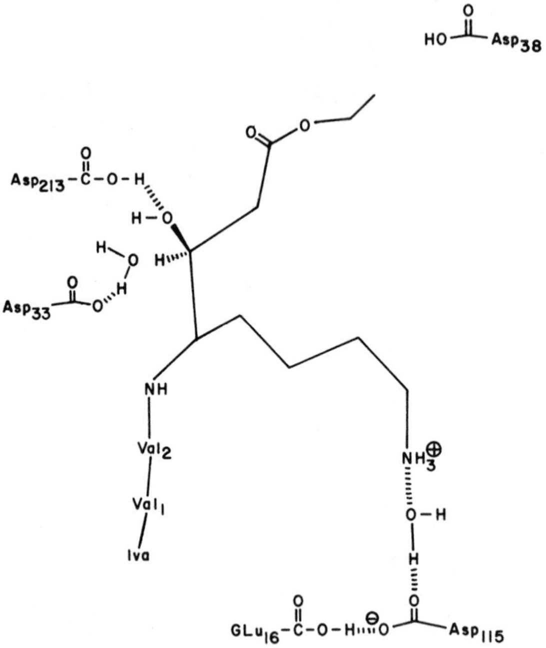

Figure 4. Schematic representation of the binding of the lysine side-chain analog of statine, Iva-Val-Val-DAHOA-OEt, 22, to penicillopepsin.

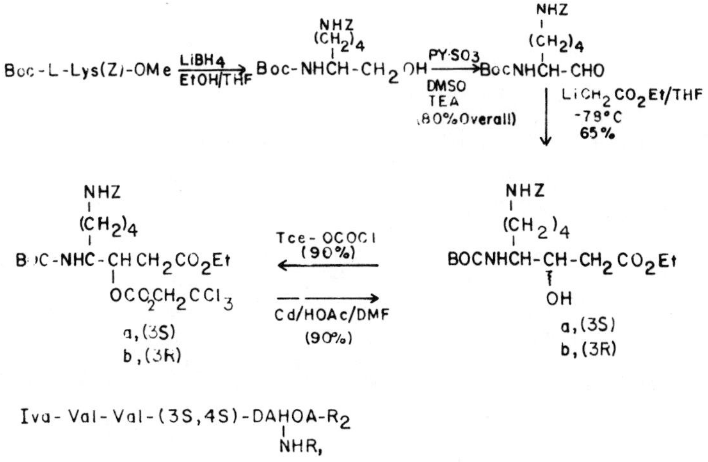

$$\text{Boc-L-Lys(Z)-OMe} \xrightarrow[\text{EtOH/THF}]{\text{LiBH}_4} \text{Boc-NHCH-CH}_2\text{OH} \xrightarrow[\substack{\text{DMSO}\\ \text{TEA}\\ (80\% \text{Overall})}]{\text{PY·SO}_3} \text{BocNHCH-CHO}$$

with substituent $\overset{\displaystyle \text{NHZ}}{\underset{\displaystyle (\text{CH}_2)_4}{|}}$ on the middle and right structures.

$$\downarrow \substack{\text{LiCH}_2\text{CO}_2\text{Et/THF}\\ -79^\circ\text{C}\\ 65\%}$$

Right product:

$$\text{BOCNHCH-CH-CH}_2\text{CO}_2\text{Et}$$

with $\overset{\displaystyle \text{NHZ}}{\underset{\displaystyle (\text{CH}_2)_4}{|}}$ and OH

a,(3S)
b,(3R)

Left product:

$$\text{BOC-NHC-CHCH}_2\text{CO}_2\text{Et}$$

with $\overset{\displaystyle \text{NHZ}}{\underset{\displaystyle (\text{CH}_2)_4}{|}}$ and $\text{OCO}_2\text{CH}_2\text{CCl}_3$

a,(3S)
b,(3R)

$$\xleftarrow[]{\substack{\text{Tce-OCOCl}\\(90\%)}}$$

$$\xrightarrow[\substack{\text{Cd/HOAc/DMF}\\(90\%)}]{}$$

Iva-Val-Val-(3S,4S)-DAHOA-R$_2$
                    |
                   NHR$_1$

25, R$_1$= Z; R$_2$ = OEt

22, R$_1$=H; R$_2$ =OEt   24, R$_1$=H; R$_2$ =Phe-OMe

Scheme II.

Effect of Pepstatin Chain Length on Specificity. Studies of
the susceptibility of peptides toward cleavage by an enzyme
have established the importance of amino acid residues distal
to the scissile amide bond (i.e., outside of the P1-P1' positions) with respect to k_{cat} and k_{cat}/K_m.(26) The close structural relationship between the statine residue and the tetrahedral intermediate for amide bond hydrolysis suggested that
more potent and more selective inhibitors might be developed
when the peptide sequences in the P2-P4 and P2'-P4' positions
were modified to inhibit a particular enzyme. As a first step
toward determining the enzyme specificity, several pepstatin
analogs (Table II) were tested for inhibition of aspartyl proteases. The results show that each enzyme is inhibited by a
particular inhibitor chain length. In the case of pepsin,
maximal inhibition requires a branched hydrophobic residue in
the P3 position with the chain length extending to the P3' position.(32,33) When these criteria are met, e.g., compound 30,
pepsin inhibitors essentially equipotent with pepstatin are
produced. Cathepsin D requires a longer inhibitor, e.g., compound 27, which spans the P4 to P3' positions. Penicillopepsin
is efficiently inhibited by analogs spanning the P4 to the P2'
positions, e.g., compound 32, but additional atoms in the P3'
position, e.g., compound 26, do not tighten the interaction
between the enzyme and the inhibitor. These results clearly
point to differences within the active sites of these closely
related aspartyl proteases and suggest that peptide sequences
that more closely resemble substrate should lead to more potent
and more selective inhibitors. This expectation was realized
in the case of renin where exceptionally potent inhibitors are
produced when statine is incorporated in place of -Leu-Leu- in
renin substrate sequences.(20,21)

Renin Inhibitors. Inhibition of the renin-angiotensin system
via converting enzyme inhibitors is now a well-established
approach to the treatment of hypertension. Inhibition of the
first enzyme in this sequence, renin, has yet to yield a therapeutically useful drug although several very potent inhibitors
of renin have been developed. Burton and coworkers (34,35)
developed the first potent inhibitors of renin, e.g. compound
35, by replacing the leucine residues in the minimal porcine
renin substrate, His-Pro-Phe-His-Leu-Leu-Val-Tyr, 33, with
phenylalanine (Table III). Szelke et al. obtained potent competitive inhibitors of canine renin by replacing the Leu 10-Leu
11 peptide bond in pig angiotensinogen(6-13) octapeptide 33
with the methylene amino isostere ($-CH_2NH-$), formed by reduc-
tion of the amide group.(36) The improved binding of compounds
36 and 37 relative to substrate 33 is thought to result from
the tetrahedral geometry of the methylene group, which obviates
the need to expend energy to distort an amide carbonyl group
from trigonal to tetrahedral geometry, although a possible

ionic bridge between Asp-32 and the methylene amino nitrogen
has not been excluded. This class of inhibitor still lacks a
hydroxyl group needed for hydrogen bonding to active site
aspartyl carboxyl groups. Boger et al. devised potent renin
inhibitors by replacing the Leu 10-Val 11 and Leu 10-Leu 11 dipeptide units in human and pig angiotensinogens with statine
and obtained both extremely potent and selective renin inhibitors 38 and 39 that have demonstrated hypotensive activity in
animal model systems.(20,21) Szelke et al. very recently
reported the synthesis of renin inhibitors designed by replacing the Leu 10-Val 11 bond in human angiotensinogen octapeptide 34 with the hydroxyethylene isostere of Leu-Val, i.e.,
Leu(CHOHCH$_2$)Val, as in compound 40.(22) The potency of this
class of inhibitor is virtually identical with that of the corresponding statine derived renin inhibitors. Evin et al. also
obtained good renin inhibitors by replacing the C-terminal tetrapeptide in the porcine angiotensin octapeptide sequence 33
with Sta-Ala-Sta to form 41.(37) All of these compounds are
much better inhibitors of human and animal renins than
pepstatin and most are enzyme selective.
      These results establish that very potent inhibitors of
renin have been designed by means of two independent approaches. The approach of Szelke begins with an assumed enzymatic mechanism and known substrate sequence to generate analogs of the tetrahedral intermediate. The approach of Boger et
al. begins with a highly promising natural product and tailors
the peptide sequence in the inhibitor to produce the desired
selectivity and potency by incorporating renin substrate sequences. Boger's structure-activity studies were facilitated
by the recognition that statine binds to aspartyl proteases as
an analog of a dipeptide tetrahedral intermediate. This concept was supported by early data for the crystal structure of
pepstatin bound to R. chinensis pepsin that were compatible
with a computer graphic molecular model of a plausible
transition-state geometry. The congruent structural features
of inhibitors generated by either strategy (Table III) is
remarkable. It is likely that modifications of naturally
occurring inhibitors of other proteases can be used to clarify
enzyme mechanisms and provide lead compounds for the inhibition
of therapeutically important proteases.

Other Types of Inhibitors of Aspartyl Proteases

An unusual inhibitor of aspartyl proteases that may be another
type of collected-substrate inhibitor, has been discovered as a
result of systematic modification of statine. Because x-ray
data (Figure 2) suggested that the pro-R hydrogen in statine
could be replaced by a methyl group without encountering steric
interactions with the enzyme, we synthesized new statine analogs in which the C-3 proton was replaced by a methyl group,

designated Me^3Sta,42, and Me^3AHPPA,43.(38) Pepstatin analogs
containing these derivatives with known chirality were synthesized and shown to be potent inhibitors of aspartyl proteases
only when the configuration of the C-3 hydroxyl group is R
(Table IV)! Because 3R-Sta and 3R-AHPPA analogs, e.g., compounds 49B and 50B, which lack the added methyl group at C-3,
and 3S-Me^3Sta and 3S-Me^3AHPPA derivatives 44A-48A, which have
the same hydroxyl configuration found in statine, are very poor
aspartyl protease inhibitors, it follows that the 3R-Me^3Sta and
3R-Me^3AHPPA derivatives 44B-48B must have a new mechanism for
stabilizing the aspartyl protease-inhibitor complex relative to
previously studied pepstatin analogs.

One explanation for this surprising result is that the 3R-
Me^3Sta and 3R-Me^3AHPPA analogs are collected-substrate inhibitors of aspartyl proteases in which the pro-S methyl group displaces the "bound" water molecule from the active site while
the pro-R hydroxyl group compensates for some of the lost hydrogen bonds between enzyme and water by hydrogen bonding to
the carboxyl group of Asp-33 (Figure 5). The poor binding of
the 3S-Me^3Sta derivatives is harder to rationalize but may suggest that placement of a pro-R methyl group adjacent to the
Asp-33 (35) carboxylate anion in these enzymes is a highly
unfavorable process.

The Catalytic Mechanism of Aspartyl Proteases

The presence of two catalytically active aspartic β-
carboxyl groups in the active sites of aspartyl proteases was
deduced from pH-dependence and alkylation experiments.(26)
These residues were subsequently assigned as Asp-32 and Asp-215
in the sequence of porcine pepsin.(31) The results of transpeptidation and ^{18}O-exchange studies led to numerous proposals
for a catalytic mechanism for aspartyl proteases which usually
featured direct nucleophilic attack by an active site carboxylate on a peptide substrate carbonyl, with the intermediacy of
either an "amino-enzyme" (usually formulated as a carboxamide)
(39-43) or of an acyl enzyme (formulated as a mixed carboxylic
anhydride).(44,45) However, amino-transfer transpeptidation is
observable only for specific substrates, suggesting that proposed mechanisms involving covalent amino-enzyme intermediates
are inconsistent with a general mechanism for peptide hydrolysis.(46) Later studies of ^{18}O-exchange during transpeptidation
reactions convincingly discounted a carboxamide derived from an
enzyme carboxyl group and an amine product as a credible intermediate.(47) The possibility that a general acid-base mechanism could be operable, that is, one in which water attacks the
carbonyl of the scissile peptide bond with the active site car-
boxylates mediating the appropriate proton transfers, gained
attractiveness after it was recognized (26) that the resynthe-
sis of peptide bonds from final hydrolysis products was an

Table IV. Inhibition of Pepsin, Penicillopepsin and Cathepsin D by Me³Sta and Me³AHPPA Analogs

		Pepsin (x 10⁹ M)	Cathepsin D (x 10⁸ M)	Penicillopepsin (x 10⁹ M)
44A	Iva-Val-(3S,4S)-Me³Sta-Ala-Iaa	10,000		
B	Iva-Val-(3R,4S)-Me³Sta-Ala-Iaa	100		
45A	Iva-Val-(3S,4S)-Me³Sta-Ala-Iaa	1,200	> 40[a]	> 5000
B	Iva-Val-(3R,4S)-Me³Sta-Ala-Iaa	1.5	21.4	80
46A	Boc-Val-(3S,4S)-Me³Sta-Ala-Iaa	> 100	> 62	
B	Boc-Val-(3R,4S)-Me³Sta-Ala-Iaa	12	3.1	
47A	Boc-Val-(3S,4S)-Me³AHPPA-Ala-Iaa	20,000	ND	
B	Boc-Val-(3R,4S)-Me³AHPPA-Ala-Iaa	72	ND	
48A	Iva-Val-(3S,4S)-Me³AHPPA-Ala-Iaa	2,000	93	
B	Iva-Val-(3R,4S)-Me³AHPPA-Ala-Iaa	2.1	1.2	
49A	Iva-Val-(3S,4S)-AHPPA-Ala-Iaa	0.12	0.096	
B	Iva-Val-(3R,4S)-AHPPA-Ala-Iaa	> 200	> 10	
50A	Iva-Val-(3S,4S)-Sta-Ala-Iaa	0.1	0.37[b]	
B	Iva-Val-(3R,4S)-Sta-Ala-Iaa	100	> 100	

a Inhibition not observed at this concentration.
b Value for N-terminal Boc group is 0.11.
c ND - not assayed.

energetically reasonable process under the appropriate conditions.(48) Thus, most of the results of transpeptidation experiments could be rationalized by invoking the microscopic
reversibility of a general acid-general base catalyzed forward
reaction, which includes a structure-dependent ordered release
of hydrolysis products.(26,49) Further evidence in support of
the latter mechanism as opposed to a covalent mechanism involving an acyl enzyme intermediate includes the failure to trap an
activated enzyme carboxyl group with nucleophiles (50) and x-
ray data which argue against a covalent mechanism on spatial
grounds.(14,49) Results from ^{18}O-exchange studies (47,51,52)
are most consistent with a general acid-base mechanism; however, all possibilities consistent with covalent catalysis are
not rigorously excluded, and more conclusive evidence is
required to support the general acid-base mechanism.

It was necessary to establish unambiguously that the
We have approached this problem by studying the interactions between pepsin and ketones with structures based on that
of pepstatin. Our strategy was to design ketones which would
serve as pseudosubstrates, that is, be subject to the catalytic
action of the enzyme, but only to the point of formation of a
tetrahedral intermediate which, because of the increased stability of a C-C vs a C-N bond, would not break down to products. Such a stable tetrahedral intermediate would then, in
principle, be amenable to study by the appropriate physical
methods. ^{13}C-NMR appeared to be an ideal method since changes
in hybridization of the susceptible carbonyl carbon could be
followed readily. The results we have obtained provide the
first direct observation of a tetrahedral adduct in the active
site of an aspartyl protease, show that the transformation from
trigonal to tetrahedral geometry is an enzyme-catalyzed process, and establish the origin of the added nucleophile as
water. Our data thus provide strong support for the general
acid-general base catalytic mechanism. Further, the methods
described here should be applicable to the study of mechanisms
of other enzymes.

The statone (4-amino-3-oxo-6-methylheptanoic acid) containing peptide Iva-Val-Sto-Ala-Iaa, 6, was synthesized via
oxidation of the statine C-3 hydroxyl group in statine peptide
4 and was found to be a good inhibitor of pepsin (K_i = 56
nM).(53) The C-3 of ^{13}C-3-Sto analog 6 is found to be >95%
trigonal in aqueous buffer by ^{13}C-NMR spectroscopy. After the
inhibitor binds to pepsin, the ^{13}C chemical shift (99 ppm)
indicates that the geometry at C-3 is tetrahedral and that the
added atom is oxygen.(54)

It was necessary to establish unambiguously that the
transformation from trigonal to tetrahedral geometry was an
enzyme-catalyzed process, as opposed to one in which the ketone
was hydrated in solution followed by binding to the enzyme.
Thus, when statone analog 6 was incubated with pepsin in 99%
H_2^{18}O for three hours, recovered ketone contained < 10% ^{18}O at

C-3 as determined by mass spectral analysis.(55) In a mechanism involving ketone hydration prior to binding, ^{18}O incorporation in recovered inhibitor should be at least 50%, a value
corresponding to that expected for a single cycle of nonstereo-
specific addition/nonstereospecific elimination of water to the
ketone carbonyl. The actual results then indicate that
addition-elimination is a highly stereospecific process and
thus enzyme-catalyzed.

   The origin of the oxygen nucleophile that adds to the Sto
C-3 carboxyl group was established by measuring the ^{13}C chemical shift for the C-3 carbon of statone peptide 6 both in $^{2}H_2O$
and $^{2}H_2{}^{18}O$.(55) In $^{2}H_2O$ the C-3 carbon resonance is shifted
upfield 0.36 ppm. Since alcohol carbon resonances are shifted
upfield 0.15 ppm per hydroxyl upon changing the solvent from
water to $^{2}H_2O$ due to the addition of one deuterium, the 0.36
ppm shift is consistent with two hydroxyl groups on the statine
C-3 carbon in the tetrahedral species bound to the enzyme.
This conclusion was verified by a ^{13}C NMR experiment carried
out in $^{2}H_2{}^{18}O$ which gave a 0.05 ppm upfield shift in the resonance for the C-3 carbon relative to the carbon resonance in
$^{2}H_2{}^{16}O$. The upfield shift in the carbon resonance establishes
that the oxygen nucleophile that adds to the C-3 carbonyl group
when 6 binds to pepsin must come from water. These labeling
results are not consistent with the addition of the Asp-32
carboxyl group to the carbonyl group to form a covalent tetrahedral species as would occur during nucleophilic catalysis.

   In order to establish that the addition process observed
for 6 in the active site of pepsin is analogous to that occurring with peptide substrates, the ^{13}C NMR experiments were
repeated using peptide 10 which contained the ketomethylene
dipeptide isostere 7 which was 99% ^{13}C enriched at C-4. The
same ~ 100 ppm upfield shift of the carbonyl resonance (from C-
4 in compound 7) was observed. In $^{2}H_2O$, the C-4 carbon resonance was shifted farther upfield by 0.30 ppm relative to a
sample run in H_2O and shifted upfield 0.04 ppm when the ^{13}C NMR
spectrum was obtained in $^{2}H_2{}^{18}O$ compared to that in $H_2{}^{16}O$.
These data unambiguously establish that a gem diol species is
formed in the active site of pepsin when the ketone analogs 6
and 10 are added to the aspartyl protease as shown in Figure 6
and exclude the formation of a covalent intermediate. Our data
strongly support the general acid-general base catalysis mechanism for aspartyl proteases that is illustrated schematically
in Figure 1.

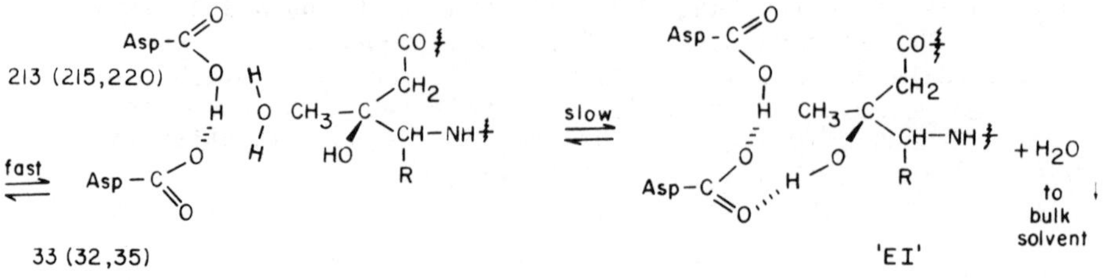

Figure 5. Postulated "collected-substrate" mechanism for inhibition of aspartyl proteases by (3R)-Me^{3}Sta and (3R)-Me^{3}AHPPA peptides.

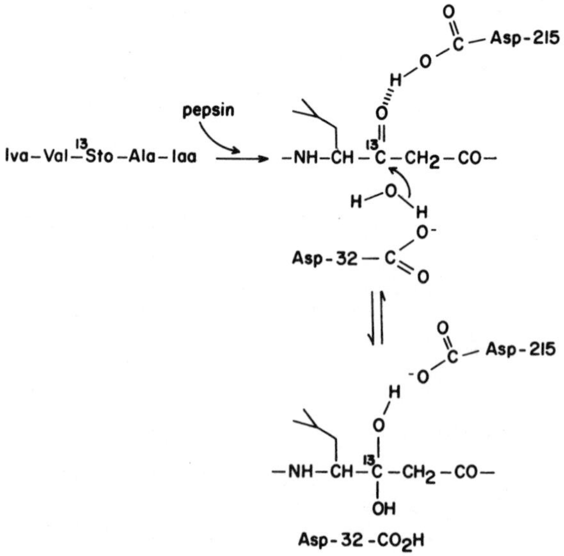

Figure 6. Schematic representation of the addition of water to the ^{13}C labeled carbonyl in statone pseudosubstrate 6. Labeling of water ($^2H_2{}^{16}O$ or $^2H_2{}^{18}O$) establishes that water not Asp-32 adds to the carbonyl group (Cf text).

Acknowledgements

This work was supported in part by grants from the National
Institutes of Health (AM20100) and from Merck Sharp and Dohme.
We thank Dr. Richard Bott and Dr. Joshua Boger for the computer
graphic data presented in Figures 2 and 3 and Drs. M.N.G. James
and Theo Hofmann for communicating their substrate modeling
studies to us prior to publication. We are also indebted to
our colleagues cited in the references who collaborated on the
early phases of this work.

Literature Cited

1.   Cushman, D. W.; Ondetti, M. A.; Progress in Medicinal
     Chemistry 1980, 17, 41.
2.   Wolfenden, R. in "Transition States of Biochemical Pro-
     cesses"; Gandour, R. D.; Schowen, R. L., Eds.; Plenum
     Press: New York, 1978; pp. 555-578.
3.   Patchett, A. A.; Harris, E.; Tristram, E. W.; Wyvratt, M.
     J.; Wu, M. T.; Taub, D.; Peterson, E. R.; Ikeler, T. J.;
     ten Broeke, J.; Payne, L. G.; Ondeyka, D. L.; Thorsett, E.
     D.; Greenlee, W. J.; Lohr, N. S.; Hoffsommer, R. D.;
     Joshua, H.; Ruyle, W. V.; Rothrock, J. W.; Aster, S. D.;
     Maycock, A. L.; Robinson, F. M.; Hirschmann, R.; Sweet, C.
     S.; Ulm, E. H.; Gross, D. M.; Vassil, T. C.; Stone, C. A.
     Nature 1980, 288, 280-3.
4.   Almquist, R. G.; Crase, J.; Jennings-White, C.; Meyer, R.
     F.; Hoefle, M. L.; Smith, R. O.; Essenburg, A. D.; Kaplan,
     H. R. J. Med. Chem. 1982, 25, 1292-1299.
5.   Galardy, R. E. Biochem. Biophys. Res. Comm. 1980, 97, 94.
6.   Jacobsen, N. E.; Bartlett, P. A. J. Amer. Chem. Soc. 1981,
     103, 654-7.
7.   Roques, B. P.; Fournie-Zaluski, M. C.; Sorola, E.;
     Lecomte, J. M.; Malfroy, B.; Llorens, C.; Schwartz, J.-C.
     Nature 1980, 288, 286-8.
8.   Aoyagi, T. in "Bioactive Peptides Produced by Micro-
     organisms" Umezawa, H.; Takita, T.; Shiba, T., Eds.;
     Halsted Press, New York, 1978, pp. 129-51.
9.   Rich, D. H.; Sun, E. T. O. Biochem. Biophys. Res. Commun.
     1980, 27, 157-62.
10. Marshall, G. R. Fed. Proc., Fed. Am. Soc. Exp. Biol. 1976,
     35, 2494.
11. Marciniszyn, M. P.; Hartsuck, J. A.; Tang, J. J. N. J.
     Biol. Chem. 1976, 251, 7088-94.
12. Rich, D. H.; Sun, E. T. O.; Ulm, E. J. Med. Chem. 1980,
     23, 27-33.
13. Rich, D. H.; Sun, E.; Singh, J. Biochem. Biophys. Res.
     Comm. 1977, 74, 762-764.
14. Bott, R.; Subramanian, E.; Davies, D. R. Biochemistry
     1982, 21, 6956-62.
15. James, M. N. G.; Sielecki, A.; Salituro, F.; Rich, D. H.;
     Hoffman, T. Proc. Natl. Acad. Sci. USA 1982, 79, 6137-41.

16. James, M. N. G.; Sielecki, A. R.; Moult, J. in "Peptides: Structure and Function. Proceedings of the Eighth American Peptide Symp."; Hruby, V. J.; Rich, D. H.; Eds.; Pierce Chem. Co., Rockford, IL in press.

17. James, M. N. G.; Sielecki, A. J. Mol. Biol. 1983, 163, 299-361.

18. Jencks, W. P. Adv. Enzymology Relat. Areas Mol. Biol. 1975, 43, 219-410.

19. Powers, J. C.; Harley, A. D.; Myers, D. V., in "Acid Proteases-Structure, Function and Biology"; Tang, J., Ed.; Plenum: New York, 1977, pp. 141-57.

20. Boger, J., in "Peptides Structure and Function. Proceedings of Eighth American Peptide Symp."; Hruby, V. J.; Rich, D. H., Eds.; Pierce Chem. Co., Rockford, IL, in press.

21. Boger, J.; Lohr, N. S.; Ulm, E. H.; Poe, M.; Blaine, E. H.; Fanelli, G. M.; Lin, T-Y.; Payne, L. S.; Schorn, T. W.; LaMont, B. I.; Vassil, T. C.; Sabilito, I. I.; Veber, D. F.; Rich, D. H.; Boparai, A. S. Nature 1983, 303, 81-4.

22. Szelke, M.; Jones, D. M.; Atrash, B.; Hallett, A.; Leckie, B., in "Peptides Structure and Function. Proceedings of Eighth American Peptide Symp."; Hruby, V. J.; Rich, D. H., Eds.; Pierce Chem. Co., Rockford, IL, in press.

23. Rich, D. H.; Salituro, F. G.; Holladay, M. W. ibid, in press.

24. Holladay, M. W.; Rich, D. H. Tetrahedron Lett. 1983, 24, 4401-4404.

25. Medzihradszky, K.; Voynick, I. M.; Medzihradszky-Schweiger, H.; Fruton, J. S. Biochemistry 1967, 9, 1154-62.

26. Fruton, J. S. Adv. Enzymol. Relat. Areas Mol. Biol. 1976, 44, 1-36.

27. Hofmann, T.; Hodges, R. S. Biochem. J. 1982, 2-3, 603-10.

28. James, M. N. G.; Hofmann, T., personal communication.

29. Hamada, Y.; Shioiri, T.; Chem. Pharm. Bull. 1982, 30, 1921-4.

30. Fersht, A. R. J. Mol. Biol. 1972, 64, 497-509.

31. Tang, J.; Sepulveda, P.; Marciniszyn, J.; Chen, K. C. S.; Huang, W. Y.; Tao, N.; Liu, D.; Lanier, J. P. Proc. Natl. Acad. Sci. USA 1973, 70, 3437-9.

32. Rich, D. H.; Bernatowicz, J. Med. Chem. 1982, 25, 791-5.

33. Rich, D. H.; Salituro, F. G. J. Med. Chem. 1983, 26, 904-10.

34. Burton, J.; Poulsen, K.; Haber, E. Biochemistry 1975, 14, 3892-8.

35. Poulsen, K.; Haber, E.; Burton, J. Biochim. Biophys. Acta 1976, 452, 533-7.

36. Szelke, M.; Leckie, B. J.; Hallett, A.; Jones, D. M.; Sueiras, J.; Atrash, B.; Lever, A. F. Nature 1982, 299, 555-7.

37. Evin, G.; Castro, B.; Devin, J.; Menard, J.; Corvol, P.;
     Guegan, R.; Diaz, J.; Demarne, H.; Cazaubon, C.; Gagnol,
     J. P. in "Peptides Structure and Function. Proceedings of
     Eighth American Peptide Symposium."; Hruby, V. J.; Rich,
     D. H., Eds.; Pierce Chem. Co., Rockford, IL, in press.
38. Kawai, M.; Boparai, A. S.; Bernatowicz, M. S.; Rich, D. H.
     J. Org. Chem. 1983, 48, 1876-9.
39. Bender, M. L.; Kezdy, F. J. Ann. Rev. Biochem. 1965, 34,
     49-76.
40. Delpierre, G. R.; Fruton, J. S. Proc. Nat. Acad. Sci.
     U.S.A. 1965, 54, 1161-1167.
41. Bruice, T. C.; Benkovic, S. "Bioorganic Mechanisms" Vol.
     I, W. A. Benjamin, Inc., New York, 1966, pp. 2-4.
42. Knowles, J. Phil. Trans. Roy. Soc. Lond. 1970, B257,
     135-146.
43. Clement, G. E. Prog. Bioorganic Chem. 1973, 2, 177-238.
44. Takahashi, M.; Wang, T. T.; Hofmann, T. Biochem. Biophys.
     Res. Comm. 1974, 57, 39-46.
45. With sulfite ester substrates: Kaiser, E. T.; Nakagawa,
     Y. in Ref. 19, pp. 159-177.
46. Silver, M. S.; Stoddard, M. Biochemistry 1972, 11,
     191-200.
47. Antonov, V. K. in Ref. 19, pp. 179-198.
48. Kozlov, L. V.; Ginodman, L. M.; Orekhovich, V. N.;
     Valueva, T. A. Biokhimiya 1966, 31, 315-321.
49. James, M. N. G.; Hsu, I-N.; Delbaere, T. J. Nature 1977,
     267, 808-813.
50. Cornish-Bowden, A. J.; Greenwell, P.; Knowles, J. R.
     Biochem. J. 1969, 113, 369-375.
51. Antonov, V. K.; Ginodman, L. M.; Kapitannikov, Y. V.;
     Barshevskaya, T. N.; Gurova, A. G.; Rumsh, L. D. FEBS
     Lett. 1978, 88, 87-90.
52. Antonov, V. K.; Ginodman, L. M.; Rumsh, L. D.;
     Kapitannikov, Y. V.; Barshevskaya, L. P.; Gurova, A. G.;
     Volkova, L. I. Eur. J. Biochem. 1981, 117, 195-200.
53. Rich, D. H.; Boparai, A. S.; Bernatowicz, M. S. Biochem.
     Biophys. Res. Comm. 1982, 104, 1127-1133.
54. Rich, D. H.; Bernatowicz, M. S.; Schmidt, P. G. J. Amer.
     Chem. Soc. 1982, 104, 3535-3536.
55. Schmidt, P. G.; Holladay, M. W.; Salituro, F. G.; Rich, D.
     H., submitted for publication.

RECEIVED December 12, 1983

Design of Peptide Analogs

Theoretical Simulation of Conformation, Energetics, and Dynamics

R. S. STRUTHERS and A. T. HAGLER

The Agouron Institute and the Peptide Biology Laboratory, The Salk Institute, La Jolla, CA 92037

J. RIVIER

Peptide Biology Laboratory, The Salk Institute, La Jolla, CA 92037

The application of modern theoretical techniques for the conformationally based design of peptide drugs is discussed. The early developments in the theoretical treatment of peptides and peptide hormones is briefly reviewed with emphasis on studies concerned with the enkephalins. A recent molecular dynamics simulation of Gonadotropin-Releasing Hormone(GnRH) is used to demonstrate the application of modern techniques. This allows us to treat highly flexible molecules such as GnRH, which is seen in the simulation to undergo large conformational fluctuations and major transitions from an extended to a folded state. The ability of a cyclic peptide to induce high energy conformational states in given residues is also discussed, and transitions in the phenylalanine residue in a molecular dynamics study of vasopressin are used to illustrate this behavior. From the wide range of conformations accessible to peptide hormones, as is found in these and other studies, it becomes clear that a rational, conformationally based approach to analog design requires supplementary information. We show how we have gone about this problem by incorporating theoretical simulations on additional constrained analogs, and developed a "template forcing" procedure to determine the conformational compatibility of these analogs. We also show how we designed a new analog, a highly constrained transannular bridged analog of a GnRH cyclic antagonist, using these methods and tested its proposed conformation theoretically. Other analogs are being designed by similar methods and routes for their synthesis are under study to test spectroscopically and biologically, the conformational predictions made through these studies.

The importance of peptide hormones has long been realized and in recent years there has been a renewed excitement, with new discoveries made almost daily on the role of peptides in the regulation of physiologic function, and the isolation and characterization of new peptide factors carrying out these roles. The fact that the

0097–6156/84/0251–0239$07.00/0
© 1984 American Chemical Society

roles served by these peptide messengers make them natural targets for development as therapeutic agents has not escaped notice, and a large research effort has been devoted to the development of useful analogs. Native peptide hormones have long played an important role as diagnostic agents. Insulin has been used for some time in the treatment of diabetes, and oxytocin for the induction of labor. Research is being carried out on the use of gonadotropin releasing hormone(GnRH) antagonists as possible contraceptive agents(1); GnRH super-agonists for the treatment of endometriosis(2), precocious puberty(3), and some forms of cancer(4); vasopressin antagonists for treating hyponatremias(5); somatostatin analogs for treating acromegaly(6), glucagonoma(7), and juvenile diabetes(8); enkephalins as improved analgesics(9); and angiotensin antagonists for control of hypertension(10); and the uses of antigenic peptides derived from viral proteins as safe synthetic vaccines(11).

Solid phase synthetic techniques coupled to high pressure liquid chromatography for purification allow for the synthesis of many analogs of new peptides almost simultaneously with the determination of the native sequence(12). A great deal of effort has been expended in trying to determine the "active" structure of each new peptide, much of it at the level of primary structure in order to define the residues necessary for receptor recognition and to systematically optimize their steric and electronic properties(13). Veber and co-workers(14) have shown that only five residues of somatostatin(the native peptide is 14 amino acids long) are sufficient for full biological activity if the five residues are held in the "correct" conformation by the proper cyclic constraint. Introducing cyclic constraints into linear peptides greatly restricts the conformational space available to the molecule and has been a powerful technique successfully applied to other peptides such as enkephalins(15), α-melanotropin(16), bradykinin(17), and GnRH(13). These are some of many examples of successful application of conformational restriction to the synthesis of bio-active peptides (for a review on the topic see Hruby(18)).

Conformational Information Required. A rational approach to the design of peptide analogs most often involves a hypothesis, sometimes implicit, about the conformation of the molecule and the relative spatial orientation of functional groups (the pharmacophore) necessary to interact with the receptor. Cyclic analogs which bind to the receptor, such as those mentioned above, yield much information about the overall folding of the molecule. Spectroscopic techniques such as NMR, IR, raman, CD, and fluorescence may be used to give still further information about the spatial relation of specific functional groups or conformational states of individual internal coordinates (such as the torsion angle phi from vicinal coupling constants from NMR). Conformational energy calculations, mainly rigid geometry calculations in which all bond lengths and angles are held fixed and torsion angles are varied to find low energy structures, have been carried out on numerous peptides and peptide hormones(19). Relatively little has been done however, in calculating a variety of analogs and formulating a methodology by which these can be compared systematically in order to derive the conformational, steric, and electrostatic properties required for binding and transduction, and then using these criteria to design new analogs for synthesis and biological evaluation. In addition the imposition of fixed bond lengths and angles, and the omission of entropic and dynamic effects in the first treatments of these molecules may introduce artifacts into the conformations obtained.

In this paper we shall review briefly some of the early developments in the theoretical treatment of peptides and peptide hormones. We shall go on to describe some recent results we have obtained in which we have applied modern theoretical techniques including molecular dynamics and valence force field minimization to the study of several peptide hormones and their analogs. In these techniques, all internal degrees of freedom of the molecule are included (allowing flexibility of bond lengths and angles), and the dynamic behavior of these flexible molecules is simulated. We will also describe the techniques we have developed for using this information to derive and compare the conformational properties of analogs, postulate the conformational requirements for activity, and design analogs for synthesis in order to test these postulated requirements.

CALCULATION OF PEPTIDE CONFORMATION

Early Techniques - Rigid Geometry Mapping and Minimization. In the early 1960's, Hendrickson (20) first proposed that the energy of a molecule could be calculated on a computer. His interest was in the conformation of cycloalkanes, but the use of computers quickly spread to biomolecules including peptides. The first application to peptides was made by Ramachandran and co-workers(21) who generated a map of the sterically allowed conformations of acetylalanine N'-methylamide(Figure 1). At that time the available computer technology forced simplifications in the expression of the potential energy in order to make the problem tractable. To calculate a conformational energy map of peptides allowing all internal degrees of freedom to vary at each value of ϕ and ψ would have been a problem requiring the computers then available to work continuously for weeks. Since the energy required to stretch bonds and distort angles is significantly greater than the energy to twist about a single bond, it was assumed that bond lengths and angles could be kept fixed at their equilibrium values. This is the so-called "rigid geometry" approximation. In Ramachandran's initial treatment the nature of the interaction between atoms was approximated by a "hard sphere" model to account for excluded volume effects. Using this approach the authors found that only certain regions of phi-psi space were sterically allowed. Further, these allowed regions accounted for the amino acid conformations known at the time from X-ray crystal studies. The "hard sphere" model was quickly superceded by the more realistic representation incorporating a softer van der Waals term and electrostatic interactions. This advance made it possible not only to calculate allowed regions of phi-psi space, but also to begin to examine the relative energetics of the various conformational states. This work has been reviewed in detail by Scheraga(22), Ramachandran and Sasisekharan (23), and Liquori (24).

Following the initial mapping work, minimization algorithms were introduced to find the energy minima as a function of ϕ, ψ, and the sidechain torsion angles χ(see Figure 1), that is to solve for the conformation where the derivative of the energy with respect to these variables is equal to zero. At this stage of development it is possible to begin considering oligopeptides of biological interest.

Rigid geometry minimization has been a useful tool for generating plausible conformations of peptides with reasonable geometries and non-bonded interactions. It may be used to generate conformations of peptide hormones which can help the peptide chemist in appreciating the three dimensional structure of the peptide(25). Rigid geometry studies of nearly all the smaller peptide hormones have been performed. Among these, the enkephalins were studied by many groups and selected examples can serve to illustrate the way in which these rigid geometry calculations have been applied to the study of peptide conformation.

Rigid Geometry Studies of Enkephalin: The enkephalins are linear pentapeptides, H-Tyr-Gly-Gly-Phe-Met-NH$_2$ (see Figure 2a.) and H-Tyr-Gly-Gly-Phe-Leu-NH$_2$, which bind to several classes of opiate receptors in the mammalian brain including the same receptor as morphine(26, 27). Enkephalins have drawn the interest of theoretical biophysicists for two reasons. First, because of their natural opiate activity, it is hoped that improved analgesics can be developed. Second, as pentapeptides, enkephalins are small enough that the molecule can be examined theoretically without excessive expense of computer time.

Isogai and coworkers(28) carried out rigid geometry minimizations of Met-enkephalin in order to search for conformations accessible to the molecule. Seventy-one conformations were chosen as starting conformations for minimization. These initial conformations were constructed from regular repeating conformations of peptides, various bend structures, combinations of amino acid and dipeptides in minimum energy conformations, and compact conformations from model building. The authors found 52 minimum energy structures within 11 Kcal/mole of their lowest energy structure. Of the 52 conformations generated, one group of conformations characterized by a type II' β-bend centered at Gly^3-Phe^4 was lower in energy ($^-$5 Kcal/mole) than other conformations. This family of conformations was stabilized significantly by a hydrogen bond from the phenolic hydroxyl of Tyr^1 to the mainchain carbonyl of either Gly^3 or Phe^4. Based on their energetic analysis and comparison to NMR results, the authors concluded that when free in solution, enkephalin exists in this preferred conformation. However, the authors also observed that because of the dependence of the stability of this conformation on the presence of the Tyr(OH) hydrogen bond, the molecule would be quite flexible in the absence of this hydrogen bond.

Subsequent experimental evidence appears to indicate that the Tyr(OH) hydrogen bond is not present in aqueous solution(29) and that the tyrosine sidechain interacts instead with the aqueous medium(30). Nevertheless, the fact that the results yield 52 minimum energy structures within 11 Kcal/mole indicates that there are a large number of conformations of the pentapeptide, which, given the possibility of enhanced stability through binding, cannot be ruled out *a priori* as being the binding conformation at the enkephalin receptor.

It is clear from the existence of a large number of accessible conformations for the native enkephalins, that if one wants to gain insight into the conformational properties required for binding, additional information is required. Loew and Burt (31) attempted to chose among conformations by comparing enkephalin to the "rigid" opiate 7-[1-phenyl-3-hydroxybutyl-3] endoethenotetrahydrothebaine or PET(See Figure 2b).(32) The authors observed that the striking common feature between enkephalins and most rigid opiates was the para-OH phenethylamine moiety circled in Figures 2a-b. Sequence activity studies had previously shown that replacement of Gly^2 in enkephalin by D-Ala^2 resulted in enhanced biological activity, (33) while the replacement with L-Ala resulted in a loss of activity(34). Their stated goal was then "...the selection of the lowest energy conformers that are local minima with at least tyramine-overlap with rigid opiates and that could accommodate both Gly^2 and D-Ala^2 (but not L-Ala^2) in similar conformations."

The authors pursued this goal by several different routes. In the first, torsion angles of Met-enkephalin were adjusted sequentially, in order to maximize overlap with corresponding functional groups on PET. Conformations were then taken at various stages of the overlapping procedure and minimized. The second method employed the 52 minimum energy conformations obtained by Isogai(28). The values for the

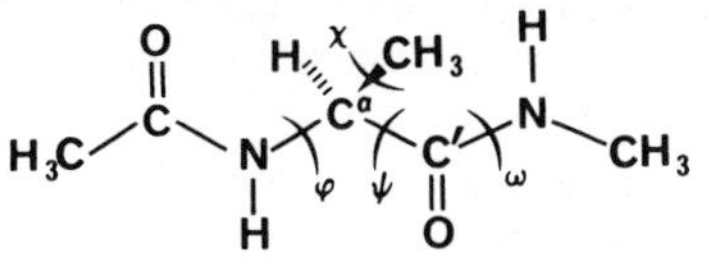

Figure 1. N–Acetylalanyl N'–methylamide.

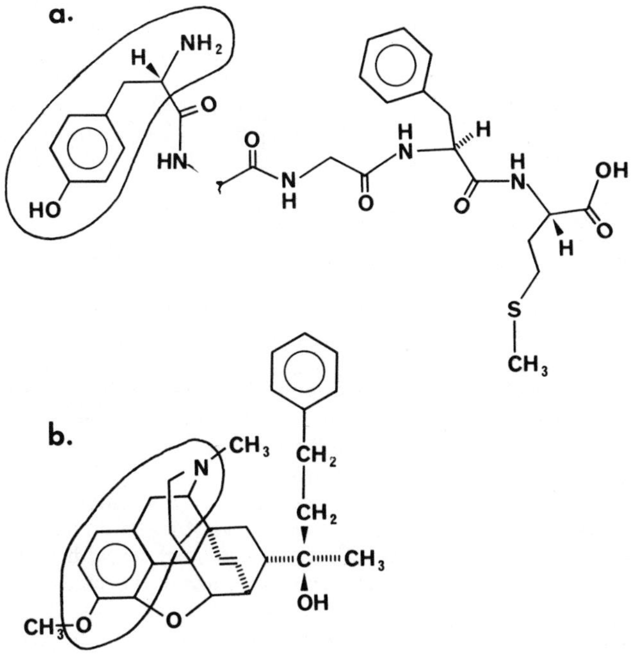

Figure 2. The native Met–enkephalin, NH_2–Tyr–Gly–Gly–Phe–Met–OH (a), and the opiate 7–[1–phenyl–3–hydroxybutyl–3]endotheno-tetrahydrothebaine, PET (b), are shown. The tyramine moiety common to enkephalins and the rigid opiates is circled.

sidechain torsion angles of Tyr[1] in these conformations were adjusted so that $\chi_1=-90°$, $\chi_2=180°$ in order to obtain overlap with the tyramine moiety of PET (ie. the terminal NH_2 and sidechain of Tyr[1]). Of the resulting conformations, those which were strained by less than 30 Kcal/mole due to this adjustment were taken as starting conformations for minimization. In the final approach, the Gly[2] residue in each of Isogai's conformations was replaced with D-Ala and the resulting molecule minimized with and without the constraint on χ_1 and χ_2 of Tyr. The D-Ala[2] in the resulting optimized conformations was then restored to Gly and the molecule optimized once more.

Using these approaches one conformation was found which satisfied the authors' criterion for tyramine overlap (Tyr[1] $\chi_1 = -90$, $\chi_2 = 180$ degrees), and where the Phe[4] sidechain also shows overlap with the phenethyl substituent of the model opiate. Conformations with the lowest energy were found to have no resemblance to PET. However, although most of the opiate is rather rigid due to the interconnected ring systems, the phenethyl C_{19} moiety, which the authors discuss, has at least four free torsion angles which control its orientation relative to the rest of the molecule. Therefore, if other conformations of PET were examined, it is possible that other conformations of enkephalin could be found which overlap the important functional groups of the opiate.

Manavalan and Momany(35) took the approach of comparing Met and Leu enkephalins with seven peptide analogs ([D-Ala[2]]Met-Enk amide, [D-Ala[2]]Met-Enk, [D-Met[2], Pro[5]]Enk amide, [D-Ala[2], D-Phe[5]]Enk, [D-Ala[2], D-Leu[5]]Enk, [D-Ala[2], NMe-Phe[4]]Met-Enk amide, and [D-Ala[2], NMe-Met[5]]Met-Enk amide), in order to determine the commonly accessible conformations.

Starting conformations for energy minimization were obtained for each analog by combining the known dipeptide minima for the component residues and excluding those resulting conformations which contained bad steric overlaps(36). Based on the conformational states of the component residues (e.g. α_r, α_l, C_7^{eq}, C_7^{ax} etc.) the authors arrived at five conformations which are common to the nine molecules. The number of conformational families was reduced to three by considering only the relative orientations of the sidechains (ie. different backbone conformations presented similar arrangements of the sidechains upon visual inspection). Although the authors note that the presence of several different types of opiate receptors may recognize several different "active" conformations of enkephalins, a more specific pharmacophore hypothesis is necessary in order for it to be useful for the conformationally based design of further analogs. Therefore, the logical next step would be to design analogs which distinguish between the three conformational classes presented.

Along these lines, the recently synthesized highly active cyclic enkephalin analogs of Dimaio and Schiller(15) and related structures(37, 38) may prove quite useful in delineating the relationship between binding and conformation of the enkephalins. The analog of Dimaio and Schiller takes advantage of the tolerance for D-amino acids at position 2 in enkephalin, in this case incorporating D-γ-diaminobutyric acid, and uses the sidechain amine to close the ring by making the amide bond with the Leu[5] carboxyl. This analog is more potent than enkephalin in the standard assays and proved to be resistant to degradation by enzymes present in rat brain suspensions. The authors subsequently examined the potencies of this analog and the corresponding linear analog, [D-aminobutyric acid[2], Leu[5]]enkephalin and found that the constraint imposed on cyclization imparted a high degree of selectivity to the cyclic analog for the μ receptor type relative to the selectivity of the linear analog. Mosberg and coworkers(37) synthesized the analog cyclo[D-penicillamine[2], D-penicillamine[5]]enkephalin and found it to be highly selective for the δ receptor class. Comparing the accessible conformations of these two selective analogs with the less selective native Leu-enkephalin could lend insight into the conformational basis for the receptor selectivity of enkephalins.

The lack of agreement between the structures calculated to date for enkephalin, and the "binding conformation" inferred from the active cyclic peptides, may be due to the intrinsic inability of the rigid geometry calculation to take into account strain in the molecule. These tight ring systems (~14 atoms) can be expected to show considerable strain, especially in Mosberg's bis-penicillamine containing analogs(37). The distortion of bond angles might be expected to play an important role in the conformation of the molecule. In fact, such distortions have been found to occur both in vasopressin and to an even greater extent in a cyclic decapeptide gonadotropin-releasing hormone antagonist (see below). Failure to account for the ability to distort bond lengths and angles, yielding excessive stiffness, could render the rigid geometry approximation impotent for intramolecular situations where these effects are an integral part of the molecular structure, such as those created by relatively strained ring systems.

Recent Techniques: Applications of a Valence Force Field. The necessity of accounting for the distortion of internal geometries has been recognized for some time(39) in the application to hydrocarbons and in the field of "molecular mechanics". As noted above, Hendrickson took (20) angle deformation into account in his pioneering study of hydrocarbons, but only recently has this occurred in the study of biologically active peptides(40-42). Treatment of all degrees of freedom is taken into account by the use of a valence type force field(43) or a related form called the Urey-Bradley force field(43) to express the energy of a molecule(Equation 1). In Equation 1 the energy is taken as the sum of the energies required to stretch and compress bonds, bend angles, twist dihedral angles, distort planar groups, and the interatomic energies of van der Waal's and coulombic interactions between non-bonded atoms. In addition there are coupling terms which reflect the fact that the energy to distort a given internal coordinate may be "coupled" to the distortion of a neighboring internal coordinate. It is only in the representation of these terms that the Urey-Bradley differs from the functional form of the Valence Force Field(43).

$$
\begin{aligned}
V = &\sum \{D_b[1 - e^{-\alpha(b-b_0)}]^2 - D_b\} + 1/2 \sum K_\theta (\theta - \theta_0)^2 \\
&+ 1/2 \sum K_\phi (1 + s \cos n\phi) + 1/2 \sum K_\chi \chi^2 \\
&+ \sum\sum F_{bb'}(b - b_0)(b' - b_0') \\
&+ \sum\sum F_{\theta\theta'}(\theta - \theta_0)(\theta' - \theta_0') + \sum\sum F_{b\theta}(b - b_0)(\theta - \theta_0) \\
&+ \sum\sum F_{\phi\theta\theta'} \cos \phi (\theta - \theta_0)(\theta' - \theta_0') + \sum\sum F_{\chi\chi'}\chi\chi' \\
&+ \sum \epsilon [2(r^*/r)^9 - 3(r^*/r)^6] + \sum q_i q_j / r
\end{aligned}
\tag{1}
$$

There are two types of quantities represented in the equation: constants characteristic of the energy required to deform a given internal coordinate $(K_b, K_\theta...F_{bb}, F_{\theta\theta}...)$, or characteristic of the strength of a given interatomic nonbonded interaction (r^*, ϵ, q); and the internal coordinates specifying the geometry of the molecule (bond lengths, b; bond angles, θ; dihedral angles, ϕ; out of plane angles, χ; and non-bonded interatomic distances, r). Therefore, given a molecular geometry and values for the potential constants, we can calculate the energy of a molecule.

Obviously, the accuracy of the calculation depends on the accuracy of the potential parameters. This is a crucial area which requires further extensive research. The parameters used in our work have been derived by fitting a wide range of experimental data including crystal structure of amides and carboxylic acids, unit cell vectors and the orientation of the molecules in the asymmetric unit, sublimation energies, molecular dipole moments, molecular structure, vibrational spectra, and strain energies of small model amides, peptides, and other organic compounds. Ab-initio molecular orbital calculations have also been used in conjunction with experimental data to give information on charge distributions, energy barriers, and coupling terms, both to supplement and confirm the results obtained from fitting the experimental data.(40, 44-51)

Properties Implicit In The Energy Surface. The ability to calculate the energy of a molecule from the atomic coordinates is the foundation of all theoretical simulation techniques.(19) Implicit in the energy surface of a molecule are all conformational and dynamic properties of interest, (except quantum properties such as rearrangement of bonds and charge transfer events). We can compare the relative energies of any two conformations of a given molecule. By calculating the first derivatives of the energy with respect to the Cartesian coordinates of the atoms and solving for the case where these derivatives are equal to zero, we can find the minimum energy structures of a molecule. Since the negative of the first derivatives gives the force on each atom, and we know the mass of each atom, we can solve Newton's equation of motion ($F=ma$) for the accelerations of the atoms. By following these accelerations for a short time, recalculating them from the new atom positions, then following the new accelerations in an iterative manner, we can follow the trajectory of the atoms and "see" the dynamic behavior of the molecule. We can also determine the second derivatives of the energy with respect to the Cartesian coordinates, and by calculating the eigenvalues and corresponding eigenvectors of the mass- weighted second derivative matrix, find the vibrational frequencies and normal modes, respectively. Furthermore, applying classical statistical thermodynamics we can use these frequencies to calculate the entropy, vibrational energy, and free energy of a given conformational state. Thus, the structure, dynamics, vibrational spectra, energetics and other properties derived from these (e.g. vicinal coupling constants for NMR) are all accessible through the ability to calculate the energy of the molecule.

We now turn to several examples where these techniques have been applied to peptide hormones, and show how we can study the conformational properties, including conformational minima and fluctuations, dynamics, and energetics of these molecules, and how these properties can in turn be used to design analogs.

Structure, Dynamics, and Energetics of Gonadotropin Releasing Hormone. Gonadotropin releasing hormone(GnRH) is a member of the class of peptide hormones secreted by the hypothalamus to regulate pituitary hormone levels. It controls the release of luteinizing hormone (LH) and follicle stimulating hormone (FSH), which in turn, are involved in the regulation of ovulation and spermatogenesis. The amino acid sequence of GnRH, pGlu-His-Trp-Ser-Tyr-Gly-Leu-Arg-Pro-Gly-NH$_2$, was elucidated some 10 years ago(52, 53), and since that time GnRH has been the subject of an extensive research effort involving the design of more than a thousand analogs. Among these, antagonists to GnRH were developed which have been shown to inhibit both ovulation and spermatogenesis and they have therefore elicited intense interest as possible contraceptive agents(1).

Conformational studies are of obvious importance. These studies, both experimental and theoretical, have been limited to date by the relatively large size of the peptide. A number of spectroscopic studies have been performed utilizing fluorescence (54), ultraviolet-visible(55), carbon-13 NMR(56), and proton NMR(57-59). Little or no consensus was reached among these authors as to the conformation of the peptide. Theoretical studies have been limited by the relatively large size of the peptide and only a few studies have been carried out(36, 60, 61).

We have recently undertaken an extensive study of the conformational and dynamic properties of GnRH and several analogs in an attempt to elucidate conformational properties which may underly binding and transduction, and to design new constrained analogs for synthesis and biological evaluation based on these features which can then serve to test putative pharmacophore models. In this work we have utilized modern theoretical techniques such as molecular dynamics, and developed a methodology for the comparison of structural features to assist in analog design. The preliminary results of this study provide an example of the use of these modern theoretical techniques in the design of drugs based on peptide conformation.

We have carried out a 15 picosecond molecular dynamics simulation of the native GnRH as a preliminary search of the conformational space accessible to the hormone.(62) At the start of the simulation the molecule was in an extended conformation and over the course of the simulation passed through various "local" minimum energy conformations. These minima were characterized by minimization of coordinates taken at one picosecond(ps) intervals along the molecular dynamics trajectory for the first 12 picoseconds of the simulation. In these minimizations all degrees of freedom in the molecule were relaxed using the valence force field in equation 1. The minimum energy conformations after 1, 4, 6, and 8 picoseconds are shown in Figure 3a-d.

The structure resulting from minimization after 1ps shows residues four through ten to be in a repeating C_7 hydrogen bonded structure, where each residue is near ϕ, ψ = -80°, +80°(the hydrogen-bonds are shown in the figure as dotted or dashed lines). An interesting feature of this conformation is the amphipathic organization of the sidechains with pGlu, Trp, Tyr, Leu, and Pro on the right side of the chain, and the hydrophilic sidechains His, Ser, Arg, Gly-NH_2 on the left. This is a relatively high energy local minimum (77Kcal/mole), being ~20Kcal/mole above the lowest energy minimum we have found for the molecule in this simulation. After 4 picoseconds, the trajectory has taken the molecule into a more compact and lower energy(69Kcal/mole) structure. Major transitions have occurred in the backbone of residues Tyr^5 and Leu^7 bringing about the turn structure. Now, instead of the amphipathic organization, there is a clustering of the hydrophobic residues (Trp, Tyr, Leu, and Pro) in the center of the molecule. After 6 ps the peptide has returned to a more extended structure, again of higher energy(74.5Kcal/mole). By 8 ps the peptide has undergone a major change in shape to a very compact conformation where the guanidinium group of Arg^8 is found in the center of the molecule and is involved in a hydrogen-bonding network with the carbonyl groups of Trp^3 and Tyr^5, and the NH groups of Tyr^5 and Leu^7. The conformational energy is now 60 Kcal/mole, or 17 kcal/mole less than the minimum energy structure after 1ps. This is due mostly to an increase in favorable coulombic interactions and a decrease in unfavorable van der Waals interactions. At one end of the molecule we have an unorthodox open turn structure involving the five residues Trp-Ser-Tyr-Gly-Leu, while at the other end we have hydrogen bonds between the NH of the terminal amide and the CO of $pGlu^1$, and between the NH of the His^2 sidechain and the CO of Gly^{10}. These two features combine to give the conformation an overall pseudo-cyclic appearance.

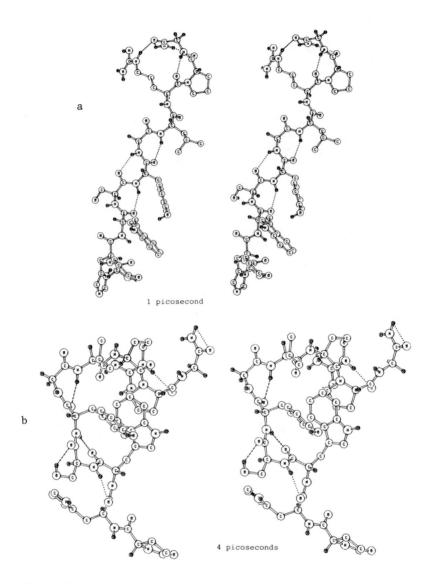

a

1 picosecond

b

4 picoseconds

Figure 3.   Minimum energy conformations of gonadotropin-
releasing hormone (GnRH), pGlu–His–Trp–Ser–Tyr–Gly–Leu–Arg–
Pro–Gly–NH$_2$, obtained by minimization of the structures
along the molecular dynamics trajectory at 1, 4, 6, and 8
picoseconds.

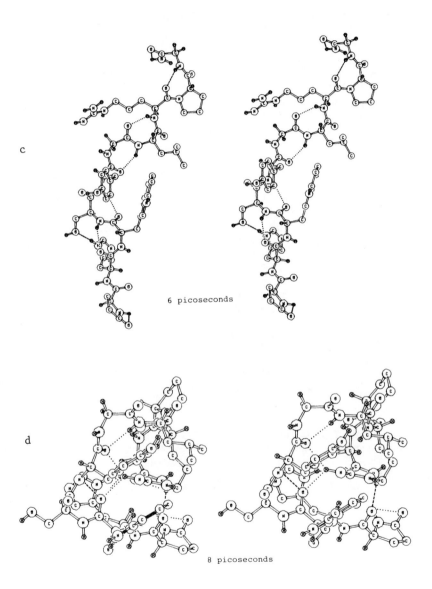

c

6 picoseconds

d

8 picoseconds

Figure 3. Continued.

These four conformations are but a few examples. The lowest minimum energy structure found was somewhat more compact and had an energy of 56.3 Kcal/mole. Each of the other minimizations from the molecular dynamics gave unique minima showing that for the 15 picoseconds of simulation the molecule was continually exploring new regions of conformational space. A complete description of these structures will be presented elsewhere(62).

Transitions of Leu[7]. Another way to appreciate the fluctuations the molecule undergoes, and the difference between a dynamic and static representation of conformation is by examining the conformational states of the individual torsion angles in the molecule. The values of ϕ, ψ and any other torsion angle can be plotted as a function of time along the dynamic trajectory in order to observe their fluctuations and transitions. The example of Leu[7] is given in Figure 4.

As can be seen from Figure 4, at the beginning of the simulation, Leu[7] is in an extended conformation, ϕ, ψ = 200°,165° (-160,165). For the first ˜6 picoseconds ϕ oscillates between values of -80° and -160°, while ψ which begins at 165° quickly drops to ˜80°, gradually returns to ˜180°, then gradually declines back to values near 80°. These fluctuations constitute excursions through most of the allowed regions in the top left hand quadrant (-,+) of the Phi-Psi map(63). At ˜6ps a sharp transition occurs in the psi angle, seen as a sharp drop in Figure 4. This transition from the C_7^{eq} (ϕ, ψ ≃ +80, -80) conformation to the α_r (ϕ, ψ ≃ -60, -60) is a step in the transition from the more extended structure at 6 picoseconds (Figure 3c) to the very compact structures such as that seen after 8 picoseconds (Figure 3d). The effect of the transition is to bring the Arg sidechain into the proximity of the Tyr carbonyl. The resulting hydrogen-bond interaction helps to pull the two ends of the molecule together to form the open turn structure mentioned above. At the conclusion of the simulation Leu has shifted to more negative phi angles visiting the α' (ϕ, ψ ≃ -160, -60) region of the map and producing more classical turn structures involving the four residues, Tyr-Gly-Leu-Arg.

Vasopressin Dynamics: Conformational Transitions in Individual Residues: Vasopressin is secreted by the posterior pituitary and acts both in the circulatory system, causing vasoconstriction, and in the kidney, causing the increased uptake of water from the collecting ducts. It is a disulfide bridged cyclic-hexapeptide with a tripeptide tail, [Cys-Tyr-Phe-Gln-Asn-Cys]-Pro-Arg-Gly-NH$_2$, and provides another example of the power of the combined application of molecular dynamics and energy minimization for studying accessible conformations of flexible biologically active peptides. It also serves to demonstrate how structural fluctuations and induced strain in portions of the molecule can be simulated by these techniques. Although the disulfide bond introduces a ring constraint, we have found that vasopressin is still a very flexible molecule(64). Part of this flexibility appears to arise from the enhanced stabilization of higher energy conformational states for a given residue by intramolecular interactions, thus lowering the energy difference between conformational states.

The energetics of Phe[3] provide an excellent example of this phenomenon. In our molecular dynamics simulation of vasopressin, we found that Phe[3] underwent conformational transitions between three regions of conformational space: the C_7^{eq} (ϕ, ψ ≃ -80, +80), α_r (ϕ, ψ ≃ -60, -60), and C_7^{ax} (ϕ, ψ ≃ +80, -80) conformations(64). These conformations in the isolated residue, taken as the N-acetyl, N'-methylamide blocked phenylalanine, are well separated energetically as can be seen in Table I. The C_7^{eq} is 3.1 Kcal more stable than the C_7^{ax}, and 4.7 Kcal more stable than the α_r. In order to compare the relative stabilities of these phenylalanine conformations in the

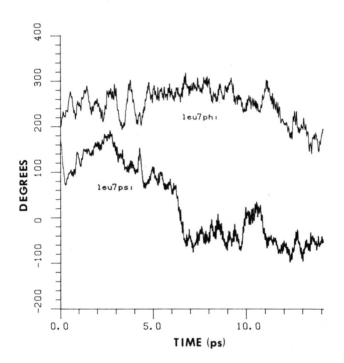

Figure 4. A history of the fluctuations in torsion angles ϕ and ψ of the leucine residue as a function of the time elapsed during the molecular dynamics simulation of GnRH.

Table I. Intra-Residue Energies of Phenylalanine in Vasopressin Minimum Energy Structures and in minimum energy conformations of Ac-Phe-NMe.

		In Vasopressin		Isolated		
Conf.	time(ps)[1]	Energy[2] (Kcal/mole)	(ϕ,ψ)	Energy (Kcal/Mole)	(ϕ,ψ)	Strain Energy[3] (Kcal/mole)
C_7^{eq}	0.2	32.7(0)	-74,69	26.2(0)	-88,97	6.5
α_r	1.4	34.7(2.0)	-57,-54	30.9(4.7)	-78,-55	3.8
C_7^{ax}	6.9	34.9(2.2)	48,-81	29.3(3.1)	75,-69	5.6

[1] The time given is that of the molecular dynamics conformation which was minimized to give the minimum energy structure of vasopressin. The energy of the Phe fragment was calculated for these structures.

[2] The energy calculated includes the $C\alpha$ and CO of the previous residue and the NH and $C\alpha$ of the subsequent residue in vasopressin. The energies in vasopressin and in the isolated residue are then directly comparable.

[3] The strain energy is calculated as the energy of the residue in the vasopressin molecule minus the energy of the isolated residue.

isolated form and when incorporated into the vasopressin molecule, we "cut" the N-acetyl, N'-methyl blocked residue from minimum energy structures of vasopressin and calculated the potential energy(Table I).

All three conformations show a significant degree of strain caused by geometric constraints imposed by the rest of the hexapeptide ring. The three conformational states are not strained to the same degree, however. The C_7^{eq} is still the most stable conformation of the residue when incorporated into vasopressin, but as is seen in the last column of Table I, it has suffered the highest degree of strain (6.5 Kcal). The α_r conformation is accommodate best in the ring, being strained by 3.8 Kcal/mole relative to its lowest energy minimum when isolated, while the C_7^{ax} is strained 5.6 Kcal/mole relative to the isolated amino acid minima. Thus in these minimum energy structures of the vasopressin molecule instead of being 4.7 Kcal more stable than α_r the C_7^{eq} is only 2.0 Kcal more stable. In addition, because of the difference in strain energies imposed on Phe[3] in the α_r and C_7^{ax} conformations, the C_7^{ax}, which was more stable than the α_r in the isolated residue (1.6 Kcal/mole), is now slightly less stable than the α_r.

These results demonstrate that intramolecular constraints, especially in a cyclic molecule, may accommodate some conformations of a residue better than others, in this case bringing the energies of the various conformations closer together. This results in an enhanced flexibility of the vasopressin molecule at this position, and serves to demonstrate that knowledge of the relative stabilities of the minimum energy conformations of the isolated residue may not be sufficient to predict the relative stabilities of these conformations when they are incorporated into a peptide. These conclusions can have serious implications for the interpretation of activities of analogs in which so-called "conformation imposing" residues such as α-methyl amino acids, N^α-methyl amino acids and others have been used(65). Simply because one of these "conformation imposing" residues prefers, or even "strongly" prefers, one conformational state over another in the isolated residue, it does not rigorously follow that this conformation is maintained when incorporated into a larger, constrained peptide, which might significantly destabilize the "preferred" conformation. An experimental observation of this effect is seen in the crystal structures of α-methyl amino acid containing peptides, where, this "α-helical" residue, although overwhelmingly found in the α-helical conformation, is also found to take up significantly different conformations(66), induced in this case either by the crystal lattice forces, or intramolecular constraints such as those discussed above. Further, both C_7 and C_5 hydrogen bonds have been observed in solution(67).

ANALOG DESIGN

In the enkephalin studies we began to see how theoretical techniques can be used to generate conformations of related molecules. With the results from GnRH and vasopressin we saw how flexible these molecules are and how the conformational fluctuations and dynamics of these molecules can be studied. We also saw how the relative stabilities of conformations of a molecular fragment can be influenced by conformational constraints of the whole molecule. In the following section we will present some ideas on how these calculations can be incorporated into a conformational based approach to drug design.

There are several levels at which the theoretical computer simulation techniques can help the medicinal chemist to design analogs incorporating such properties as increased potency, selectivity, etc. The first involves observation of the conformations visited in movies of dynamic trajectories and stereographic figures of minimum energy structures of the molecule of interest. The knowledge of the accessible structures and spatial relationships of the functional groups in the native peptide, observable from these movies or figures, may allow the chemist to postulate the importance of a given conformation in interacting with the receptor. Analogs then may be designed based on these structures in order to "lock" in or enhance the stability of these conformations.

The second level at which the theoretical analysis may be used is to extend the use of the computational techniques to analyze the results of the simulation and characterize similarities and differences between the conformational and energetic properties of various analogs. Several tools are used at this level including: a least squares superposition which gives the best overlap between specified atom sets of two analogs; the calculation of the root mean square distance (RMS) between corresponding atoms in the superposed analogs to quantitatively characterize the similarities of the conformations; energetic analysis to yield relative stabilities of classes of conformations in different analogs and to locate differential strains due to modifications in sequence; and "template forcing", a technique which we developed to force one analog along a minimum energy path into the conformation of another. With these tools we can then examine the similarity and difference between analogs quantitatively as well as displaying molecules which have been optimally superposed to observe differences systematically. From the template forcing we can look for common conformations of two analogs directly, and also begin to ask why a desired conformation is inaccessible to a given analog and propose modifications which could alleviate unfavorable interactions precluding the target conformation. Template forcing is emerging as an extremely powerful technique for analog comparison and design. Finally, observations of given structural features in these common conformations can lead to putative analogs which can then be simulated theoretically to determine if the desired features are maintained, before any synthesis takes place.

Comparison of GnRH Conformations With Those of a Cyclic Antagonist: As we saw above, GnRH has a high degree of flexibility, and if we want to understand the conformational requirements for binding and transduction of the message, it is necessary to gain additional information. This is done by considering the conformational properties of other analogs, especially constrained analogs, and comparing the allowed conformational states of these analogs to one another and to the native molecule.

The most powerful constraints, from the point of view of restricting the accessible conformational space available to the peptide, are ring constraints introduced by linking residues well separated in the sequence. We therefore decided to look at the cyclic antagonist   cyclo[Δ^3-Pro-D-Phe(p-Cl)-D-Trp-Ser-Tyr-D-Trp-NMe-Leu-Arg-Pro-β-Ala], which is the most active cyclic antagonist reported to date.(13) In cultured pituitary cells a 3.5 fold excess of the antagonist is required, relative to GnRH, to reduce GnRH induced secretion of LH by 50%, indicating that the binding of this analog is somewhat weaker than that of GnRH. By defining the conformations accessible to this molecule, and then determining those conformations that are available to GnRH as well, we hoped to further define putative binding conformations, which could form the basis for new conformationally constrained analogs whose synthesis and binding assays can, in an iterative fashion, ultimately establish the binding conformation(s), and lead to new therapeutic agents.

In order to search the accessible conformational space of this molecule, a molecular dynamics simulation over a trajectory spanning a time of 24 ps. was carried out. As with the native GnRH, configurations were taken from the resultant trajectory at 1 ps intervals and minimized. Several identical structures were found from these minimizations leaving 18 distinct conformations. The fluctuations are much smaller than for native GnRH and in fact only in going from the initial minimized structure to the structure after 1 ps. does any residue undergo a transition to a different conformational state (e.g. $\Delta^{3,4}$-Pro from the α_r region (ϕ,ψ = -84°, -74°). to the C_7^{eq} (ϕ,ψ -78°, +93°) and D-Phe^2 from the C_7^{eq} (ϕ,ψ = -79°,63°) to the α_l (ϕ,ψ = 69°,40°)). This difference in conformational flexibility of the cyclic antagonist and GnRH is dramatic. Basically one conformational family (in this case one backbone conformation with several variations in sidechain conformations) is observed. In fact this cyclic decapeptide antagonist appears more constrained and rigid than the six residue ring in vasopressin. These preliminary results are the subject of further study in our laboratory. One of the low energy members of this family can be seen Figure 5a. The structure is characterized by a hydrogen bonded turn at the level of Tyr-D-Trp-NMe-Leu-Arg (shown at the top of the figure) and a second chain reversal in the bridge region, β-Ala-Δ^3-Pro-D-Phe-D-Trp.

Several of the folded structures of GnRH appeared to have conformations similar to the cyclic antagonist. In order to compare the calculated conformations quantitatively, we superposed residues 4-9 of GnRH (Ser^4-Tyr^5-Gly^6-Leu^7-Arg^8-Pro^9) onto residues 4-9 of the cyclic antagonist (Ser^4-Tyr^5-D-Trp^6-NMe-Leu^7-Arg^8-Pro^9), with the exception of the sidechain of D-Trp^6 in the antagonist (Gly^6 in GnRH) and the methyl group on the nitrogen of NMe-Leu^7 (Leu^7 in GnRH). This was done by first translating GnRH so that the center of mass of the selected atoms coincided with that for the selected atoms of the cyclic antagonist, and subsequently minimizing the root-mean-square distance between corresponding atoms with respect to the three rotational degrees of freedom of GnRH. This preliminary choice of residues was made since it is the most common sequence to the two analogs and, not coincidentally, important to high binding affinity. A measure of the similarity between the conformations is given by the resulting optimized RMS distance between corresponding atoms in each pair of conformations. The best fit is obtained between the GnRH minimum energy conformation after 11 picoseconds and the cyclic antagonist minimum energy conformation after 18 picoseconds with an RMS deviation of ˜2.6Å. On the other hand, as would be expected, more extended conformations of GnRH have much poorer fits to the cyclic antagonist (e.g. the GnRH minimum energy conformation at 1 picosecond has an RMS distance to the cyclic antagonist minimum energy conformation after 18 picoseconds of ˜6.4Å) To put these fits in some perspective, we note that the corresponding superpositions of the different conformations of GnRH itself range up to 6.4Å, while the RMS deviation for this region of the cyclic antagonist were found only as high as 2.7Å. These results indicate that GnRH can adopt conformations which are close to those adopted by the cyclic antagonist, at least in the region 4-9.

Template Forcing. In order to answer the general question of how closely the relative spatial orientations of corresponding functional groups in two flexible molecules can be, we have recently developed the technique of "template forcing" to solve for the conformation which optimizes the overlap of these functional groups while maintaining the lowest potential energy cost to the molecule. In template forcing we minimize the energy of the molecule to be superposed onto an analog (the template), along with a penalty function which is proportional to the RMS distance between the common atoms

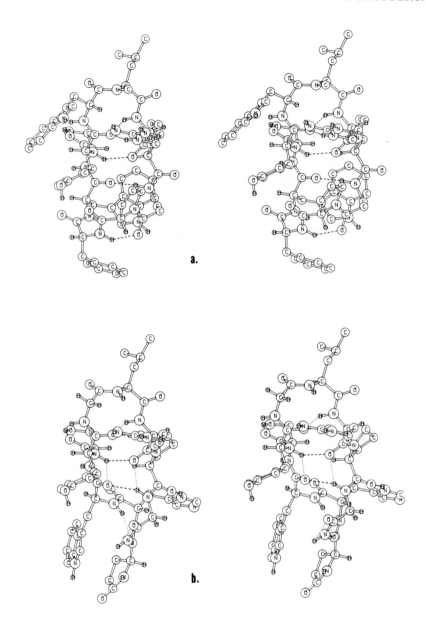

Figure 5. A minimum energy structure for the GnRH cyclic antagonist cyclo[Δ^3-Pro-D-Phe(p-Cl)-D-Trp-Ser-Tyr-D-Trp-NMeLeu-Arg-
Pro-β-Ala] (a) is compared with the conformation of GnRH obtained by "template forcing" to the cyclic antagonist (b).
See text for a discussion of template forcing.

to be superposed. That is, we minimize the energy of the molecule, subject to an external force which forces the common atoms together (equation 2).

$$F = V + K[\sum_{i}^{N}(x_i - x_i^0)^2/N]^{1/2} \qquad (2)$$

In this equation, F is a function which is the sum of the the energy V from the normal valence force field (equation 1) plus the penalty function, a constant, K, times the root-mean-square deviation between the coordinates of the corresponding atoms of the template (x_i^0) and the forced molecule (x_i) (N is the total number of atoms forced). As the distance between the atoms of the forced molecule and the template goes to zero the contribution of this penalty function vanishes. The balance between the degree to which the superposed molecule is forced onto the template and strain energy caused by the forcing is governed by the value of the constant K, which can be chosen arbitrarily to give any desired degree of fit.

We have applied this technique to force GnRH into a conformation which best superposed the residues 4-8 and 4-9 onto the corresponding residues of the cyclic antagonist. The superposition of residues 4-8 is shown in Figure 5. A very close fit (0.29Å and 0.38Å) can be achieved at a relatively low cost in energy as can be seen from Table II.

Table II. Template Forcing of GnRH onto the Cyclic Antagonist

Residues Forced	RMS	Energy of GnRH in forced Conformation[1]
4-8	0.29Å	61.5 (5.2)[2] Kcal/mole
4-9	0.38Å	61.2 (4.9) Kcal/mole

[1] A stiffness constant of K = 10 was used for this forcing.

[2] The number in parenthesis is the difference in energy between the forced conformation and the lowest energy GnRH conformation found so far.

One of the powers of this technique is that we are not limited solely to the comparison or consideration of minimum energy structures. Indeed, the dynamic fluctuations of a molecule are fluctuations about minimum energy conformations and the actual minimum energy structure itself may seldom be adopted. More importantly, binding to the receptor may well induce limited strain into the ligand(68) and possibly into the receptor as well. Therefore, we see that when comparing two molecules it may be important not only to compare the geometric distance between minima, but the difference between conformations close to but not necessarily located at local minima. In this regard it is also important to consider the energetic distance between the minima and strained conformations. Template forcing gives us a method by which we can directly find the common conformations of two molecules and compare their relative stabilities. In the example above we are limited to having one fixed structure acting as a "template", but in fact one could simultaneously minimize the energy of both molecules, together with the superposition function, and remove this limitation. (This modification to the technique is currently being developed.)

Design of a Transannular Bridged Analog of the Cyclic Antagonist: Testing the Putative Binding Conformation. The next step after adopting a hypothesized binding conformation, is to design covalently bridged analogs based on close spatial relationships which exist in the postulated conformation and which, ideally, are far removed sequentially. Inspection of the low energy conformations of the cyclic antagonist (ie. Figure 5b) reveal that the α-hydrogens of Ser[4] and Pro[8] are directed into the center of the ring, roughly across from each other (~ 2.5Å). It follows that we should be able to bridge these α-carbon atoms with two or three methylene groups ($-CH_2-CH_2-$ or $-CH_2-CH_2-CH_2-$), without introducing any large perturbations into the structure. We have built these hypothetical analogs on the computer and minimized their energy with respect to all degrees of freedom. As postulated, the cyclic structure can easily accommodate the proposed modification according to the calculation, with only minor perturbations of the structure. This may be seen by inspecting the resultant minimized structures shown in stereo for the ethylene bridged analog in Figure 6. The RMS deviations of these structures from the parent cyclic antagonist are only .3Å($-CH_2-CH_2-$) and .6Å($-CH_2-CH_2-CH_2-$).

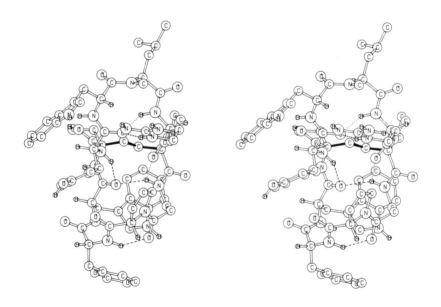

Figure 6. A minimum energy structure of the transannular bridged analog of the GnRH cyclic antagonist designed to constrain the conformation to that found for the parent cyclic antagonist. The α-carbons of Ser[4] and Pro[4] have been linked by an ethylene bridge to accomplish this.

Thus through these techniques we have now found a putative binding conformation, and based on this conformation designed a transannular bridge which results in an even more constrained analog. A key feature is that the conformation of this analog has been analyzed theoretically, and preliminary results indicate that the target conformation will be maintained. This prediction can be tested by synthesis of the analog and spectroscopic analysis (which should result in essentially equivalent spectra for the two analogs). The equivalence of the conformations of the two molecules would be strong evidence for the hypothesized binding conformation. If, in addition, the transannular bridged analog itself were active, then this would essentially prove this to be the binding conformation. This analog presents a non-classical synthetic peptide problem and we are investigating possible synthetic routes. We are also in the process of designing more readily synthesizable analogs with similar objectives in mind.

Acknowledgments: This work was supported in part by contract N01-HD-2-2807 and grant HD-13527 from the National Institutes of Health, and grant PCM-8204908 from the National Science Foundation. Support from Smith Kline and French Laboratories is also gratefully acknowledged.

Literature Cited

1. in *LHRH Peptides as Male & Female Contraceptives*, ed. G.I. Zatuchni, J.D. Shelton, & J.J. Sciarra, Harper & Row, Philadelphia (1981).

2. D.R. Meldrum, R.J. Chang, J. Lu, W. Vale, J. Rivier, and H.L. Judd, *J. of Clin. Endo. Metab.*, **54**, 1081 (1982).

3. W.F. Crowley Jr., F. Comite, W. Vale, J. Rivier, D.L. Loriaux, and G.B. Cutler, *J. Clin. Endo. Metab.*, **52**, 370 (1981).

4. A. Corbin, *Yale J. Biol. Med.*, **55**, 27 (1982).

5. M. Manning and W.H. Sawyer, *Ann. Int. Med.*, **96**, 520 (1982).

6. C.A. Meyers, D.H. Coy, W.A. Murphy, T.W. Redding, A. Arimura, and A.V. Schally, *Proc. Natl. Acad. Sci. USA*, **77**, 577 (1980).

7. C.R. Kahn, S.J. Bhathena, L. Recant, and J. Rivier, *J. Clin. Endo. Metab.*, **53**, 543 (1981).

8. J.E. Gerich, *Metabolism*, **27**, 1283 (1978).

9. S.H. Snyder, *Nature*, **279**, 13 (1979).

10. D.T. Pals, G.S. Denning Jr., and R.E. Keenan, *Kidney Int.*, **15**, pp. S-7 (1979).

11. J.G. Sutcliffe, T.M. Shinnick, N. Green, and R.A. Lerner, *Science*, **219** (1983).

12. W. Vale, J. Spiess, C. Rivier, and J. Rivier, *Science*, **213**, 1394 (1981).

13. J. Rivier, C. Rivier, M. Perrin, J. Porter, and W. Vale, in *LHRH Peptides as Male & Female Contraceptives*, ed. G.I. Zatuchni, J.D. Shelton, & J.J. Sciarra, Harper & Row, Philadelphia (1981).

14. D.F. Veber et al., *Nature*, **292**, 55 (1981).

15. J. Dimaio and P. Schiller, *Proc. Natl. Acad. Sci. USA*, **77**, 7126 (1980).

16. J.J. Knittel, T.K. Sawyer, V.J. Hruby, and M.E. Hadley, *J. Med. Chem.*, **26**, 125 (1983).

17. G.I. Chipens F.K. Mutulis B.S. Katayev V.E. Klusha I.P. Misina N.V. Mysh-lyiakova, *Int. J. Pept. Prot. Res.*, **18**, 302 (1981).

18. V.J. Hruby and H. Mosberg, *Peptides*, **3**, 329 (1982).

19. A.T. Hagler, in *Physical Methods in Peptide Conformational Studies'' (Vol. 6 of " The Peptides'')*. in press

20. J.B. Hendrickson, *J. Am. Chem. Soc.*, **83**, 4537 (1961).

21. G.N. Ramachandran, C. Ramakrishnan, and V. Sasisekharan, *J. Mol. Biol.*, **7**, 95 (1963).

22. H.A. Scheraga, *Adv. in Phys. Org. Chem.*, **6**, 103 (1968).

23. G.N. Ramachandran and V. Sasisekharan, *Adv. Protein Chem.*, **23**, 283 (1968).

24. A.M. Liquori, *Quart. Rev. Biophys.*, **2**, 65 (1969).

25. P. Gund, J.D. Andose, J.B. Rhodes, and G.M. Smith, *Science*, **208**, 1425 (1980).

26. J.A.H. Lord, A.A. Waterfield, J. Hughes, and H.W. Kosterlitz, *Nature*, **267**, 495 (1977).

27. K-J Chang and P. Cuatrecasas, *J. Biol. Chem.*, **254**, 2610 (1979).

28. Y. Isogai, G. Nemethy, and H.A. Scheraga, *Proc. Natl. Acad. Sci. USA*, **74**, 414 (1977).

29. P.W. Schiller and C.F. Yam, in *Peptides''*, *Proc. Fifth Am. Pept. Symp.*, ed. J. Meienhofer, p. 92, John Wiley & Sons (1977).

30. M.A. Spirtes, R.W. Schwartz, W.L. Mattice, and D.H. Coy, *Biochem. Biophys. Res. Comm.*, **81**, 602 (1978).

31. G.H. Loew and S.K. Burt, *Proc. Natl. Acad. Sci. USA*, **75**, 7 (1978).

32. A.P. Feinberg, I. Creese, and S.H. Snyder, *Proc. Natl. Acad. Sci. USA*, **73**, 4215 (1976).

33. J.M. Walker, G.G. Bernston, C.A. Sandman, D.H. Coy, A.V. Schally, and A.J. Kastin, *Science*, **196**, 86 (1977).

34. C.B. Pert, A. Pert, J.K. Chang, and B.T.W. Fong, *Science*, **194**, 330 (1976).

35. P. Manavalan and F.A. Momany, *Int. J. Pept. Prot. Res.*, **18**, 256 (1981).

36. F.A. Momany, *J. Am. Chem. Soc.*, **98**, 2990 (1976).

37. H.I. Mosberg, R. Hurst, V.J. Hruby, K. Gee, H.I. Yamamura, J.J. Galligan, and T.F. Burks, *Proc. Natl. Acad. Sci. USA*, **80**, 5870 (1983).

38. J.M. Berman, M. Goodman, Thi M.-D. Nguyen, and P.W. Schiller, *Biochem. Biophys. Res. Comm.*, **115** (1983).

39. in *Proceedings of NRCC Workshop on "Computer Simulation of Organic and Biological Molecules''*, ed. A.J. Olson (1981).

40. A.T. Hagler, P.S. Stern , R. Sharon, J. Becker, and F. Naider, *J. Am. Chem. Soc.*, **101**, 6842 (1979).

41. P.S. Stern, M. Chorev, M. Goodman, and A.T. Hagler, *Biopolymers*, **22**, 1885 (1983).

42. P.S. Stern, M. Chorev, M. Goodman, and A.T. Hagler, *Biopolymers*, **22**, 1901 (1983).

43. O. Ermer, *Structure and Bonding*, **27**, 161, Berlin (1976).

44. P. Dauber and A.T. Hagler, *Accts. of Chem Res.*, **13**, 105 (1980).

45. S. Lifson, A.T. Hagler, and P. Dauber, *J. Am. Chem. Soc.*, **101**, 5111 (1979).

46.   A.T. Hagler, S. Lifson, and P. Dauber, *J. Am. Chem. Soc.*, **101**, 5122 (1979).

47.   A.T. Hagler, P. Dauber, and S. Lifson, *J. Am. Chem. Soc.*, **101**, 5131 (1979).

48.   A.T. Hagler, P.S. Stern, S. Lifson, and S. Ariel, *J. Am. Chem. Soc.*, **101**, 813 (1979).

49.   A.T. Hagler and A. Lapiccirella, *Biopolymers*, **15**, 1167 (1976).

50.   A.T. Hagler, E. Huler, and S. Lifson, *J. Am. Chem. Soc.*, **96**, 5319 (1974).

51.   A.T. Hagler and S. Lifson, *J. Am. Chem. Soc.*, **96**, 5327 (1974).

52.   H. Matsuo, Y. Baba, R.M.G. Nair, A. Arimura, and A.V. Schally, *Biochem. Biophys. Res. Comm.*, **43**, 1334 (1971).

53.   R. Burgus, M. Butcher, M. Amoss, N. Ling, M. Monahan, J. Rivier, R. Fellows, R. Blackwell, W. Vale, and R. Guillemin, *Proc. Natl. Acad. Sci. USA*, **69**, 278 (1972).

54.   M. Shinitzki and M. Fridkin, *Biochim. Biophys. Acta*, **434**, 137 (1976).

55.   B. Donzel, J. Rivier, and M. Goodman, *Biochemistry*, **16**, 2611 (1977).

56.   R. Deslauriers, G.C. Levy, W.H. McGregor, D. Sarantakis, and I.C.P. Smith , *Biochemistry*, **14**, 4335 (1975).

57.   K.D. Kopple, in *Peptides-Synthesis-Structure-Functions-Proceedings of the 7th American Peptide Symposium*, ed. D.H. Rich E. Gross, p. 295, Pierce Chemical Co., Rockford, Ill. (1981).

58.   R.F. Sprecher and F.A. Momany, *Biochem. Biophys. Res. Comm.*, **87(1)**, 72 (1979).

59.   P.L. Wessels, J. Feeney, H. Gregory, and J.J. Gormley, *J. Chem. Soc. Perkin Trans. 2*,, 1691 (1973).

60.   F.A. Momany, *J. Med. Chem.*, **21(1)**, 63 (1978).

61.   F.A. Momany, *J. Am. Chem. Soc.*, **98**, 2996 (1976).

62.   R.S. Struthers, J. Rivier, and A.T. Hagler, *Manuscript in Preparation.*

63.   S.S. Zimmerman, M.S. Pottle, G. Nemethy, and H.A. Scheraga, *Macromolecules*, **10**, 1 (1977).

64.   A.T. Hagler, P. Dauber, D.J. Osguthorpe, and J. Hempel, *Manuscript in preparation* (1983).

65.   F.A. Momany, in *Topics in Current Physics: Crystal Cohesian and Conformational Energies*, ed. R.M. Metzger, p. 41, Springer-Verlag (1981).

66.   C. Toniolo, G.M Bonora, A. Bavoso, E. Benedetti, B. DiBlasio, V. Pavone, and C. Pedone, *Biopolymers*, **22**, 205 (1983).

67.   C.H. Pulla Rao, P. Balaram, and C.N.R. Rao, *Biopolymers*, **22**, 2091 (1983).

68.   A.S.V. Burgen, G.C.K. Roberts, and J. Feeney, *Nature*, **253**, 753 (1975).

RECEIVED January 6, 1984

INDEXES

Author Index

Subject Index

Production by Frances Reed
Indexing by Robin Giroux
Jacket design by Anne G. Bigler

Elements typeset by Hot Type Ltd., Washington, D.C.
Printed and bound by Maple Press Co., York, Pa.

RECENT ACS BOOKS

"Ultrahigh Resolution Chromatography"
Edited by Satinder Ahuja
ACS SYMPOSIUM SERIES 250; 230 pp.; ISBN 0-8412-0835-2

"Chemistry of Combustion Processes"
Edited by Thompson M. Sloane
ACS SYMPOSIUM SERIES 249; 286 pp.; ISBN 0-8412-0834-4

"Geochemical Behavior of Disposed Radioactive Waste"
Edited by G. Scott Barney, James D. Navratil, and W. W. Schulz
ACS SYMPOSIUM SERIES 248; 470 pp.; ISBN 0-8412-0831-X

"NMR and Macromolecules:
Sequence, Dynamic, and Domain Structure"
Edited by James C. Randall
ACS SYMPOSIUM SERIES 247; 282 pp.; ISBN 0-8412-0829-8

"Geochemical Behavior of Disposed Radioactive Waste"
Edited by G. Scott Barney, James D. Navratil, and W. W. Schulz
ACS SYMPOSIUM SERIES 246; 413 pp.; ISBN 0-8412-0827-1

"Size Exclusion Chromatography: Methodology and
Characterization of Polymers and Related Materials"
Edited by Theodore Provder
ACS SYMPOSIUM SERIES 245; 392 pp.; ISBN 0-8412-0826-3

"Industrial-Academic Interfacing"
Edited by Dennis J. Runser
ACS SYMPOSIUM SERIES 244; 176 pp.; ISBN 0-8412-0825-5

"Characterization of Highly Cross-linked Polymers"
Edited by S. S. Labana and Ray A. Dickie
ACS SYMPOSIUM SERIES 243; 324 pp.; ISBN 0-8412-0824-9

"Polymers in Electronics"
Edited by Theodore Davidson
ACS SYMPOSIUM SERIES 242; 584 pp.; ISBN 0-8412-0823-9

"Radionuclide Generators: New Systems
for Nuclear Medicine Applications"
Edited by F. F. Knapp, Jr., and Thomas A. Butler
ACS SYMPOSIUM SERIES 241; 240 pp.; ISBN 0-8412-0822-0

"Archaeological Chemistry--III"
Edited by Joseph B. Lambert
ADVANCES IN CHEMISTRY SERIES 205; 324 pp.; ISBN 0-8412-0767-4

"Molecular-Based Study of Fluids"
Edited by J. M. Haile and G. A. Mansoori
ADVANCES IN CHEMISTRY SERIES 204; 524 pp.; ISBN 0-8412-0720-8